Dentistry: A Case-Based Approach

Dentistry: A Case-Based Approach

Editor: Kailey Corbyn

AMERICAN
MEDICAL PUBLISHERS
www.americanmedicalpublishers.com

AMERICAN
MEDICAL PUBLISHERS
www.americanmedicalpublishers.com

Cataloging-in-Publication Data

Dentistry: a case-based approach / edited by Kailey Corbyn.
p. cm.
Includes bibliographical references and index.
ISBN 979-8-88740-633-6
1. Dentistry. 2. Dentistry--Case studies. 3. Oral medicine. 4. Teeth.
I. Corbyn, Kailey.
RK51 .D46 2023
617.6--dc23

American Medical Publishers,
41 Flatbush Avenue,
1st Floor, New York,
NY 11217, USA

ISBN 979-8-88740-633-6 (Hardback)

Contents

Preface

Dentistry is a vital branch of healthcare that focuses on the diagnosis, prevention, and treatment of oral health conditions. It plays a crucial role in maintaining overall well-being by promoting good oral hygiene and preventing dental diseases. One of the key aspects of dentistry is preventive care. It includes regular check-ups to detect and address oral health issues at an early stage. Restorative and cosmetic dentistry are other important aspects of dentistry. Restorative dentistry includes use of various techniques to restore damaged teeth and improve their functionality. This may involve treatments such as fillings, crowns, bridges, or dental implants to replace missing teeth and restore oral health and aesthetics. Cosmetic dentistry focuses on enhancing the appearance of the teeth and smile. The book aims to shed light on some of the unexplored aspects of dentistry and the recent researches in this field. It will provide comprehensive knowledge to the readers.

The information shared in this book is based on empirical researches made by veterans in this field of study. The elaborative information provided in this book will help the readers further their scope of knowledge leading to advancements in this field.

Finally, I would like to thank my fellow researchers who gave constructive feedback and my family members who supported me at every step of my research.

Editor

Preface

Dentistry is a vital branch of healthcare that focuses on the diagnosis, prevention, and treatment of oral health conditions. It plays a crucial role in maintaining overall well-being by promoting good oral hygiene and preventing dental diseases. One of the key aspects of dentistry is preventive care. It includes regular check-ups to detect and address oral health issues at an early stage. Restorative and cosmetic dentistry are other important aspects of dentistry. Restorative dentistry includes use of various techniques to restore damaged teeth and improve their functionality. This may involve treatments such as fillings, crowns, bridges, or dental implants to replace missing teeth and restore oral health and aesthetics. Cosmetic dentistry focuses on enhancing the appearance of the teeth and smile. The book aims to shed light on some of the unexplored aspects of dentistry and the recent researches in this field. It will provide comprehensive knowledge to the readers.

The information shared in this book is based on empirical researches made by veterans in this field of study. The elaborative information provided in this book will help the readers further their scope of knowledge leading to advancements in this field.

Finally, I would like to thank my fellow researchers who gave constructive feedback and my family members who supported me at every step of my research.

Editor

1

Incidental Findings of Asymptomatic Fungal Infection

Nisha Manila,[1] **Madhu Nair**,[2] **and Hui Liang**[3]

[1]*Oral and Maxillofacial Radiology, Department of Diagnostic Sciences, Louisiana State University School of Dentistry, New Orleans, Louisiana, USA*
[2]*Oral and Maxillofacial Radiology, Director of Imaging Center, Texas A&M College of Dentistry, Dallas, Texas, USA*
[3]*Director of Oral and Maxillofacial Radiology Resident Program, Department of Diagnostic Sciences, Texas A&M College of Dentistry, Dallas Texas, USA*

Correspondence should be addressed to Nisha Manila; nmanil@lsuhsc.edu

Academic Editor: Darko Macan

Fungal sinusitis of the paranasal sinuses is a rare infection in healthy individuals but is relatively common in immunocompromised patients. It is often misdiagnosed and frequently a severe disease, as a few forms of it are linked with a higher mortality rate. Effective handling necessitates a speedy analysis and often counts on radiological findings. On cone-beam computed tomography (CBCT) analysis, a bulky polypoid-shaped lesion with a density close to that of soft tissue in CBCT was visualized in the right ethmoid and sphenoid sinuses. There was a significant expansion of the borders of the right ethmoid sinus, and discontinuity or perforation of the sphenoid sinus floor was suspected from CBCT images. Non-contrasted multi-detector computed tomography (MDCT) exhibited opacification and extension of the lesion into the majority of sinuses with dense inspissated materials in the center, which resembled radiographic features of invasive fungal sinusitis. Computed tomography (CT) scan of the maxillofacial region, specifically paranasal sinuses, plays a considerable role in diagnosing fungal sinusitis. In a majority of cases, fungal sinusitis is noticed and diagnosed in immunocompromised patients. However, it is also seen in healthy patients in very rare circumstances, similar to the patient in this report. If the patient is treated rapidly, the prognosis is fair. We present a case of fungal sinusitis in an otherwise healthy young male patient to increase awareness among dental professionals.

1. Introduction

Fungal sinusitis or pansinusitis is considered an uncommon inflammatory process of the paranasal sinuses, and it primarily affects immunocompromised patients and occasionally immunocompetent individuals. The recent increase in the reporting of this condition is attributed to advanced diagnostic techniques, immunodeficiency caused by cancer treatment, diabetes, overuse of antibiotics, and post-transplant therapy [1].

Fungal infection of the paranasal sinuses is broadly classified as noninvasive or invasive based on the non-appearance or appearance of the fungal hyphae in tissue, submucosa, mucosa, blood, or bone of the paranasal sinus. Noninvasive infection is further sub-categorized as allergic fungal sinusitis and fungal mycetoma (fungal ball). Invasive type is further sub-divided into acute, chronic, and granulomatous invasive fungal sinusitis [2]. A retrospective audit study conducted between January 2000 and August 2007 revealed that 63% were affected by allergic fungal sinusitis, and 34% had an invasive form of fungal infection. *Rhizopus arrhizus* remained the primary causative agent of acute invasive sinusitis, whereas *Aspergillus fumigates* was the primary contributing factor for allergic fungal sinusitis [3].

The acute invasive form is an aggressive infection observed mainly in poor diabetic control and immunocompromised patients. It reports a mortality rate of 50–80%, making it the most lethal variant [2]. To differentiate between the two primary forms of fungal sinusitis, it is integral to (a) collect appropriate amounts of exudates and other contents from sinuses, (b) biopsy samples of unaffected and affected mucosa, and (c) biopsy the bone adjacent to parts of necrosis [2]. This type of fungal infection cannot be stained with regular stains. Distinct silver-infused fungal dyes and fungal cultures are mandatory for explicit confirmation and further sub-classification of this condition. Effective treatment requires accurate and early investigation, which frequently depends on diagnostic imaging, precisely computed tomography (CT) and magnetic resonance (MR) imaging. CT evaluates bone changes accurately, and MR imaging identifies intraorbital and intracranial extensions. The prevalent knowledge indicates that invasive variant is often seen in immunodeficient patients, whereas noninvasive primarily occurs in immunocompetent individuals [4]. The treatment strategies vary for each subtype, and so as their prognoses. It is crucial to have a deeper insight into the various forms of fungal infections and their radiographic manifestations. These diagnostic imaging features are the red flag alerts that help the radiologist notify the clinician. It will also support the use of appropriate final diagnostic techniques for confirmation of the disease and help play an integral role in patient care. Apt diagnosis and instigation of proper care are needed to avoid an undesirable fatal outcome.

We report an incidental finding of fungal sinusitis in a healthy 21-year Caucasian male, contrary to the usual findings. We aim to highlight the role played by radiologists in the early detection of this case and emphasize the importance of interpreting each CBCT image by a trained radiologist It also alerts the dental community to be observant about the disease to undertake the right diagnosis and precise treatment planning, and avoidance of unexpected complications.

2. Case Report

A 21-year-old male reported to the radiology department for evaluation of the potential site for implant placement [5]. The patient was asymptomatic and medically healthy, and presented no known conditions or medications to report on history. There was no related dental history. His social history indicated the absence of smoking or substance abuse.

On examination, missing right maxillary lateral incisor and third molars were noted (Figure 1). A full field of view cone-beam computed tomography (CBCT) analysis was performed to assess the prospective implant site. The axial slice CBCT images revealed a huge mass with a polypoid shape and soft density that occupied the right ethmoid sinus and sphenoid sinus (Figure 2(a)) [5]. There was a noteworthy enlargement or bulging of the lateral and the medial wall of the right ethmoid sinus. Due to the infiltration or penetration of the lesion to the sphenoid sinus, focal bone erosion of the sphenoid sinus floor was suspected on the sagittal section CBCT images (Figure 2(c)). In addition, this lesion also had progressed into the region of the nose and right maxillary sinus (Figure 2(b)). A significant deviation of the nasal septum was observed. The coronal CBCT images of the right maxillary sinus portrayed significant soft tissue opacification/mucosal thickening involving up to the superior confines of the sinus. In addition, displacement of the inferior medial wall of the right orbit was speculated with no evidence of erosion. There was complete obstruction of the osteomeatal complex on the right side. The middle concha was displaced and was entirely obliterated by the lesion; variation in size of inferior concha was observed as well (Figure 2(b)).

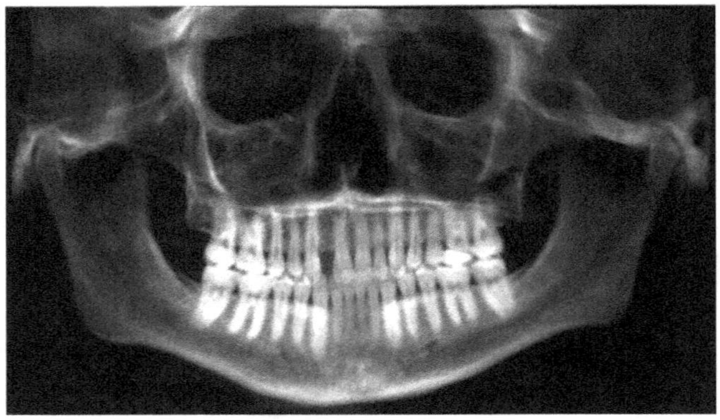

Figure 1: Reconstructed panoramic image.

Contrary to the clinical finding that the patient was asymptomatic, radiographic features were aggressive, which may downgrade the inflammatory course in the differential diagnosis. The patient was directed to an otolaryngologist for further assessment. Further, a non-contrasted multidetector computed tomography (MDCT) was performed, and the images in all three planes showed inclusive soft tissue opacification in the affected sinuses (Figure 3). Expansion of multiple sinus walls with centrally dense inspissated material with different densities suggested the lesion is more likely to be chronic (Figure 3(a)). The base of the skull and the extraocular muscles were intact, and there was no evidence of this lesion infiltrating into adjacent fat or soft tissue (Figures 3(b), 3(c)) [5]. The internal carotid artery and cavernous sinus were observed within normal limits. The differential radiological diagnosis included sinonasal polyposis, eosinophilic mucin rhinosinusitis, sinus fungal mycetoma, acute rhinosinusitis with complication, and sinonasal squamous cell carcinoma. These radiographic findings were consistent with pathologic findings of chronic invasive fungal sinusitis. Later, the patient was cured with surgical intervention without complications.

3. Discussion

This case report presents an incidental finding of fungal sinusitis in a patient who was supposed to undergo a routine dental procedure. Timely radiological diagnosis and appropriate intervention saved the patient from subsequent complications. This case has two significant points of reasoning. First, it stresses the importance of radiological screening before surgical procedures and the application of appropriate imaging for a judicious diagnosis. Second, this study emphasizes the awareness of different life-threatening fungal diseases among dental professionals.

The presentation of fungal colonies in a sinonasal tract is not uncommon and necessarily does not mean an infection. Humans are exposed to a variety of omnipresent fungi and usually do not cause any disease. The immunity of a person plays a significant role in determining the individual's susceptibility to the disease [6, 7]. Depending on the nature of this lesion, it can be a very rapid onset and can cross mucosa to involve vasculature,

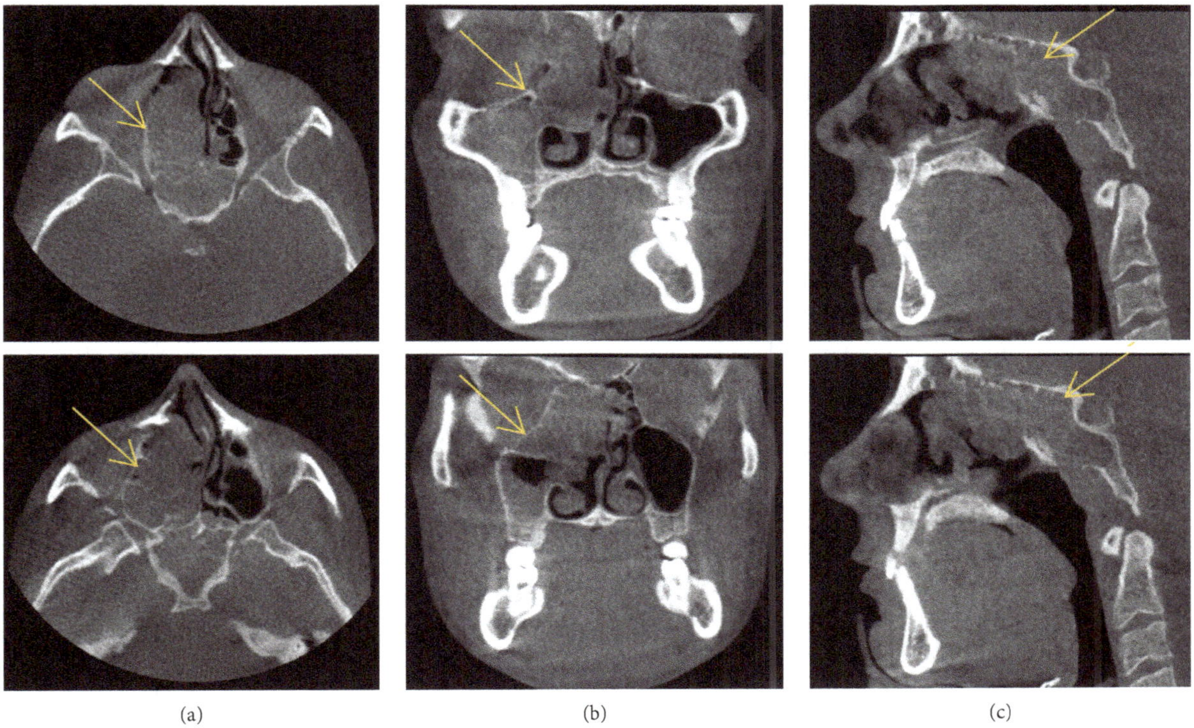

FIGURE 2: CBCT axial (a), coronal (b), and sagittal (c) images show a large mass occupying the right ethmoid sinus.

bone, adjoining soft tissues, orbit, and cranial contents [8]. Timely diagnosis is crucial as it helps treat the patients early to avoid any fatal complications arising due to this. The normal clues of a fungal infection include headaches, nasal congestion, and purulent rhinorrhea [9]. Occasionally it can also show as malaise, fever, bleeding from the nose aka epistaxis, discomfort in the sinus, cough, mucosal ulcerations, and crusting. In serious cases, the presentation will be periorbital swelling, proptosis, and mental status changes [9]. Early detection and appropriate treatment help avoid fatal complications. However, the patient discussed in this case report presented without any symptoms conferred. Hence, the clinician and the radiologist need to affirm that the patient can be asymptomatic. Fungal sinusitis commonly traits complete or partial opacification of the sinus and can portray areas of bone erosion and contiguous soft tissue infiltration. The characteristic location is the maxillary and ethmoid sinuses, but it is observed in the sphenoid sinuses and frontal sinuses, which is rare [10].

Radiographic evaluations are an invaluable tool for early diagnosis and effective management of the disease. CBCT is one of the methods used to assess bony erosion and other osseous changes. Erosion of bone, sinus, and nasal cavity involvement, and mucosal thickening can be found in other diseases, too; however, when found in the immunocompromised patient, one of the differential diagnoses must be invasive fungal sinusitis [11]. Infiltration of soft tissue with fat stranding is poorly recognized in CBCT, and in such cases, multidetector computed tomography (MDCT) or magnetic resonance imaging (MRI) offers superior imaging [11]. In the present report, the patient was asymptomatic and had no relevant medical history. Moderate to severe fungal lesions can precede enlargement and erosion of involved bone spreading to the surrounding cranial and orbital region. It could advance into a potentially deadly consequence if left undiagnosed or untreated. Judicious diagnosis with prompt referral to an otolaryngologist could circumvent grave situations such as loss of sight, and extensive spread of infection leading to unalterable outcomes, even in silent and gradual, asymptomatic development [5].

The hyperattenuating soft-tissue collection could be seen in a non-contrast CT within one or more of the paranasal sinuses. Due to the destructive nature of lesions towards borders of sinuses and expansion beyond the sinus boundaries may resemble malignancy. On contrasted CT, periantral soft tissue and adjacent musculature may enhance depending on the duration of fungal invasion.

Surgical–medical therapy is of paramount importance since it rapidly spreads invasive disease; otherwise, the condition can be fatal. If only the sinus is involved, the prognosis is fair, while it is poor with intracranial involvement. The treatment of choice is radical debridement, anti-fungal therapy, and the treatment of any underlying condition.

With the growing popularity of CBCT and its diagnostic worth, the numbers of dental health professionals utilizing this advanced imaging technology in their practice are sure to increase. Presurgical implant planning and orthodontic and prosthodontic evaluations often include paranasal sinuses; however, the majority of these scans are not evaluated entirely. It is desirable that all the CBCT images

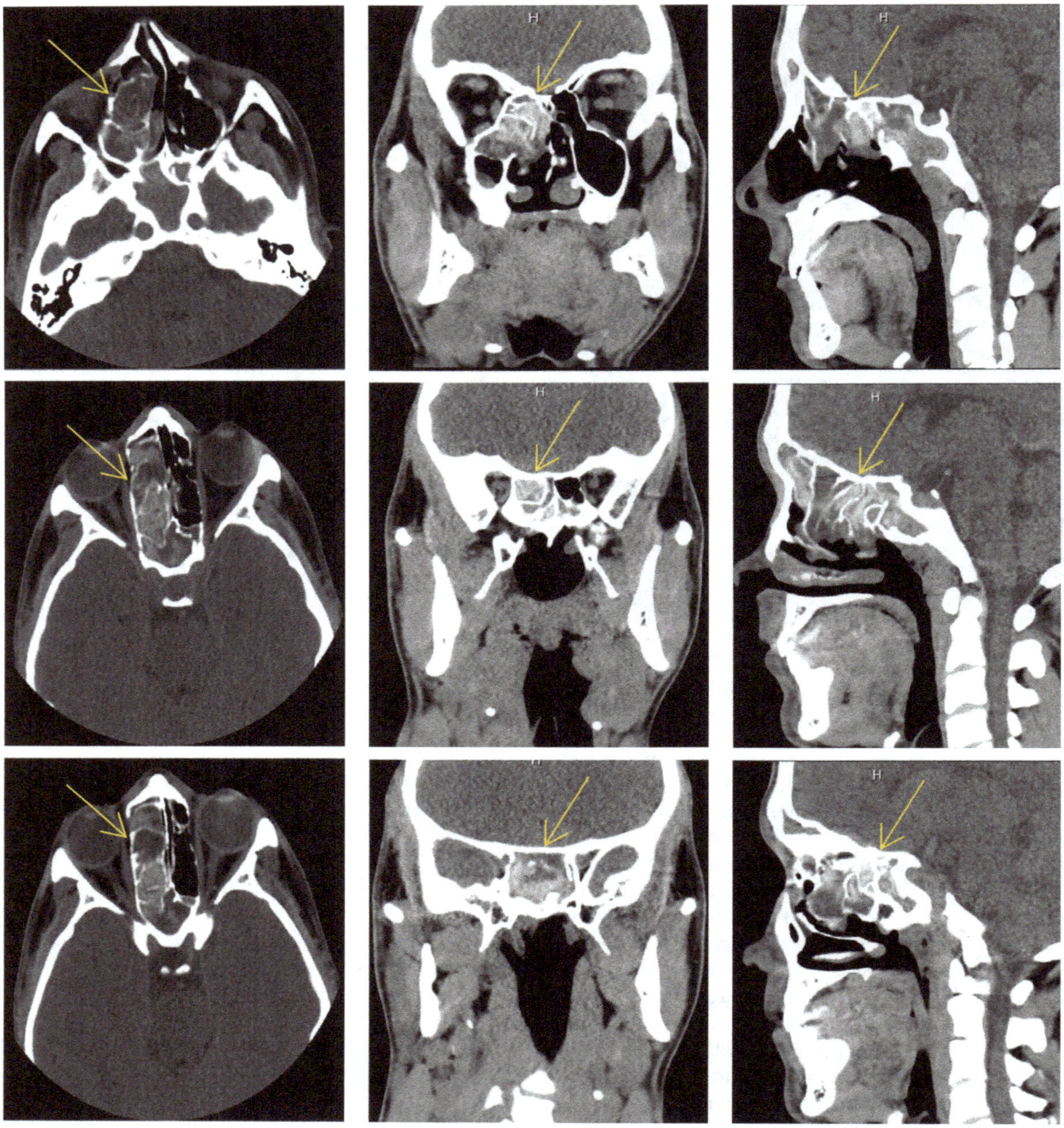

(a) (b) (c)

FIGURE 3: MDCT axial (a), coronal (b), and sagittal (c) images showing opacification and expansion of multiple sinuses with centrally dense inspissated materials.

are read by a trained oral and maxillofacial radiologist. According to the American Academy of Oral and Maxillofacial Radiology (AAOMR) executive opinion statement, "It is the practitioners' responsibility to examine the entire image dataset" [12]. Eluding the expert interpretation of acquired images might end up in a lawsuit and other legal complications in some countries. Hence, it is essential that there must be awareness among the clinicians and an effort must be made for evaluating each scan by a radiologist. Because if such findings are diagnosed at an early stage and treated radically, the patient will have a good prognosis.

in *Oral Surgery, Oral Medicine, Oral Pathology and Oral Radiology* as a conference abstract in 2021.

Acknowledgments

We would like to thank Drs. Bender, Ehlers, and Tahmasbi for referring the patient for radiological evaluation and pertinent discussion.

References

[1] H. Akhondi, B. Woldemariam, and V. Rajasurya, *Fungal Sinusitis*, StatPearls Publishing, Treasure Island, FL, 2022.

[2] P. Karthikeyan and C. V. Nirmal, "Incidence and presentation of fungal sinusitis in patient diagnosed with chronic rhinosinusitis," *Indian Journal of Otolaryngology and Head & Neck Surgery*, vol. 62, no. 4, pp. 381–385, 2010.

[3] R. C. Michael, J. S. Michael, R. H. Ashbee, and M. S. Mathews, "Mycological profile of fungal sinusitis: an audit of specimens over a 7-year period in a tertiary care hospital in Tamil Nadu," *Indian Journal of Pathology & Microbiology*, vol. 51, no. 4, pp. 493–496, 2008.

[4] C. E. Reddy, A. K. Gupta, P. Singh, and S. B. Mann, "Imaging of granulomatous and chronic invasive fungal sinusitis: comparison with allergic fungal sinusitis," *Otolaryngology-Head and Neck Surgery*, vol. 143, no. 2, pp. 294–300, 2010.

[5] N. Manila, E. A. Scott, S. Bender, M. A. Tahmasbi, M. K. Nair, and H. Liang, "Incidental findings of asymptomatic fungal infection in paranasal sinuses: a case report and literature review to increase awareness among dental professionals," *Oral Surgery, Oral Medicine, Oral Pathology and Oral Radiology*, vol. 132, no. 3, article e116, 2021.

[6] H. Takahashi, Y. Hinohira, N. Hato et al., "Clinical features and outcomes of four patients with invasive fungal sinusitis," *Auris, Nasus, Larynx*, vol. 38, no. 2, pp. 289–294, 2011.

[7] J. Gavito-Higuera, C. B. Mullins, L. Ramos-Duran, H. Sandoval, N. Akle, and R. Figueroa, "Sinonasal fungal infections and complications: a pictorial review," *Journal of Clinical Imaging Science*, vol. 6, p. 23, 2016.

[8] J. Kwon, K. H. Park, S. I. Park, and S. Y. Jin, "Aspergillosis of the paranasal sinuses: diagnostic significance of the computed tomography," *Yonsei Medical Journal*, vol. 30, no. 3, p. 294, 1989.

[9] M. Mossa-Basha, A. T. Ilica, F. Maluf, O. Karakoc, I. Izbudak, and N. Aygun, "The many faces of fungal disease of the paranasal sinuses: CT and MRI findings," *Diagnostic and Interventional Radiology*, 2012.

[10] M. H. Dahniya, R. Makkar, E. Grexa et al., "Appearances of paranasal fungal sinusitis on computed tomography," *The British Journal of Radiology*, vol. 71, no. 843, pp. 340–344, 1998.

[11] G. R. Thompson and T. F. Patterson, "Fungal disease of the nose and paranasal sinuses," *Journal of Allergy and Clinical Immunology*, vol. 129, no. 2, pp. 321–326, 2012.

[12] L. Carter, A. G. Farman, J. Geist et al., "American Academy of Oral and maxillofacial radiology executive opinion statement on performing and interpreting diagnostic cone beam computed tomography," *Oral Surgery, Oral Medicine, Oral Pathology and Oral Radiology*, vol. 106, no. 4, pp. 561–562, 2008.

2

Fiber Post Removal using a Conservative Fully Guided Approach: A Dental Technique

Abdullah Alfadda,[1] **Abdulmohsen Alfadley**,[2] **and Ahmed Jamleh**[2]

[1]*Endodontic Division, Dental Services, Central Region, King Abdulaziz Medical City, Ministry of National Guard Health Affairs, Riyadh, Saudi Arabia*
[2]*Department of Restorative and Prosthetic Dental Sciences, College of Dentistry, King Saud Bin Abdulaziz University for Health Sciences, King Abdullah International Medical Research Center, Ministry of National Guard Health Affairs, Riyadh, Saudi Arabia*

Correspondence should be addressed to Ahmed Jamleh; aojamleh@gmail.com

Academic Editor: Andrea Scribante

This report describes the usefulness of an endodontic template for the removal of a fiber post. A 40-year-old man presented with discomfort in the maxillary left canine. Clinical and radiographic examinations showed tooth #23 with a permanent core material retained with fiber post along with a persistent apical radiolucency. Among the various treatment modalities, nonsurgical root canal retreatment with fiber post removal using a conservative fully guided approach was proposed. After obtaining both the cone-beam computed tomographic images and the cast surface scan, their data were merged using implant planning software (ImplaStation for Windows x64 Bit Beta Version, ProDigiDent, Miami, Florida, USA) and superimposed. The drilling space was planned based on the location, diameter, and apical extent of the fiber post and was virtually overlapped and transferred clinically using a resin template to drill through the fiber post. With guides in position over the rubber dam, drilling was made with increments of 2 mm using a size 4 long-shank round bur (Thomas, Bourges, France) until it exposed the coronal gutta-percha. As soon as the canal was located, K3 rotary files (Sybron Endo, Orange, USA) were used along with chloroform to remove the old obturating materials. Then, additional shaping and cleaning were done with ProTaper Next rotary files (Dentsply Sirona, Ballaigues, Switzerland), sizes X2 and X3, and 5.25% NaOCl irrigation, respectively. The root canal was then dried with paper points and obturated with gutta-percha and AH Plus sealer (Dentsply Sirona, Ballaigues, Switzerland) using the continuous-wave compaction technique. Finally, the tooth was temporarily restored using the double seal technique with zinc oxide and zinc sulfate-based temporary material (Cavit W; 3M ESPE, St. Paul, MN, USA) and resin-modified glass ionomer material (Photac Fil; ESPE, Norristown, PA, USA) filling materials and referred for the final restoration.

1. Introduction

Recurring periapical pathology can develop after inadequate nonsurgical root canal treatment. A common procedure for clinicians to encounter is the retreatment of endodontically treated teeth with posts [1]. Metal posts retained with traditional types of cement such as zinc phosphate can usually be removed; however, in recent years, adhesively bonded glass [2], carbon [3], or quartz fiber [4] posts have become popular, replacing metal posts. The fiber posts are bonded into the root canal space with adhesive materials such as composite resins or glass ionomers, which are reported to be more difficult to remove [5, 6]. It is reported that the fiber posts can be fragmented and removed by using a microscope along with drilling with long-shank round burs, ultrasonic tips, and/or special removal kits [7, 8]. Nevertheless, currently used post removal techniques frequently result in procedural errors such as excessive removal of intraradicular dentin, deviation from the root axis, and perforation of the root structure [9]. Furthermore, these techniques are time-consuming and dependent on the clinician's experience [7, 9–12]. Post removal requires fragmentation within a limited anatomic area that is difficult to visualize, which may result in excessive substance loss leading to iatrogenic errors that compromise stability and hence compromise the tooth prognosis [13].

Cone-beam computed tomographic (CBCT) imaging has been recently recommended in endodontics as a diagnostic aid in root canal treatment planning [14, 15]. It lays the foundation for the 3D printing of endodontic templates [16]. In guided endodontics, the combined use of CBCT imaging and intraoral scanning allows the manufacturing of a 3D endodontic template. This template facilitates a straight access cavity to the root canal by guiding the endodontic bur to the exact area [17, 18]. The use of guided endodontics has been previously performed and reported in the literature as a safe [19] and predictable technique [20] which, in turn, leads to an improved long-term prognosis as they help to preserve the dental structure and avoid accidents such as deviations and perforations [18]. The present case report proposes a fully guided preparation as an attempt to minimize dentin loss and eliminate iatrogenic errors during fiber post removal.

2. Case Report

A 40-year-old normal healthy male patient, ASA I (According to the American Society of Anesthesiologists), presented to the postgraduate endodontic clinic at King Abdulaziz medical city, complaining of discomfort in the upper left anterior area for the past month. After clinical examination, tooth #23 exhibited sensitivity to percussion while the mobility was normal (grade I) as tested using two ends of metallic instruments. The periodontal probing depths were checked with a periodontal probe and were found within normal limits. Radiographic interpretation revealed a permanent core retained with a fiber post of unknown sources with an inadequate root canal filling and periapical radiolucency (Figure 1). A CBCT was taken using Planmeca ProMax 3D S (Planmeca OY, Helsinki, Finland) operated at 80 kV, 3.0 mA, and voxel size of 0.15 mm to fully assess the anatomy of tooth #23 and surrounding structures. The imaging revealed apical root resorption and a radiolucent area with intact buccal and palatal plates. The obturation was found to be 2.15 mm short from the apex and the fiber post was located up to the middle third (Figure 2). Based on these, a diagnosis of a previously root canal-treated tooth with symptomatic apical periodontitis was reached. Among the various treatment modalities, nonsurgical root canal retreatment with fiber post removal using a conservative fully guided approach was proposed. The procedure's benefits and risks were explained to the patient, and consent was obtained.

An impression of the upper arch was made using polyvinyl siloxane material (Imprint 4, 3 M, Saint Paul, Minnesota, USA) and poured to fabricate a diagnostic cast. The cast was then scanned by using the desktop laser scanner R700 Desktop (3Shape, Copenhagen, Denmark). Then, both the DICOM file from CBCT images and the cast surface scan file were merged using implant planning software (ProDigiDent, ImplaStation for Windows x6464 Bit Beta Version) and superimposed by selecting three reference landmarks in both files. The template was made with 3.5 mm thickness and 0.15 mm offset, which was extended to cross the midline for maximal stability. The drilling space was planned based on the location, diameter, and apical extent of the fiber post in the sagittal view. It was found to be 20.74 mm long with a 1.48 mm diameter apically. The space was virtually overlapped over the fiber post to drill through it with minimal dentin loss (Figure 3). The endo-guide template was then created and exported for printing using a digital light processing (DLP) (M-One; MAKEX Technology, Zhejiang, China) technology. A 3D printer (MiiCraft 125; MiiCraft, Jena, Germany) was used with a photo-polymerized biocompatible polymer resin (Freeprint Temp; DETAX GmbH & Co., Ettlingen, Germany) to print the template. The printer settings included 50 μm thickness, 405 nm wavelength, and a curing time of 2.40 s per layer. To guide the bur in the created drilling space, a guiding sleeve with 3.0 mm external diameter, 1.7 mm internal diameter, and 5 mm length was virtually customized using CAD software (Google SketchUp) (SketchUp, Trimble Navigation, Sunnyvale, California, USA) and printed using a selective laser melting system (GE Additive company, Boston, MA, USA) with standard parameters. Both the custom sleeve and endo-guide template were integrated to fully guide the bur during

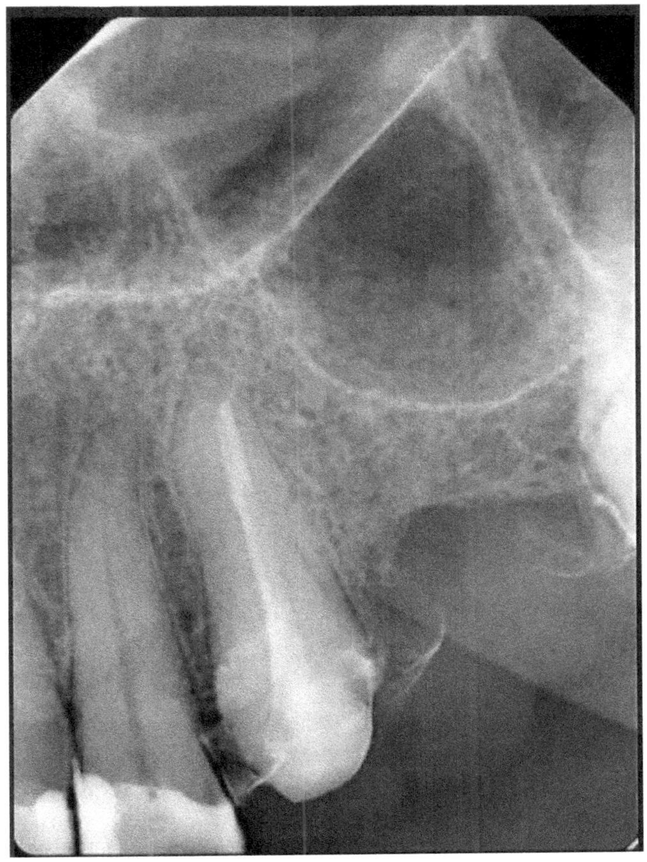

Figure 1: Preoperative radiographic assessment showing tooth #23 with permanent core retained with a fiber post and inadequate root canal filling.

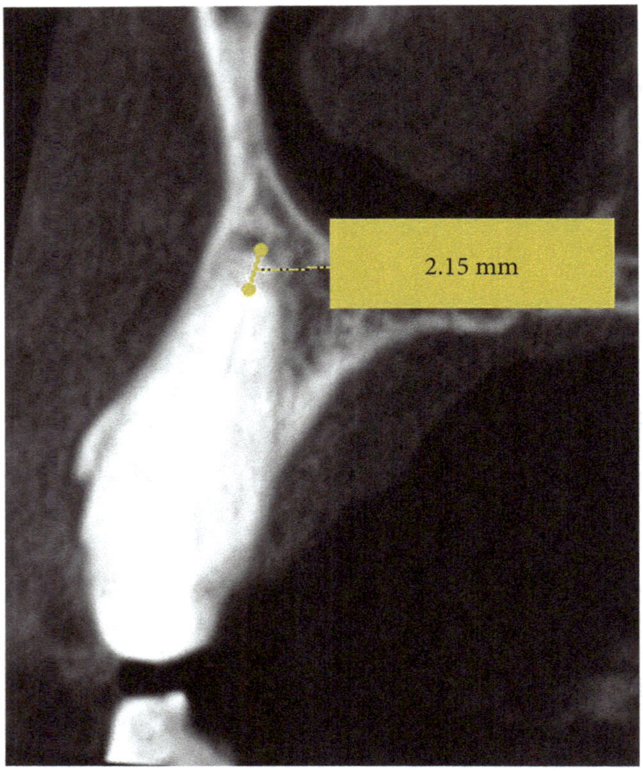

Figure 2: Preoperative CBCT assessment. Sagittal slice of tooth #23 confirms apical root resorption with the radiolucent area, 2.15 mm short obturation, and fiber post cemented up to the middle third.

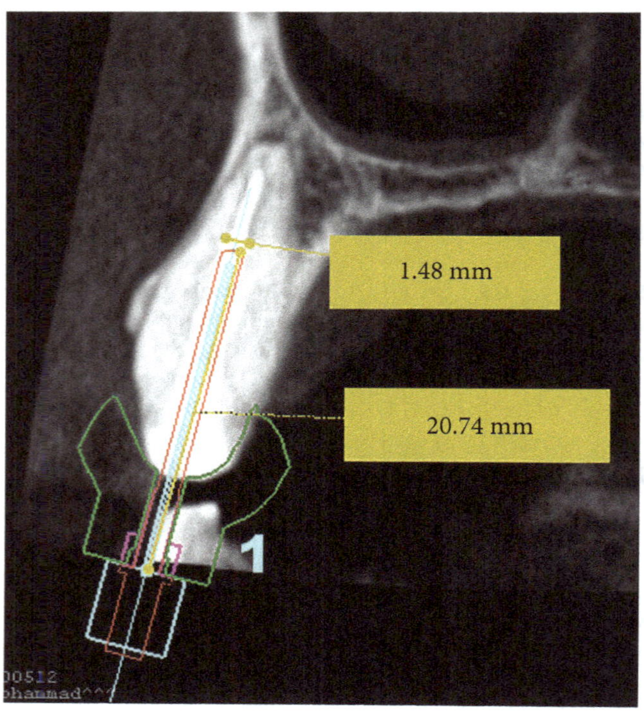

Figure 3: Virtual planning of fiber post removal. The drill was positioned along the long axis of the fiber post set up to its apical tip.

the fiber post removal. In the second visit, the tooth was anesthetized using 2% lidocaine with 1:80,000 epinephrine (Lignospan Special; Septodont, Saint-Maur-des-fossés, France) and isolated with a rubber dam. The endo-guide template was fitted inside the patient's mouth (Figure 4(a)). After a satisfactory assessment of the fit and stability, with pumping movement, drilling was made with increments of 2 mm using a high-speed handpiece with a size 4 long-shank round bur (Thomas, Bourges, France), which has a 1.4 mm head diameter, 1.6 mm shank diameter and 28 mm shank length. The full procedure was performed by an endodontic resident and recorded under a dental operating microscope (ZEISS OPMI pico; Carl Zeiss Meditec AG, Oberkochen, Germany). The procedure took 14 min and 55 s to expose the coronal gutta-percha inside the canal (Figure 4(b) and 4(c)). Then, K3 rotary files (Sybron Endo, Orange, USA) sizes 25 06 taper and 30 06 taper were used along with chloroform to remove the old obturating materials. A size 30 K-file was then inserted to verify the working length with an electronic apex locator (Root ZX; J Morita, Tokyo, Japan) and confirm it radiographically (Figure 5(a)). Then, additional shaping and cleaning were done with ProTaper Next rotary files (Dentsply Sirona, Ballaigues, Switzerland) sizes X2 and X3, and 5.25% NaOCl irrigation, respectively. The root canal was then dried with paper points and obturated with gutta-percha and AH Plus sealer (Dentsply Sirona, Ballaigues, Switzerland) using the continuous-wave compaction technique. Finally, the tooth was temporarily restored using the double seal technique with zinc oxide and zinc sulfate-based temporary material (Cavit W; 3 M ESPE, St. Paul, MN, USA) and resin-modified glass ionomer material (Photac Fil; ESPE, Norristown, PA, USA) filling materials and referred for final restoration (Figure 5(b) and 5(c)).

3. Discussion

The present case report describes a guided technique for the removal of fiber post during nonsurgical endodontic retreatment using CBCT and a 3D printer. Evaluation of the preoperative periapical radiograph of tooth #23 confirmed the presence of a fiber post that extended to the middle third of the root. Overall, fiber posts can be removed using one or a combination of several techniques such as ultrasonic vibrations, drilling with long-shank burs, and using special post removal kits [8]. Nevertheless, currently used post removal techniques frequently result in procedural errors such as excessive removal of intraradicular dentin, deviation from the root axis, and perforation of the root structure [9]. The difficulty of post removal varies according to post type, design, material, length, and cementing material [5].

CBCT is a reliable and noninvasive tool that has gained widespread use in the diagnosis and treatment planning of dentoalveolar conditions. The American Association of Endodontists and the American Academy of Oral and Maxillofacial Radiology have published a joint position statement related to the use of CBCT [21]. The need for a CBCT scan can be considered if careful evaluation of differently angled periapical radiographs failed to yield conclusive information or if further information in the buccolingual dimension is

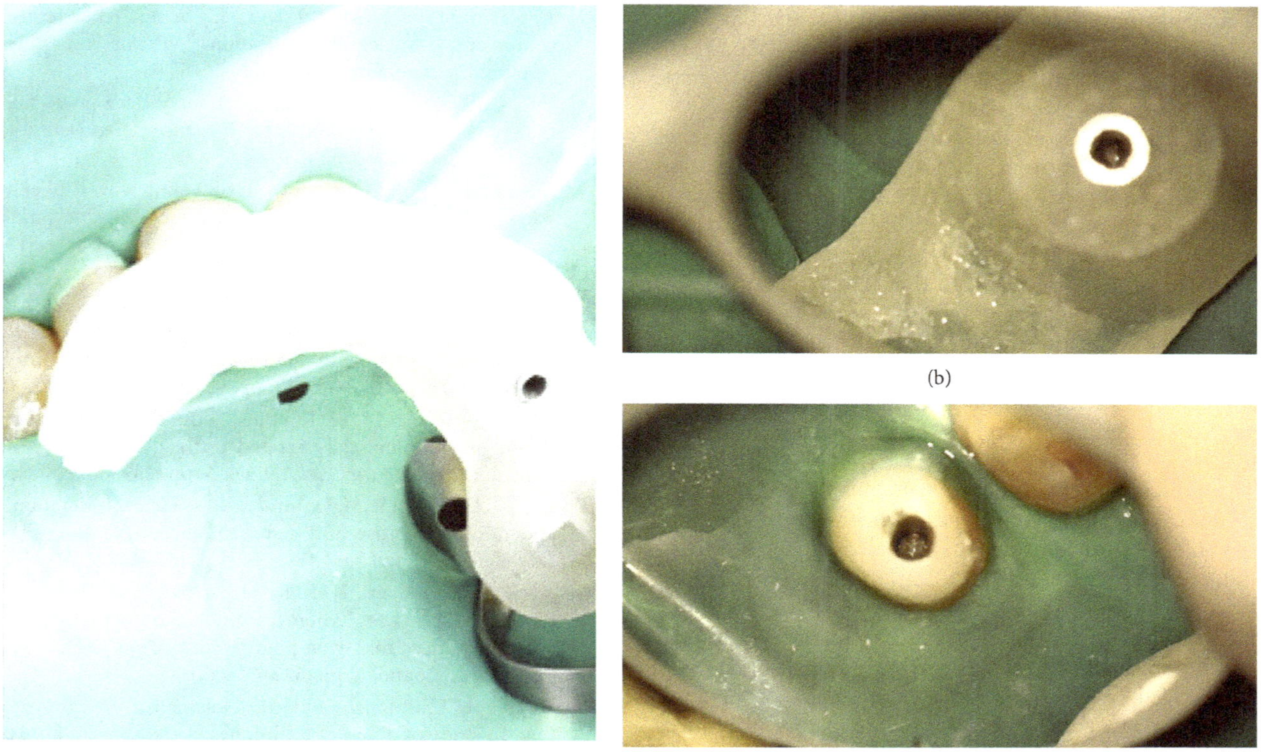

(a) (b) (c)

Figure 4: (a) Under rubber dam isolation, the guide was positioned on the teeth to check the correct fitting. (b, c) Intracanal space following complete removal of the fiber post with coronal gutta-percha exposure.

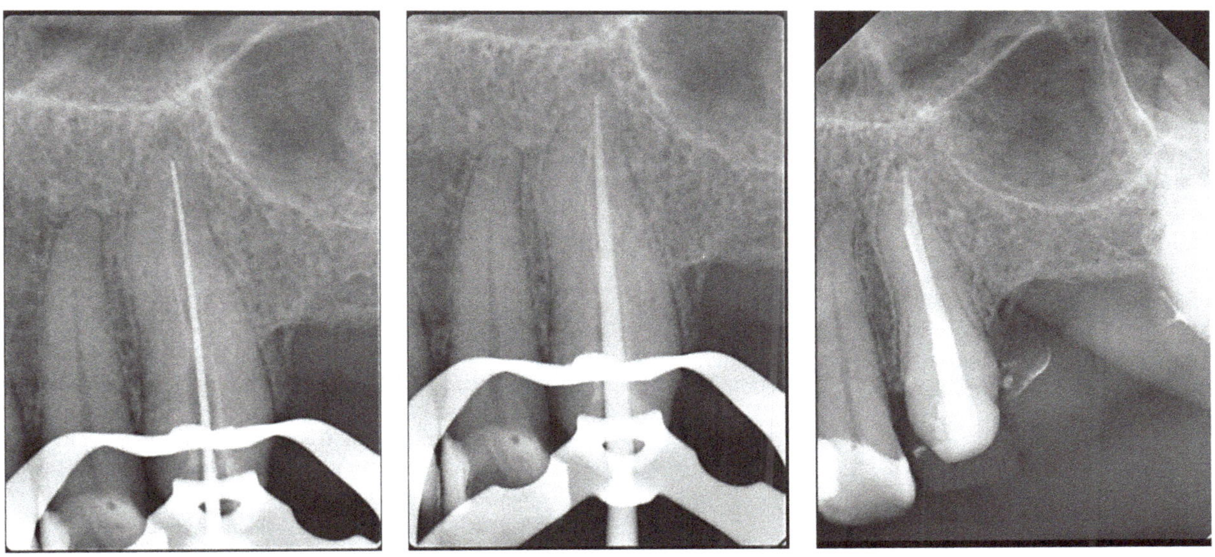

(a) (b) (c)

Figure 5: (a) Working length determination radiograph. (b) Master gutta-percha cone radiograph. (c) Final radiograph.

still required. In cases deemed appropriate for the scan, a narrow field of view that is associated with reduced radiation dose and higher spatial resolution is advisable [21]. Hence, CBCT should only be used as an adjunctive tool in certain clinical situations such as assessment of teeth with suspected complex morphology, localization of obliterated canals, evaluation of the endodontic treatment outcome, and planning of nonsurgical and surgical endodontic retreatment as well as dentoalveolar trauma and resorptive defects [21, 22]. Furthermore, CBCT is frequently used in oral implantology for three-dimensional planning to quantify the alveolar bone levels and to localize vital anatomic structures [23] as well as in guided implant surgery to help with implant site preparation and implant placement [24].

Zehnder and his colleagues introduced the concept of "guided endodontics" to facilitate access cavity preparation for teeth with root canal obliteration and reported that deviations of planned and prepared access cavities were ranging from 0.17 to 0.47 mm at the tip of the bur, while the mean of angle deviation was 1.81° [18]. In this case, a custom sleeve was fabricated and integrated with the endo-guide template to adequately guide the drilling pathway without the risk of resin being damaged by over-heating or undesirable resin drilling [25]. Therefore, in comparison to guided implant surgery, the accuracy of guided endodontics is considered relatively high [26].

The guided preparation that was used to remove the fiber post in our study conserved as much tooth substance as possible. A previous study revealed that the mean amounts of prepared dentin in traditional and conservative guided approaches to access root canal systems were 49.9 and 9.8 mm^3, respectively. Moreover, unlike traditional access preparations, the success of the guided approach is not influenced by the operator's experience [27]. Hence, the conservative guided technique significantly reduces access cavity size, follows a clear path, and preserves the tooth structure [28].

The guided approach presented in this case report has some limitations. For instance, the technique requires prior training for the clinician with an associated learning curve. Also, guided endodontic procedures require the use of CBCT to permit 3D evaluation of the target area. CBCT is associated with more ionizing radiation than conventional radiographs [15], which might be concerning for some patients. Moreover, the presented approach is sensitive to distortions or errors made during intraoral scanning, 3D virtual planning, and printing of the guide. Another limitation of guided endodontics is that it does not enable immediate intervention due to the need for CBCT imaging and intraoral scanning in advance.

The speedy progress of digital dentistry workflows, supported by the evolving technology, will continue to improve the accuracy of guided endodontics. This progress will give rise to the widespread implementation of this digitally supported technique in dental practice.

4. Conclusion

A guided endodontics template created with virtual planning facilitated complete removal of the fiber post with no iatrogenic errors observed and shortened treatment time. Furthermore, to produce predictable results, this approach does not necessitate specialized training or extensive clinical experience.

References

[1] C. J. Ruddle, "Nonsurgical retreatment," *Journal of Endodontics*, vol. 30, no. 12, pp. 827–845, 2004.

[2] A. Scribante, P. K. Vallittu, and M. Özcan, "Fiber-reinforced composites for dental applications," *Biomedical Research International*, no. article 4734986, 2018.

[3] C. J. Goodacre, "Carbon fiber posts may have fewer failures than metal posts," *The Journal of Evidence-Based Dental Practice*, vol. 10, no. 1, pp. 32–34, 2010.

[4] J. Su and S. Cai, "Effects of quartz splint woven fiber periodontal fixtures on evaluating masticatory efficiency and efficacy," *Medicine (Baltimore)*, vol. 97, no. 44, article e13056, 2018.

[5] A. P. M. Gomes, C. H. Kubo, R. A. B. Santos, D. R. Santos, and R. Q. Padilha, "The influence of ultrasound on the retention of cast posts cemented with different agents," *International Endodontic Journal*, vol. 34, no. 2, pp. 93–99, 2001.

[6] R. S. Schwartz and J. W. Robbins, "Post placement and restoration of endodontically treated teeth: a literature review," *Journal of Endodontics*, vol. 30, no. 5, pp. 289–301, 2004.

[7] P. S. McCabe and P. M. Dummer, "Pulp canal obliteration: and endodontic diagnosis and treatment challenge," *International Endodontic Journal*, vol. 45, no. 2, pp. 177–197, 2012.

[8] J. J. Kim, S. Alapati, K. L. Knoernschild, Y. H. Jeong, D. G. Kim, and D. J. Lee, "Micro-computed tomography of tooth volume changes following post removal," *Journal of Prosthodontics*, vol. 26, no. 6, pp. 522–528, 2017.

[9] F. Haupt, J. Pfitzner, and M. Hülsmann, "A comparative in vitro study of different techniques for removal of fibre posts from root canals," *Australian Endodontic Journal*, vol. 44, no. 3, pp. 245–250, 2018.

[10] N. Scotti, E. Bergantin, M. Alovisi, D. Pasqualini, and E. Berutti, "Evaluation of a simplified fiber post removal system," *Journal of Endodontics*, vol. 39, no. 11, pp. 1431–1434, 2013.

[11] N. Haji-Hassani, M. Bakhshi, and S. Shahabi, "Frequency of iatrogenic errors through root canal treatment procedure in 1335 charts of dental patients," *Journal of International Oral Health*, vol. 7, Suppl 1, pp. 14–17, 2015.

[12] D. F. Alhekeir, R. A. Al-Sarhan, H. Mokhlis, and S. Al-Nazhan, "Endodontic mishaps among undergraduate dental students attending King Saud University and Riyadh Colleges of Dentistry and Pharmacy," *Saudi Endodontic Journal*, vol. 3, no. 1, pp. 25–30, 2013.

[13] H. Lang, Y. Korkmaz, K. Schneider, and W. H.-M. Raab, "Impact of endodontic treatments on the rigidity of the root," *Journal of Dental Research*, vol. 85, no. 4, pp. 364–368, 2006.

[14] F. Abella, S. Patel, F. Durán-Sindreu, M. Mercadé, R. Bueno, and M. Roig, "An evaluation of the periapical status of teeth with necrotic pulps using periapical radiography and cone-beam computed tomography," *International Endodontic Journal*, vol. 47, no. 4, pp. 387–396, 2014.

[15] S. Patel, C. Durack, F. Abella, H. Shemesh, M. Roig, and K. Lemberg, "Cone beam computed tomography in endodontics - a review," *International Endodontic Journal*, vol. 48, no. 1, pp. 3–15, 2015.

[16] C. Moreno-Rabié, A. Torres, P. Lambrechts, and R. Jacobs, "Clinical applications, accuracy and limitations of guided endodontics: a systematic review," *International Endodontic Journal*, vol. 53, no. 2, pp. 214–231, 2020.

[17] J. Buchgreitz, M. Buchgreitz, D. Mortensen, and L. Bjørndal, "Guided access cavity preparation using cone-beam computed tomography and optical surface scans—an ex vivo study,"

International Endodontic Journal, vol. 49, no. 8, pp. 790–795, 2016.

[18] M. S. Zehnder, T. Connert, R. Weiger, G. Krastl, and S. Kühl, "Guided endodontics: accuracy of a novel method for guided access cavity preparation and root canal location," *International Endodontic Journal*, vol. 49, no. 10, pp. 966–972, 2016.

[19] G. Krastl, M. S. Zehnder, T. Connert, R. Weiger, and S. Kühl, "Guided endodontics: a novel treatment approach for teeth with pulp canal calcification and apical pathology," *Dental Traumatology*, vol. 32, no. 3, pp. 240–246, 2016.

[20] W. J. van der Meer, A. Vissink, Y. L. Ng, and K. Gulabivala, "3D Computer aided treatment planning in endodontics," *Journal of Dentistry*, vol. 45, no. 2, pp. 67–72, 2016.

[21] "AAE and AAOMR Joint Position Statement: Use of Cone Beam Computed Tomography in Endodontics 2015 Update," *Journal of Endodontics*, vol. 41, no. 9, pp. 1393–1396, 2015.

[22] G. Gambarini, L. Piasecki, G. Miccoli, G. Gaimari, D. D. Nardo, and L. Testarelli, "Cone-beam computed tomography in the assessment of periapical lesions in endodontically treated teeth," *European Journal of Dentistry*, vol. 12, no. 1, pp. 136–143, 2018.

[23] M. E. Guerrero, R. Jacobs, M. Loubele, F. Schutyser, P. Suetens, and D. van Steenberghe, "State-of-the-art on cone beam CT imaging for preoperative planning of implant placement," *Clinical Oral Investigations*, vol. 10, no. 1, pp. 1–7, 2006.

[24] G. Yatzkair, A. Cheng, S. Brodie, E. Raviv, B. D. Boyan, and Z. Schwartz, "Accuracy of computer-guided implantation in a human cadaver model," *Clinical Oral Implants Research*, vol. 26, no. 10, pp. 1143–1149, 2015.

[25] M. C. Santiago, M. M. Altoe, C. P. de Azevedo Mohamed, L. A. de Oliveira, and L. P. Salles, "Guided endodontic treatment in a region of limited mouth opening: a case report of mandibular molar mesial root canals with dystrophic calcification," *BMC Oral Health*, vol. 22, no. 1, p. 37, 2022.

[26] A. Tahmaseb, D. Wismeijer, W. Coucke, and W. Derksen, "Computer technology applications in surgical implant dentistry: a systematic review," *International Journal of Oral and Maxillofacial Implants*, vol. 29, Suppl, pp. 25–42, 2014.

[27] T. Connert, R. Krug, F. Eggmann et al., "Guided endodontics versus conventional access cavity preparation: a comparative study on substance loss using 3-dimensional-printed teeth," *Journal of Endodontics*, vol. 45, no. 3, pp. 327–331, 2019.

[28] L. M. Maia, V. de Carvalho Machado, N. da Silva et al., "Case reports in maxillary posterior teeth by guided endodontic access," *Journal of Endodontics*, vol. 45, no. 2, pp. 214–218, 2019.

3

A Rare Case of Concrescence of Mandibular Third Molar and Supernumerary Fourth Molar

Jiao Wang,[1] Errui Wang,[1] Xin Yang,[1] Lu Yuan,[1] Zhige Li,[1,2] Jie Zhang,[1,2] and Baoping Zhang[1,2]

[1]*School of Stomatology, Lanzhou University, Lanzhou 730000, China*
[2]*Department of Oral and Maxillofacial Surgery, Lanzhou University, Lanzhou 730000, China*

Correspondence should be addressed to Zhige Li; lizhige0106@163.com, Jie Zhang; zhangjie@lzu.edu.cn, and Baoping Zhang; zhangbp@lzu.edu.cn

Jiao Wang and Errui Wang contributed equally to this work.

Academic Editor: Maria Beatriz Duarte Gavião

Concrescence reveals a rare developmental anomaly in which two fully formed teeth are joined along the root surfaces by cementum, and generally occurs in maxillary molars, especially in a third molar and a supernumerary tooth. Very few cases have been reported about the concrescence of a third molar and a supernumerary fourth molar. Based on our available knowledge, this case report described a rare presentation in which concrescence is observed between a third molar and a supernumerary fourth molar in the mandible by diagnosing with cone-beam CT and histological examination.

1. Introduction

Aberrant gene regulation from ectodermal and mesenchymal tissues leads to developmental tooth abnormalities. According to morphological diversification, they are generally classified gemination, fusion, concrescence, syndontia and double teeth [1, 2]. For depth profiling phenotypes for these abnormalities, a previous study has found that tooth development depends on the interaction between the dental epithelium and the underlying ectomesenchyme [3].

Concrescence is a twinning anomaly involving the union of two teeth by cementum only. Such cases were frequently noted in maxillary molars, but were rarely found in the mandible, especially in a third molar and a supernumerary fourth tooth [2]. Previous research studies reported that the incidence of supernumerary fourth molar is 0.32%, not significantly different between the sexes [4], and the concrescence of teeth shared similar anatomic morphology with normal molars; usually it might not be erupted [5]. For clinical applications, it is important to establish a normative diagnosis so that proper treatment can be provided at the earliest time possible. This case reported a rare presentation in which concrescence was observed in a third molar and a supernumerary fourth molar of the mandible, and through appropriate treatment, it will provide a kind of standardized diagnosis code and acceptable therapeutic strategy.

2. Case Report

One year ago, a 21-year-old man extracted his right upper wisdom tooth in another hospital and found his third molar combination with fourth molar in the left mandibular after diagnosing with cone-beam computed tomography (CBCT). One day, he came to the Department of Oral and Maxillofacial Surgery of Hospital of Stomatology, Lanzhou University, with the chief complaint of hurt when chewing with the lower left posterior tooth. His medical history revealed no important health problems or traumas. His family members declared that they did not have any dental anomalies. Gingivitis and class I molar relationship was detected in intraoral examination. No wisdom teeth eruption, bleeding, or purulent secretion in mouth was observed. CBCT

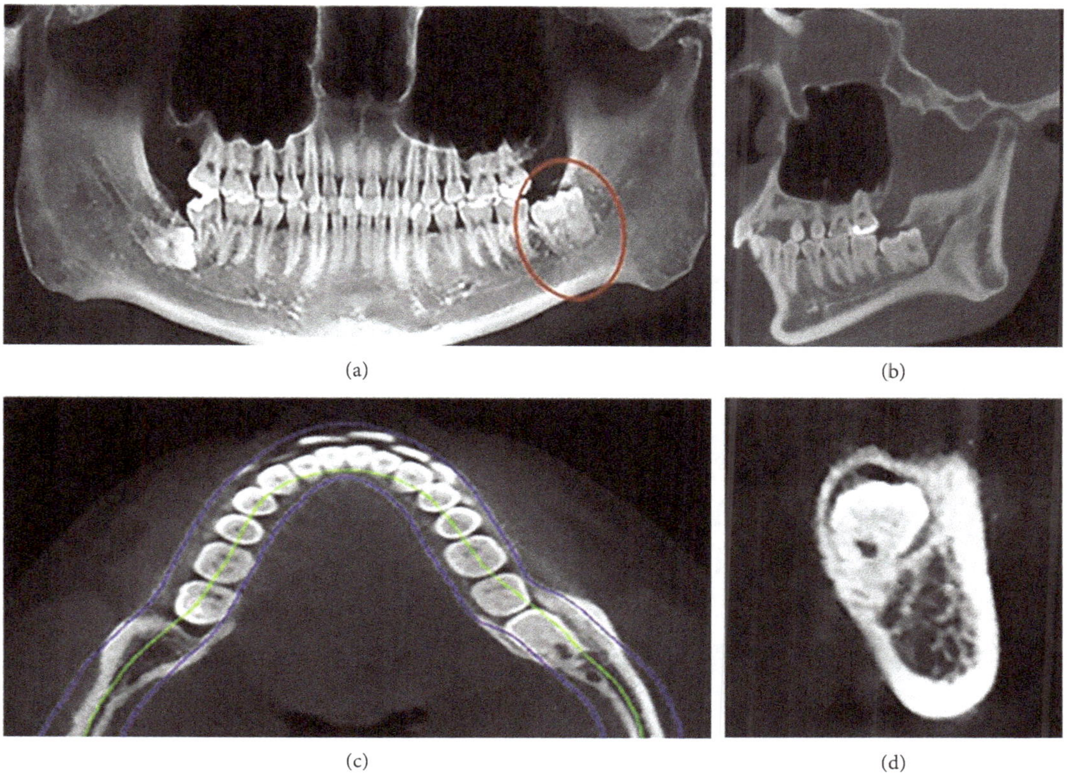

Figure 1: Preoperative CBCT examination. (a) A fourth molar in the mandible left third molar distal; (b–d) the relationship between roots and mandibular canal in coronal, transversal, and sagittal planes.

Table 1: Construction of a scoring system for predicting preoperative risk of inferior alveolar nerve injury (IANI).

Variable	Classification	Score	
		Temporary IANI	Permanent IANI
Age	<25 years old	1	1
Gender	Female	0	0
Contact relationship between mandibular third molar and IAC	Contact	2	2
The vertical contact position of the mandibular third molar with IAC	Middle 1/2 of the root to the neck of the tooth	0	0
Impaction depth	Low-level hindrance	0	0
Root number	Single/multiple	1	1
Total		4	4

Note: IAC, inferior alveolar canal. Risk factors for IANI include the number of roots of mandibular third molars ($P < 0.01$), the impacted depth ($P < 0.05$), and the contact relationship between the roots and the IAC ($P < 0.01$) and vertical contact location ($P < 0.05$). Age <25 years was an independent risk factor for temporary IANI ($P < 0.001$), being female is a risk factor for permanent IANI ($P < 0.05$).

radiograph revealed that teeth 38# and 39# were vertical median impaction in the left mandibular region, and showed a concrescence between an impacted third molar and a supernumerary fourth molar (Figure 1) they shared similar shape but self-governed root canal system. Besides, teeth 48# was impacted at horizontal-low level (Figure 1).

2.1. Preoperative Preparation. Before surgery, we conducted a comprehensive assessment of the risk of surgery based on the patient's general condition and CBCT examination. The evaluation criteria were based on the Chinese Stomatological Association's assessment of the risk factors for lower alveolar nerve injury related to the extraction of mandibular third molars [6] (Table 1). The patient's temporary inferior alveolar nerve injury (IANI) score was divided into 4 levels, permanent IANI was scored as 4 points, and the surgical risk of this case was high hazard classification. The risks of IANI include low hazard classification (≤2 points), moderate hazard classification (3 points) and high hazard classification according to the score (≥4 points and ≤6 points) [6].

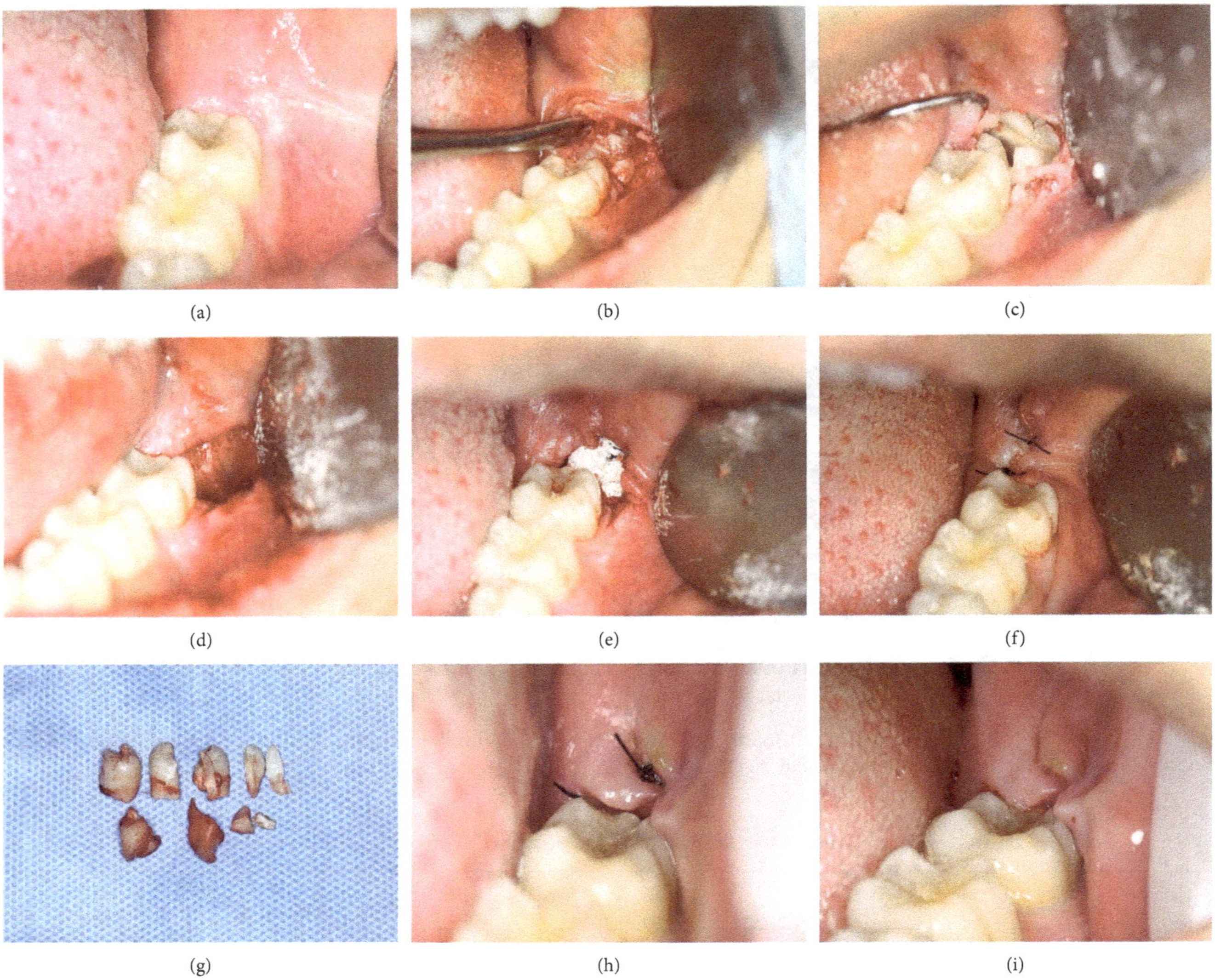

FIGURE 2: Surgery process and follow-up. (a) No wisdom teeth erupting, bleeding, or purulent secretion in the mouth. (b–f) Teeth extraction and alveolar reconstruction. (g) The fragment of teeth. (h, i) Removed stitches without severe complication and the defect of the alveolar socket healed well.

Furthermore, according to the preoperative discussion on flap design and incision design, we finally chose the envelope flap, which was proposed by Gustav Otto Kruger [7]. During surgery, a gingival sulcus incision was made from the mesial side of the mandibular second molar to the mesial surface of the mandibular second molar near the buccal tip, and then the incision was extended 45° obliquely to the mandibular ramus, which was helpful to reduce postoperative swelling and pain [8] and in turn beneficial to postoperative recovery.

2.2. Treatment Process. The patient enrolled for removal of the concrescence teeth. Surgery was carried out under local lidocaine hydrochloride (2%, 2107301, Tianjin Jinyao Pharmaceutical Co, China) and articaine (4%, S-124, Acteon group France, France)-based anesthesia blocking the inferior alveolar, lingual, and buccal nerve. A mucoperiosteal flap was prepared and raised, and then ostectomy and odontomy were performed using handpiece (Figure S1) and sterile saline irrigation. The third and fourth molars were removed. The entire procedure went very smoothly with minimal bleeding and no exposure of the inferior alveolar nerve. After curettage of the cavity, the socket was flushed with saline, and stuffed large alveolar fossa defects with artificial bone material (20201216101B, Beijing Aojing Pharmaceutical Technology Co, China). Finally, the flap was repositioned with 2-0 silk sutures (220103, Ningbo Medical Suture Co, China) (Table S1). Antiflogistic and analgesics therapy were applied for 3–5 days (Figures 2(a)–2(g)).

2.3. Postoperative Follow-Up. After 7 days, the sutures were removed without severe complications (Figures 2(h)–2(i)). The envelope flap incision design mentioned above significantly reduced postoperative swelling. In the intraoral photograph one week after the operation, we could see the soft tissue coverage of the 37# distal gingival without obvious swelling.

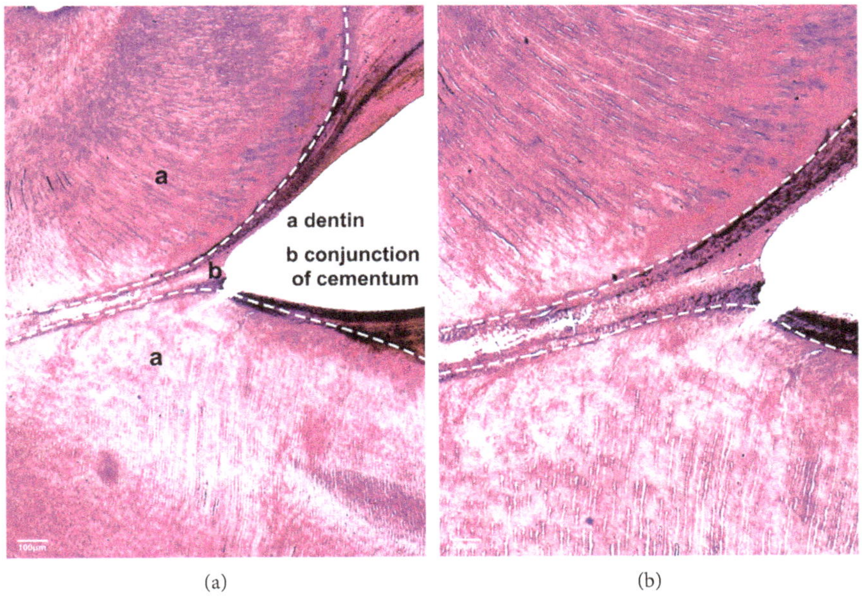

FIGURE 3: Photomicrographs of histological sections stained with the hematoxylin–eosine stain exhibiting the point of cementum fusion, revealing a real concrescence. Images obtained using (a) a 10x microscope and (b) a 20x microscope.

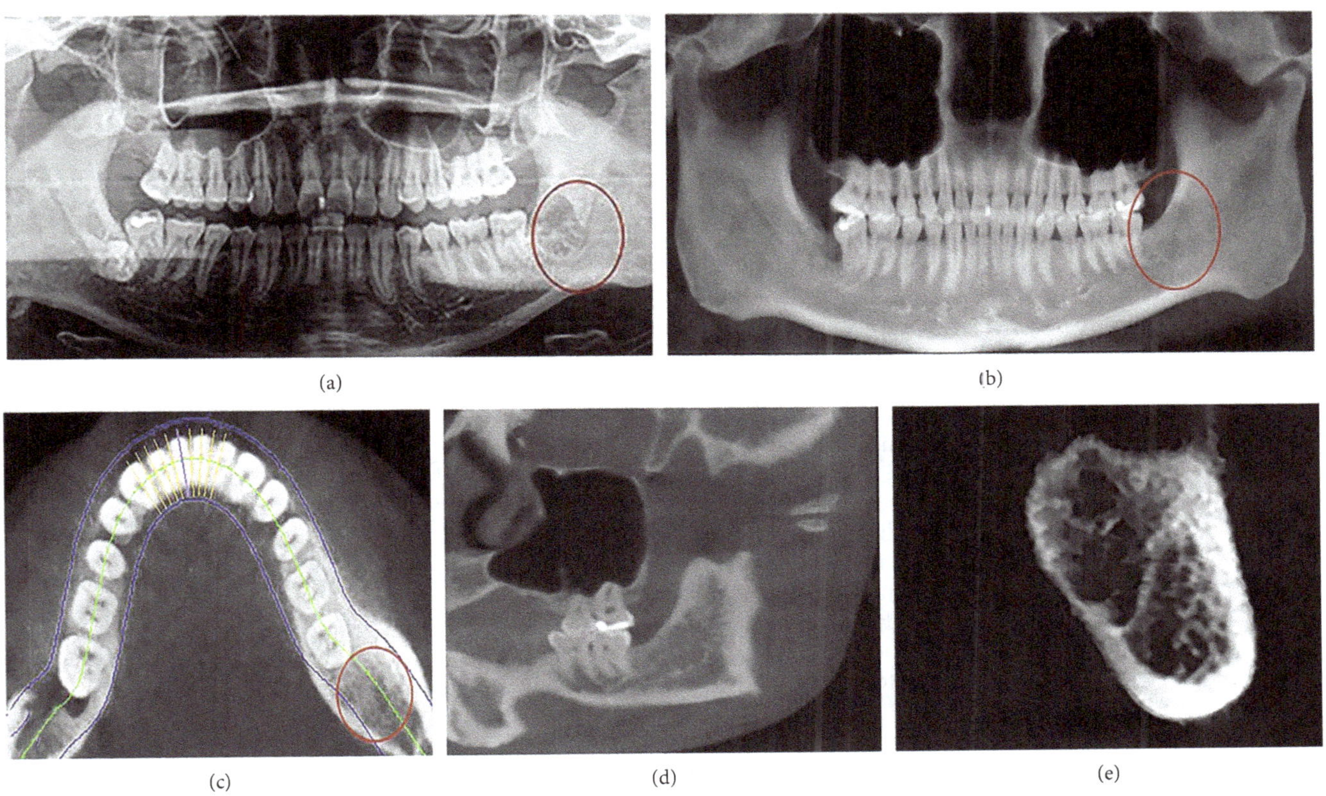

FIGURE 4: (a) Immediate postoperative panoramic examination showed the empty tooth socket; (b) after six months, CBCT examination showed good bone formation, and the alveolar bone healed well. (c) Transverse section shows increased bone density in empty alveolar bone; (d, e) Coronal and sagittal plane shows increased height of the alveolar bone.

Oral clinical examination: no numbness, paresthesia, pain, and loss of touch were noted in the left lower lip and jaw. There is also no numbness in the ipsilateral half tongue.

Histological sections were employed to evaluate which odontogenic tissues were involved in the affected teeth. The histological examination revealed fusion of cementum between the mandibular third molar and supernumerary fourth molar which is diagnostic for concrescence (Figure 3).

Oral clinical examination after 6 months: there was no swelling in the distal mucosa of the 37# and the 37# distal periodontal attachment was in good condition. CBCT examination showed increased bone density (Figure 4).

3. Discussion

Concrescence may occur during root formation or after the radicular phase of development is completed. From the stages of tooth development, different degrees union of cementum, dentine, and enamel are possible [2], and the cause of tooth development abnormalities is hyperactivity of odontogenic epithelium [9]; the failure of the process of degeneration of the residual dental lamina cells leads to further reaction and over-proliferating and eventually develops into supernumerary teeth [10].

Teeth fusion is a condition in which two separate tooth buds have a joined crown that resembles a bifid crown, but concrescence is a form of fusion in which the union is in the cementum alone without confluence of the underlying dentine. In practice, there are very few cases about the concrescence of a third molar and a supernumerary tooth [11]. CBCT radiograph in the case showed that the roots of 38# and 39# seem to be connected, but their dentin was separated and their root canal system was independent. Histological examination revealed fusion of cementum between the mandibular third molar and supernumerary forth molar. In summary, concrescence of teeth (38# and 39#) was diagnosed. Slight bone defects were found in the distal of 37#. According to these findings, a surgical treatment option was provided to deal with concrescence of teeth.

Based on a plenty of the literature studies, it was found that the maxillary fourth molar is more common than those in the mandible, most of which cannot erupt, have none symptoms, and can be found by radiology examinations accidently [12]. Local infection factors, trauma, space restriction in the development, or excessive occlusal force plays crucial roles in phenotypic anomalies. It is very difficult to detect concrescence clinically, and radiographic examination is a means to distinguish between concrescence and other pathological state. When the clinical examination points to affecting aesthetics, causing crowded dentition, eruption pathologies or tooth displacement, periodontal disease, pericoronitis, root resorption of adjacent teeth, bone resorption, or cyst formation [13], treatment is required, or subjective to wishes of the patient, the teeth are supposed to be removed in time.

Several approaches are available for the treatment of supernumerary concrescence. The treatment can be performed in two means: (a) surgical extraction or (b) maintenance of the asymptomatic tooth and periodic monitoring at least once a year [9]. In this case, the impacted teeth led to pericoronitis sometimes, and they might cause the absorption and destruction of the distal neck bone in 37#. Also, the patient had the subjective willingness of extraction. Therefore, we extracted the 38# with 39# and reconstructed the alveolar with artificial bone material to preserve the bone in the distal second molar. The defected alveolar socket appeared well-healed in CBCT examination six months after treatment. In the literature, there have been rare case reports of successful surgical division of concrescent teeth, or selected shaping with or without placement of full crowns has been used for the special cases. This case report is rarely found in the mandible in which concrescence has been observed between a third molar and a supernumerary fourth molar with the space-occupying bone filling materials, restoring the massive bone defect after extraction, and it will provide a reference for the management of similar cases of supernumerary fourth molars.

Consent

Written consent obtained for clinical photographs. Published with the patient's consent.

Acknowledgments

We would like to thank the funding for assistance and the authors also cordially thank Jianlong Yang, MD, from the Institute of Pathology, Lanzhou University, for technical assistance. This study is supported by the Clinical Research Center for Oral Diseases, the Scientific and Technological Foundation of Gansu Province (20JR10FA670); Chinese Stomatological Association Western Stomatology Clinical Research Fund (CSA-W2021-06); The School/Hospital of Stomatology, Lanzhou Univesity(lzukqky-2020-t10; lzukqky-2020-t01)

References

[1] Z. Liu, T. Chen, D. Bai, W. Tian, and Y. Chen, "Smad7 regulates dental epithelial proliferation during tooth development," *Journal of Dental Research*, vol. 98, no. 12, pp. 1376–1385, 2019.

[2] K. Gunduz, M. Sumer, A. P. Sumer, and O. Gunhan, "Concrescence of a mandibular third molar and a supernumerary fourth molar: report of a rare case," *British Dental Journal*, vol. 200, no. 3, pp. 141–142, 2006.

[3] T. Nakamura, L. Jimenez-Rojo, E. Koyama et al., "Epiprofin regulates enamel formation and tooth morphogenesis by controlling epithelial–mesenchymal interactions during tooth development," *Journal of Bone and Mineral Research*, vol. 32, no. 3, pp. 601–610, 2017.

[4] A. Lao, S. Bi, H. Cheng, T. Lai, S. Huang, and S. Zhao, "A combination of kissing molars, maxillary bilateral supernumerary teeth and macrodontia: a rare case report," *BMC Oral Health*, vol. 20, no. 1, p. 112, 2020.

[5] B. O. Bamgbose, S. Okada, M. Hisatomi et al., "Fourth molar: a retrospective study and literature review of a rare clinical entity," *Imaging Science in Dentistry*, vol. 49, no. 1, pp. 27–34, 2019.

[6] J. Qianrui and Z. Xie, "Evaluation of risk factors for lower alveolar nerve injury related to mandibular third molar extraction," *Chinese Journal of Stomatology*, vol. 57, no. 3, pp. 258–265, 2022.

[7] J. S. Sifuentes-Cervantes, F. Carrillo-Morales, J. Castro-Nunez, L. L. Cunningham, and J. E. Van Sickels, "Third molar surgery:

past, present, and the future," *Oral Surgery, Oral Medicine, Oral Pathology, Oral Radiology*, vol. 132, no. 5, pp. 523–531, 2021.

[8] O. Erdogan, U. Tatli, Y. Ustun, and I. Damlar, "Influence of two different flap designs on the sequelae of mandibular third molar surgery," *Oral and Maxillofacial Surgery*, vol. 15, no. 3, pp. 147–152, 2011.

[9] M. Ye, L. Xu, M. Fu et al., "Gene-targeted deletion in mice of the Ets-1 transcription factor, a candidate gene in the Jacobsen syndrome kidney "critical region," causes abnormal kidney development," *American Journal of Medical Genetics. Part A*, vol. 179, no. 1, pp. 71–77, 2019.

[10] Y. Wu, Y. Ke, C. Siyu, H. Nengwen, and W. Liao, "Supernumerary teeth and its theranostics," *International Journal of Stomatology*, vol. 47, no. 3, pp. 311–317, 2020.

[11] P. Dabrowski, D. Nowakowski, A. Gawlikowska-Sroka, I. Maciuszczak, and S. Gronkiewicz, "A case of concrescent tooth—a developmental anomaly in a 19th century skull from Uganda," *International Journal of Paleopathology*, vol. 18, pp. 21–25, 2017.

[12] R. S. Cunha, A. Junaid, and I. Mello, "Unilateral fusion of a supernumerary tooth to a maxillary permanent lateral incisor: a report of a rare case," *Journal of Endodontia*, vol. 41, no. 3, pp. 420–423, 2015.

[13] S. Kumar, V. K. Sharma, P. Gupta, and T. P. Chaturvedi, "Management of non-syndromic multiple impacted supernumerary teeth: a rare case report," *Indian Journal of Science Research*, vol. 8, no. 2, pp. 165–168, 2018.

4

Surgical Management of Extrafollicular Variant of Adenomatoid Odontogenic Tumor in the Maxillary Posterior Region

Gerardo La Monaca,[1] Nicola Pranno,[2] Cira Rosaria Tiziana di Gioia,[3] Giorgio Pompa,[2] Iole Vozza,[2] and Maria Paola Cristalli[4]

[1]*Department of Sense Organs, Sapienza University of Rome, Rome, Italy*
[2]*Department of Oral and Maxillo-Facial Sciences, Sapienza University of Rome, Rome, Italy*
[3]*Department of Radiological, Oncological and Pathological Sciences, Sapienza University of Rome, Rome, Italy*
[4]*Department of Biotechnologies and Medical Surgical Sciences, Sapienza University of Rome, Rome, Italy*

Correspondence should be addressed to Gerardo La Monaca; gerardo.lamonaca@uniroma1.it and Nicola Pranno; nicola.pranno@uniroma1.it

Academic Editor: Eugenio Maiorano

Background. Adenomatoid odontogenic tumor (AOT) is a relatively uncommon benign neoplasm of odontogenic epithelial origin, accounting for less than 5% of odontogenic tumors. *Case Report.* The reported case describes morphological characteristics, clinical course, radiographic and histopathological features, and surgical therapy of an extrafollicular variant of AOT in the maxillary posterior region. An asymptomatic swelling on the left side in the posterior region of the maxilla, gradually increased since approximately 12 months, developed in a 16-year-old Caucasian female patient. Radiographic images revealed a well-defined, unilocular radiolucency, with some small foci of radiopacity inside, and root resorption of the first and second molars. On the base of the histological examination of the specimen retrieved by incisional biopsy, the diagnosis of AOT was made, and the conservative surgical enucleation of the lesion was performed. *Discussion.* The present case was reported in agreement with an extensive review, in which it was recommended to discontinue reporting classic follicular cases because their clinicopathological profile was well-known, but to continue reporting well-documented cases of the extrafollicular variant, with indication of the exact position. *Conclusion.* The present case was reported in order to expand the knowledge about the clinical behavior and surgical treatment of the extrafollicular variant of AOT.

1. Introduction

Adenomatoid odontogenic tumor (AOT) is a relatively uncommon benign neoplasm of odontogenic epithelial origin, accounting for less than 5% of odontogenic tumors [1–3].

The currently used name of "adenomatoid odontogenic tumor" (AOT) was proposed by Philipsen et al. [2] in 1969 and adopted for the first time in the1971 first edition of the World Health Organization (WHO) classification of histological typing of odontogenic tumor, jaw cysts, and allied lesion and retained in the 1992 second edition [4].

Later in the WHO third edition (2005) of Head and Neck Tumors, AOT was defined as an odontogenic tumor "composed of odontogenic epithelium in a variety of histoarchitectural patterns, embedded in a mature connective tissue stroma, and characterized by slow but progressive growth" [5]. Recently, in the WHO 4th edition (2017) of Head and Neck Tumors, AOT was defined as "a benign epithelial tumor that shows duct-like structures" [1].

The reported case describes morphological characteristics, clinical course, radiographic and histopathological features, and surgical therapy of an extrafollicular AOT, which

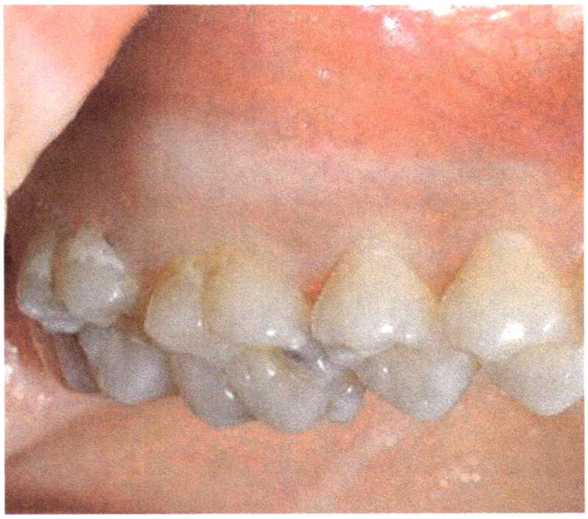

FIGURE 1: Intraoral view showing a swelling in the buccal fold of the left maxillary posterior region.

developed in the maxillary posterior region of a 16-year-old Caucasian female patient.

2. Case Presentation

A young patient (female, 16 years old) was referred to the Oral Surgery Unit of the Policlinico Umberto I Hospital–Sapienza University of Rome with the chief complaint of asymptomatic swelling in the left side in the posterior region of the maxilla, gradually increased to the present size of 3.5 cm since approximately 12 months.

Medical history and extraoral examination were noncontributory, and there was no regional lymphadenopathy.

Intraoral examination revealed, in the buccal fold of the left maxillary posterior region, a swelling extending from behind the canine up to the tuberosity, covered by normal oral mucosa (Figure 1). On palpation, the buccal cortical plate was expanded, and the swelling was smooth, nontender, and nonfluctuant, and its consistency was bony hard.

The involved teeth were sound, positive at cold sensitivity test, and without mobility.

Panoramic radiograph showed in the left maxillary posterior region a well-defined, unilocular radiolucency, root resorption of the first and second molars, and presence of an unerupted third molar (Figure 2).

Panorex view of the Computed Tomography (CT) revealed a hypodense intrabony, unilocular lesion circumscribed by radiopaque border, extending from the mesial margin of the first premolar to the distal margin of the second molar and apicocoronally from the sinus floor to the alveolar ridge. The resorption of the first molar roots and the second molar mesial root and the unerupted third molar not related to the lesion were also detectable (Figure 3(a)).

In the axial view of the CT, a limited expansion and thinning of the buccal and palatal cortical plates, limited cortical perforation in the vestibular wall upper the first molar, and

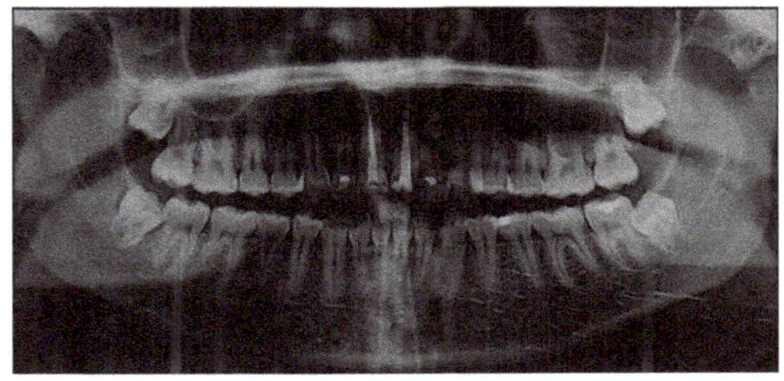

FIGURE 2: Panoramic radiograph showing in the left maxillary posterior region a radiolucent, unilocular lesion, resorptions of 2.6 roots and 2.7 mesial root, and presence of unerupted third molar.

small foci of radiopacity near the mesial root of the first molar were observed (Figure 3(b)).

The resorption of the first molar roots was also evident in the coronal view of the CT (Figure 3(c)).

Based on the clinical and radiographic findings, different pathologic conditions, such as dentigerous cyst, calcifying odontogenic cyst, odontogenic keratocyst, central giant cell granuloma, unicystic ameloblastoma, calcifying epithelial odontogenic tumor, ameloblastic fibroma, and ameloblastic fibroodontoma, were considered, and the preventive histological diagnosis was needed for treatment planning.

Incisional biopsy was performed under local anesthesia (Figure 4).

Histological examination showed a nodular proliferation of polyhedral epithelial cells of probable odontogenic origin, organized either in small cystic spaces with intraluminal basophilic PAS-positive material or in syncytial and trabecular nests. The stroma was poorly cellular, either intensely eosinophilic or amorphous like dentin, with some calcifications (Figure 5). A diagnosis of AOT was made.

Conservative surgical enucleation of the lesion, extraction of the first molar, and apicectomy of the involved teeth, previously endodontically-treated, were planned.

The surgery was performed under general anesthesia. Surgical access was obtained through a full-thickness trapezoidal intrasulcular buccal flap, extending from the mesial aspect of the canine to the distal aspect of the second molar (Figure 6(a)). The flap was detached, and the cortical bone was exposed (Figure 6(b)).

After the first molar extraction, ostectomy was performed under sterile saline irrigation with a round tungsten carbide burr mounted on a low-speed handpiece used with a tangential movement not to involve the underlying lesion. The fibrotic capsule surrounding the tumor was dissected from the bony wall, and the mass was completely enucleated (Figures 6(c) and 6(d)).

Before flap repositioning, amputation of the resorbed mesial root of the second molar, and apicectomy of the premolars and the remaining roots of the second molar, thorough debridement of the bony cavity and trimming of the rough bony edges were carried out.

A releasing periosteal incision was made at the bottom of the buccal flap to enhance its elasticity and to achieve tension-free primary closure, the tumor cavity was packed with absorbable gelatin sponge (Gelfoam®, Pfizer, New

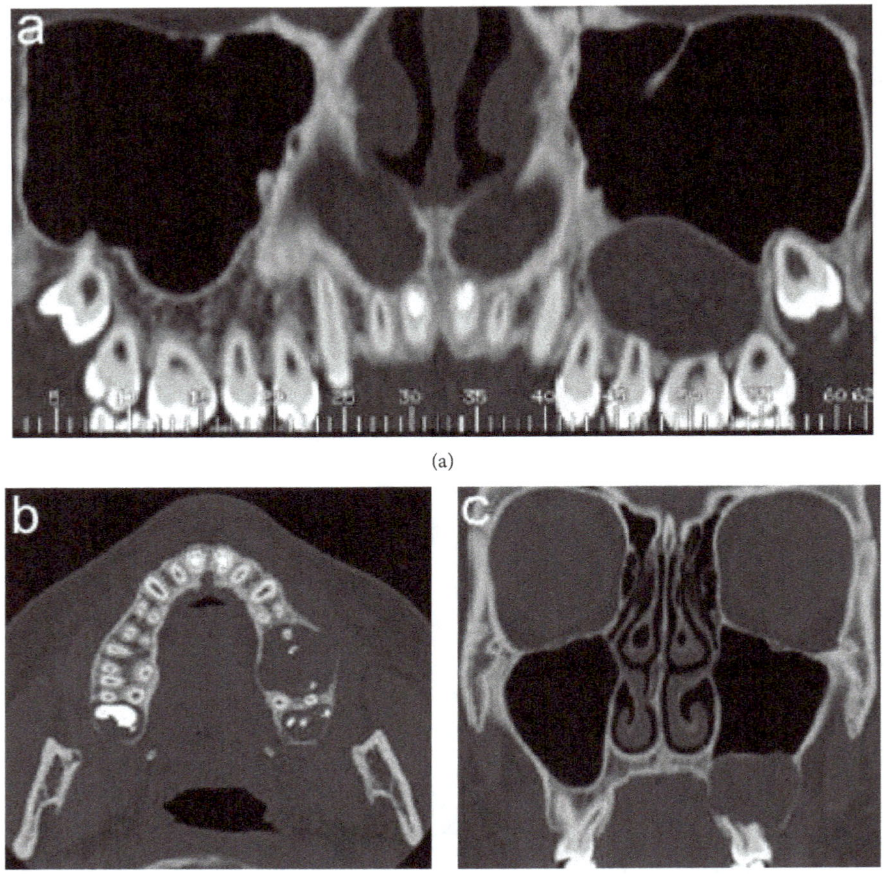

(a) (b) (c)

Figure 3: Computed tomography scan: (a) panorex view: unilocular, well defined, hypodense area extending from the mesial root of 2.4 up to the distal root of 2.7 and in the apicocoronal direction from the sinus floor to the alveolar ridge; (b) axial view: limited expansion and thinning of the buccal and palatal cortical plates, erosion of the buccal wall, and some small foci of radiopacity; and (c) coronal view: root resorption of the first molar.

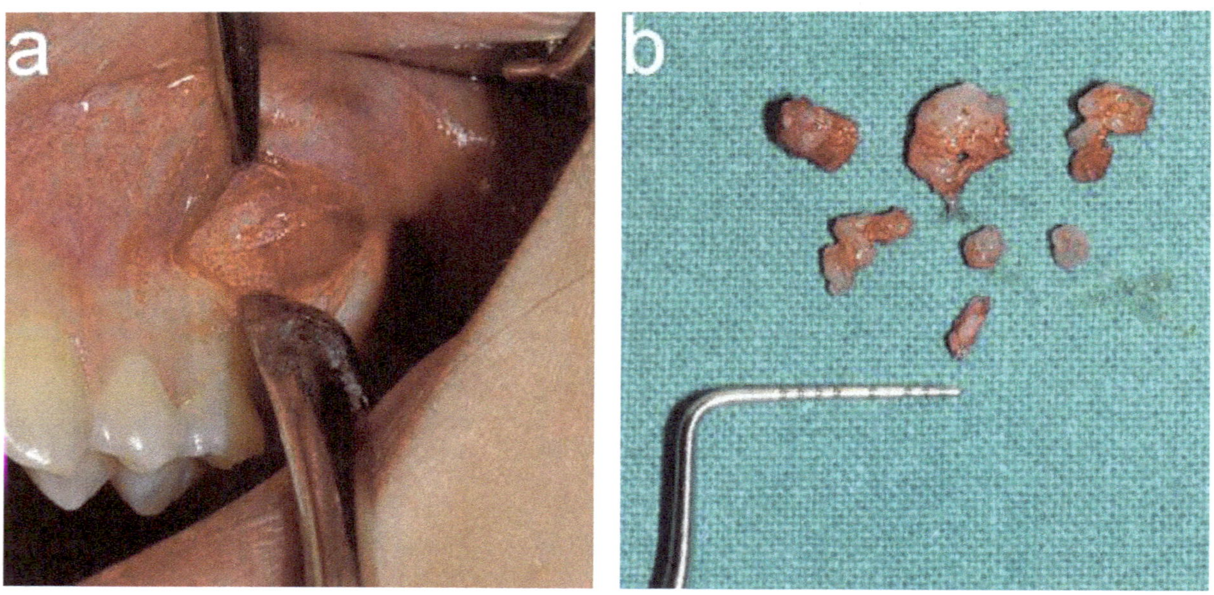

(a) (b)

Figure 4: Incisional biopsy: (a) incision in the buccal fold and (b) retrieved specimen.

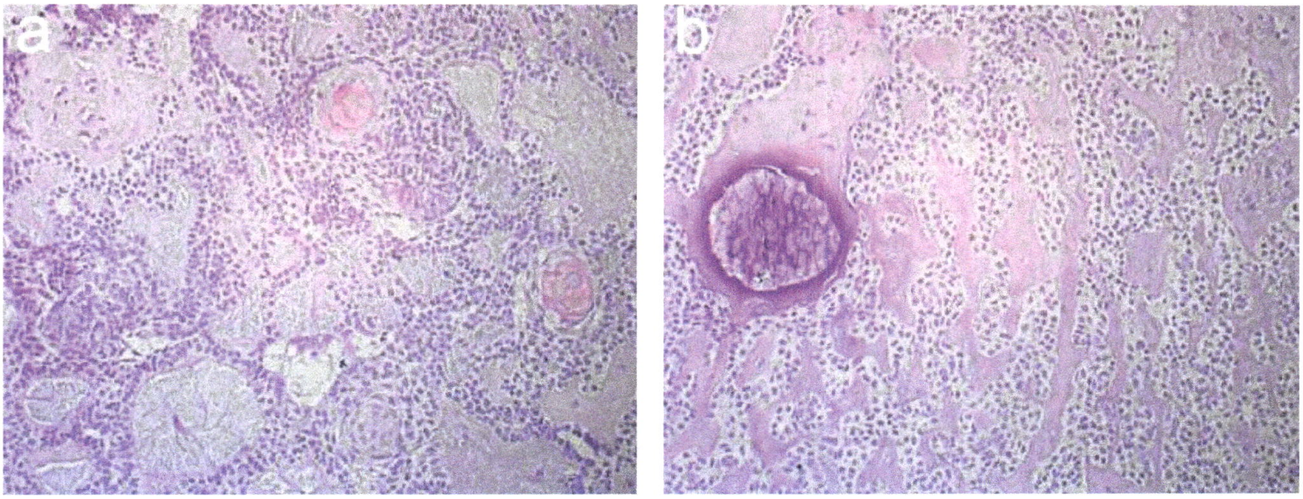

(a) (b)

Figure 5: Histopathological sections of incisional biopsy specimen: (a) characteristic of nodular epithelial proliferation composed of polyhedral to spindle cells with lobular or syncytial arrangement of cells (hematoxylin and eosin, 20X) and (b) foci of PAS-positive material and some.

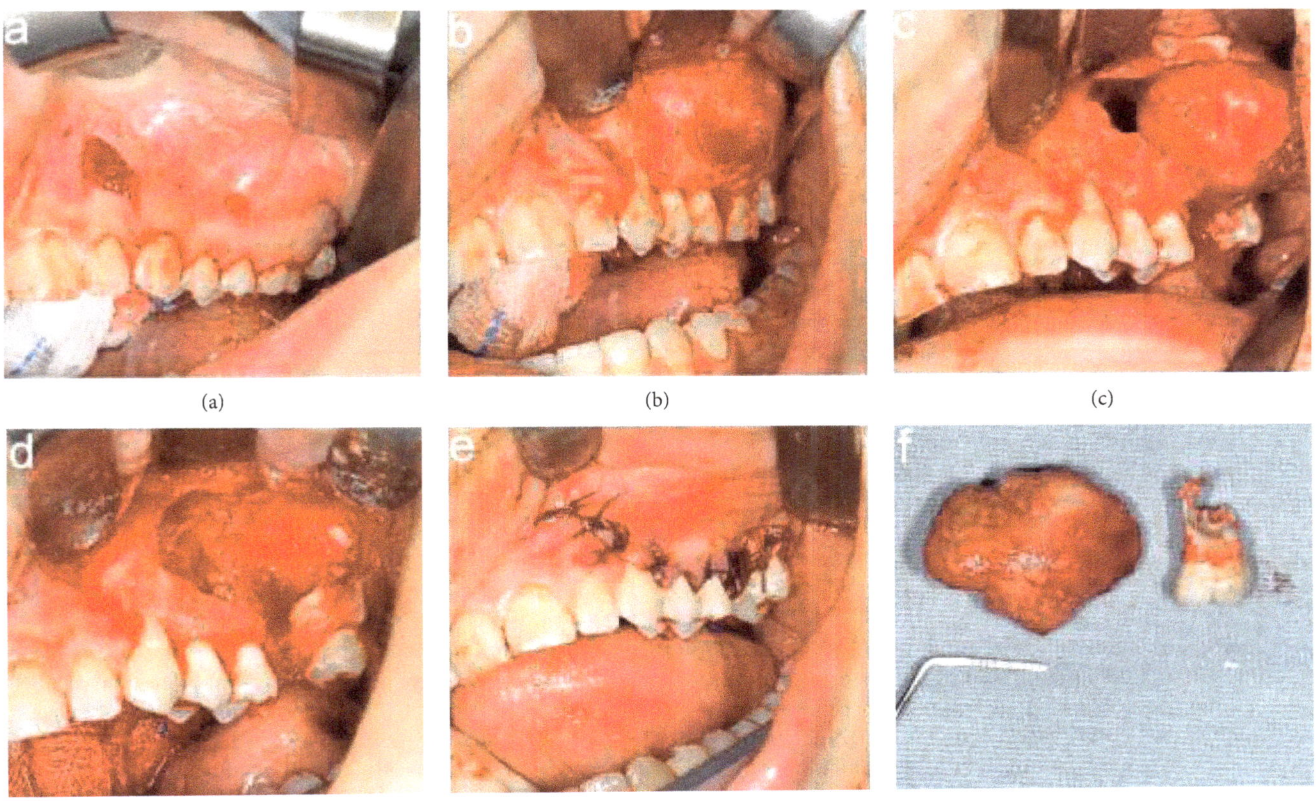

(a) (b) (c)

(d) (e) (f)

Figure 6: Surgical treatment: (a) a full-thickness intrasulcular trapezoidal buccal flap, (b) detaching of the flap, (c) ostectomy and dissection of the lesion from the bony walls, (d) bony cavity, (e) suture, and (f) surgical specimen.

York, USA), and the interrupted sutures were placed (4-0 Vicryl, Johnson & Johnson Medical, Norderstedt, Germany) (Figure 6(e)).

The surgical specimen was submitted for histopathological examination, and the diagnosis confirmed the previous incisional biopsy (Figure 6(f)).

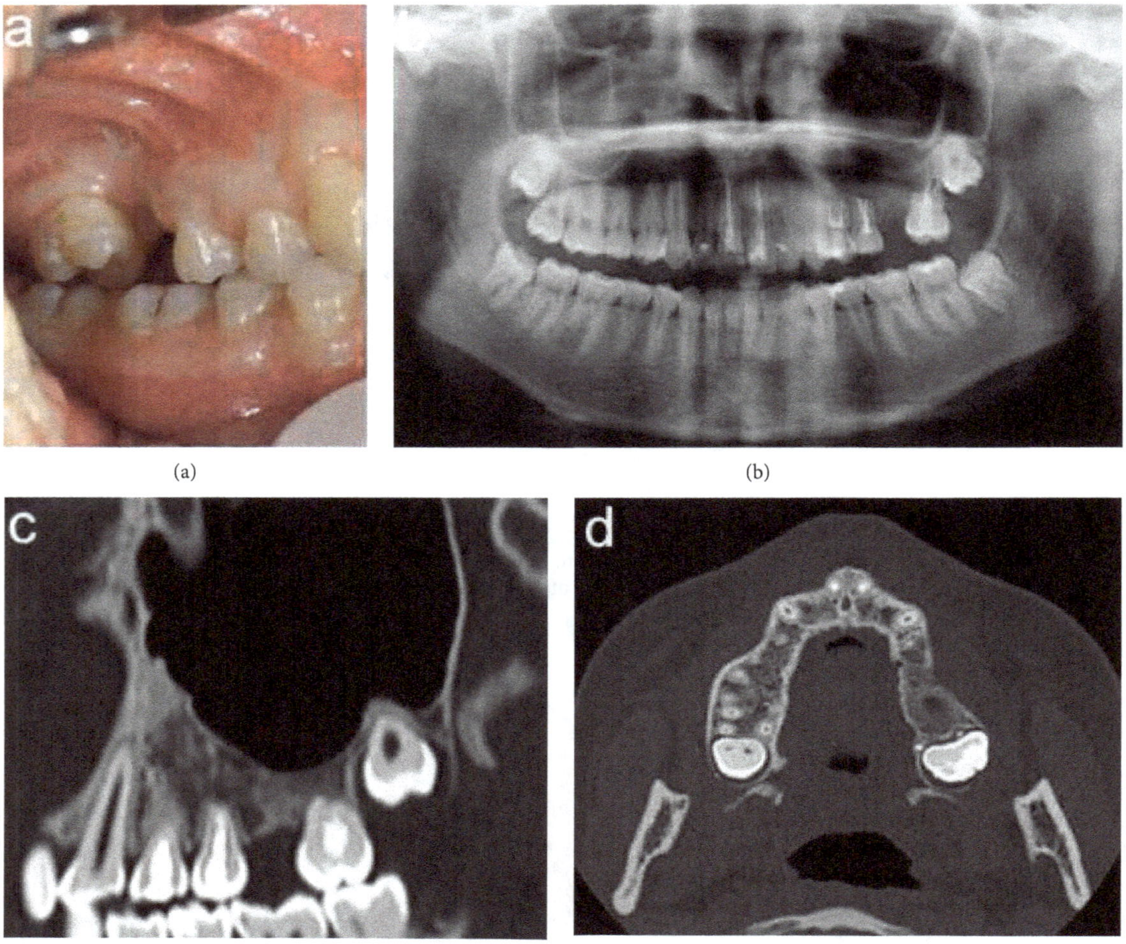

(a) (b) (c) (d)

FIGURE 7: Twelve-month follow-up: (a) intraoral view, (b) ortopantomography, (c) CT sagittal view, and (d) CT axial view.

Healing was uneventful without any complications and follow-up was performed at 3, 6, and 12 months.

One year after the surgery, clinical examination and radiographs showed restitutio ad integrum both of the bone and the soft tissues and no local recurrence (Figure 7).

3. Discussion

An extrafollicular case of AOT in the posterior maxillary region was described, as suggested in the review by Philipsen et al. [2]. The authors recommended to discontinue reporting classical follicular cases but to continue reporting well-documented cases of the extrafollicular variant, with indication of the exact position.

AOT is relatively rare, with only 1558 cases reported in a total of 436 publications retrieved in a recent updated analysis of the literature undertaken without time restrictions up to July 2018 [6].

AOT affects more frequently the second and third decade of life (range: 1-83 years), female patients (male : female ratio 1 : 1.9), and maxilla over the mandible (ratio: 2.1 : 1), with a preference for the anterior portion of the jaws [1, 2, 5–7].

AOT has three distinct clinicopathological variants without any relevant clinical and radiographic differences between them: intraosseous follicular (73% of all cases), related to retained tooth, most often a canine; intraosseous extrafollicular (24%), which is subdivided into E1 no relation to tooth structure either erupted or unerupted, E2 intraradicular adjacent roots, E3 superimposed on the root apex, and E4 superimposed on the midroot level; and peripheral (3%), in the soft tissue overlying the tooth-bearing area [5, 6, 8–10].

For the follicular variant, there is histologic and immunohistochemical evidence that it arises from the reduced enamel epithelium of the dental follicle, whereas origin of the extrafollicular variant is less clear [11, 12]. Philipsen et al. [2] argued that the identical histology in all AOT variants points towards a common origin and implicate the dental lamina or its remains.

The lesion ranges from 2 to 7 cm in size, has a slow growing pattern which can result in a painless expansion of the jaws, and often leads to the displacement of the adjacent teeth, whereas root resorption is more rare [6, 10]. The aggressive behavior of the AOT is quite exceptional, with only a few cases reported in the literature, mainly in the mandible [13].

In this report sex, age, and clinical and histopathologic appearance were consistent with the literature, but the location in the posterior region of the maxillary jaw and some features, such as root resorption, cortical perforation, and small radiopaque foci inside the radiolucent lesions, were less frequent.

Conservative surgical approach with complete enucleation of the lesion is the treatment of choice, justified by the benign behavior, presence of clear demarcation, and low rates of recurrence [6, 14].

In the present case, in addition to excision of the lesion, surgical management required the extraction of the first upper molar, mesial root amputation of the second molar, and apicectomy of the premolars and the remaining roots of the second molar.

4. Conclusion

The present case was reported to increase the knowledge about morphological characteristics, clinical course, radiographic and histopathological features, and surgical therapy of an extrafollicular AOT arising in the posterior maxilla.

Consent

Written informed consent was obtained from the patient's parents both for therapeutic approach and publication of data and images for educational and scientific purposes.

References

[1] A. K. El-Naggar, J. K. C. Chan, J. R. Grandis, T. Takata, and P. W. H. O. Slootweg, *Classification of Head and Neck Tumours*, IARC WHO Classification of Tumours, No 9, 4th edition, 2017.

[2] H. P. Philipsen, P. A. Reichart, C. H. Siar et al., "An updated clinical and epidemiological profile of the adenomatoid odontogenic tumour: a collaborative retrospective study," *Journal of Oral Pathology & Medicine*, vol. 36, no. 7, pp. 383–393, 2007.

[3] M. Marrelli, A. Pacifici, G. di Giorgio et al., "Diagnosis and treatment of a rare case of adenomatoid odontogenic tumor in a young patient affected by attenuated familial adenomatosis polyposis (aFAP): case report and 5 year follow-up," *European Review for Medical and Pharmacological Sciences*, vol. 18, no. 2, pp. 265–269, 2014.

[4] I. R. Kramer and J. J. Pindborg, "Histological typing of odontogenic tumours, jaw cysts and allied lesions," in *WHO International Histological Classification of Tumors No. 5*, Springer, Verlap, Berlin, Germany, 1971.

[5] L. Barnes, J. W. Eveson, P. Reichart, and D. Sidransky, *World Health Organization Classification of Tumours. Pathology and Genetics of Head and Neck Tumours*, IARC Press, Lyon, France, 2005.

[6] B. R. Chrcanovic and R. S. Gomez, "Adenomatoid odontogenic tumor: an updated analysis of the cases reported in the literature," *Journal of Oral Pathology & Medicine*, vol. 48, no. 1, pp. 10–16, 2019.

[7] F. Al-Shimari, S. Chandra, and D. Oda, "Adenomatoid odontogenic tumor: case series of 14 with wide range of clinical presentation," *Journal of Clinical and Experimental Dentistry*, vol. 9, no. 11, pp. 1315–1321, 2017.

[8] V. Shivali, A. Pandey, V. D. Khanna, P. Khanna, A. Singh, and T. Ahuja, "A rare case of extrafollicular adenomatoid odontogenic tumour in the posterior region of the mandible: misdiagnosed as residual cyst," *Journal of international oral health: JIOH*, vol. 5, no. 5, pp. 124–128, 2013.

[9] M. R. Oliveira, M. A. Gabrielli, M. F. Gabrielli, C. R. Andrade, B. N. Silva, and V. A. Pereira-Filho, "Unusual adenomatoid odontogenic tumor," *The Journal of Craniofacial Surgery*, vol. 27, no. 2, pp. 139–141, 2016.

[10] N. Karam Genno, N. Aoun, and S. El Toum, "Adenomatoid odontogenic tumor associated with an impacted maxillary lateral incisor: a case report with five-year follow-up," *Case Reports in Dentistry*, vol. 2017, Article ID 1709492, 5 pages, 2017.

[11] A. Thakur, J. V. Tupkari, T. Joy, and A. V. Hanchate, "Adenomatoid odontogenic tumor: what is the true nature?," *Medical Hypotheses*, vol. 97, pp. 90–93, 2016.

[12] F. Ide, T. Muramatsu, Y. Ito et al., "An expanded and revised early history of the adenomatoid odontogenic tumor," *Oral Surgery, Oral Medicine, Oral Pathology, Oral Radiology*, vol. 115, no. 5, pp. 646–651, 2013.

[13] S. Shaikh, S. Bansal, R. S. Desai, and I. Ahmad, "Aggressive adenomatoid odontogenic tumor of the mandible: a rare case report and review of the literature," *Journal of Oral and Maxillofacial Pathology*, vol. 22, no. 4, Supplement 1, pp. 11–S15, 2018.

[14] D. Virupakshappa, B. S. Rajashekhara, B. S. Manjunatha, and N. Das, "Adenomatoid odontogenic tumour in a 20-year-old woman," *BML Case Reports*, vol. 2014, article bcr2013010436, 2014.

5

Multilayered Connective Tissue Grafting Technique to Improve Aesthetics after Failed GBR: A Clinical Case Report of 16 Months Follow-Up

Gabriele Villa,[1,2] Gionata Bellucci,[1] Simone Magnolo,[1] and Farah Asa'ad[3]

[1]*Unit of Periodontology, Fondazione IRCCS Ca' Granda Ospedale Maggiore Policlinico, University of Milan, Milan, Italy*
[2]*Private Practice, Biella, Italy*
[3]*Department of Biomaterials, Institute of Clinical Sciences, The Sahlgrenska Academy, University of Gothenburg, Göteborg, Sweden*

Correspondence should be addressed to Farah Asa'ad; farah.asaad@gu.se

Academic Editor: Gavriel Chaushu

Objective. This case report describes soft-tissue management after a failed GBR procedure to enhance the soft-tissue quality, quantity, and aesthetic outcomes. *Case Presentation.* A 38-year-old patient visited the Dental Clinic of the Ospedale Maggiore Policlinico, University of Milan, Milan, Italy, for a chief complaint of unsatisfactory aesthetics of the anterior maxillary area. Dental history disclosed failed preimplant vertical bone augmentation with GBR procedure in the area of the left maxillary central incisor resulting in a severe gingival recession of adjacent teeth and compromised soft-tissue quantity and quality and severe ridge atrophy (class III). Multilayered connective tissue grafting technique, in a two-step mucogingival surgery, was used to cover the gingival recessions, reach even gingival margin, and reconstruct the defect. Frenectomy was done after the second mucogingival surgery to relieve the muscle attachment. A definitive cantilever bridge was placed to restore the left and right maxillary central incisors, and a satisfactory aesthetic outcome was reached. *Conclusions.* Multilayered connective tissue grafting technique might be successful in correcting soft-tissue quantity and quality in class III ridge defects.

1. Introduction

Bone augmentation procedures are routinely applied in cases of alveolar ridge deficiency, in order to achieve sufficient vertical and/or horizontal bone volume, which ensures successful outcomes of dental implant therapy [1]. In general, vertical bone augmentation [2] procedures are more challenging than horizontal bone augmentation procedures and employ various techniques: vertical guided bone regeneration (GBR), onlay grafting, inlay grafting, split bone block technique, and distraction osteogenesis [3–5]. These procedures are frequently associated with high complication rates, reportedly up to 45% [4], such as soft-tissue dehiscence and subsequent exposure of the bone grafting material into the oral cavity [6]. Although most of bone augmentation procedures require autogenous bone and/or bone graft substitutes to achieve successful outcomes of dental implant therapy [5], soft-tissue augmentation might also be necessary to enhance the final outcomes, especially in the anterior maxilla [7].

Management of vertical bone augmentation failures can be quite challenging, not only because of a more pronounced bone deficiency afterwards but also due to compromised quantity and quality of soft tissues at the surgical site and gingival recessions/loss of attachment on adjacent teeth. Therefore, management of bone augmentation failures frequently requires enhancement of soft-tissue quantity and quality through soft-tissue grafting procedures. Specifically, subepithelial connective tissue grafts [8, 9] and deepithelialized free gingival grafts [10] can be utilized for the purposes of increasing soft-tissue volume and covering gingival recessions around adjacent teeth.

In the present case report, we describe for the first time the application of a novel multilayered soft-tissue grafting technique, with multiple connective tissue grafts, obtained by deepithelializing multiple free gingival grafts, to augment

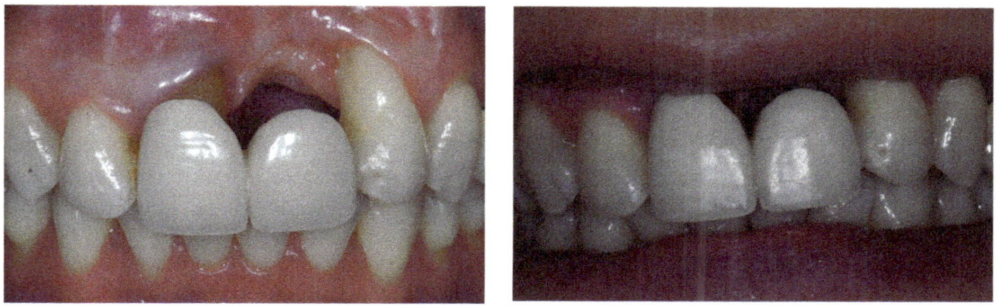

(a) (b)

FIGURE 1: (a, b) Site of chief complaint revealing unsatisfactory aesthetic appearance.

a class III Seibert defect [11] in the anterior maxilla that resulted from a previously failed vertical GBR. Since the patient was completely unsatisfied with the poor aesthetic appearance in the anterior maxilla and refused to undergo another bone augmentation procedure, soft-tissue grafting was adopted to correct the vertical GBR failure.

2. Case Presentation

In 2017, a 38-year-old Caucasian female visited the Dental Clinic of the Ospedale Maggiore Policlinico, University of Milan, Milan, Italy, with a chief complaint of unsatisfactory aesthetic appearance of the anterior maxillary area.

Intraoral examination revealed severe vertical bone loss and scarred soft tissues in the area of the left maxillary central incisor, which was replaced by a pontic (Figures 1(a) and 1(b)).

Severe gingival recession was evident on the left maxillary lateral incisor and the right maxillary central incisor, both of which had degree II mobility.

Dental history revealed that the left maxillary central incisor was extracted due to periodontal disease (Figure 2) and that a preimplant vertical GBR utilizing a titanium-reinforced nonresorbable high-density e-PTFE membrane with autogenous graft/xenograft of a 1 : 1 ratio was performed in the area four months prior to the patient's visit to the university's dental clinic.

The PTFE membrane was exposed and infected, but the patient was away on vacation and could not visit the dentist to manage the case. Therefore, the infected membrane stayed in situ for one month, which resulted in complications in soft-tissue healing, scarred soft tissues in the region of the left maxillary central incisor and severe gingival recessions of the adjacent teeth, resulting in a compromised soft-tissue quantity and quality in the anterior maxillary area. The patient was unsatisfied with the overall aesthetic appearance. The patient did not report any pain in the area of chief complaint. Cone-beam computed tomography (CBCT) revealed a severe vertical bone defect. Due to the ridge defect and lack of soft-tissue quantity, the discrepancy in the location of the gingival margin was about 1 cm (Figure 1(a)).

To manage this case, enhancement of the soft-tissue quantity and quality and improvement of the aesthetic outcomes were planned in a multistep soft-tissue reconstruction surgery.

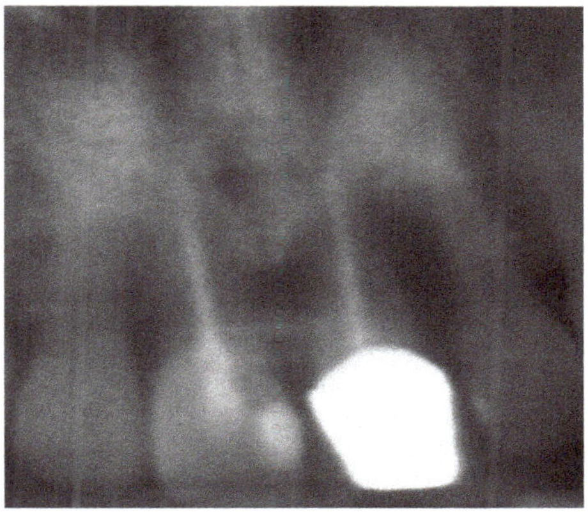

FIGURE 2: Section from panoramic radiograph representing the site of chief complaint, prior to the attempted extraction of the left maxillary central incisor. Severe vertical bone defect around the left maxillary central incisor is evident.

3. Case Management

3.1. First Mucogingival Surgery. The flap design applied to manage this case is presented in Figure 3. The flap design followed the one described by Zucchelli and De Sanctis [12, 13] to manage multiple gingival recessions with coronally advanced flap adding two vertical releasing incisions, one distal to the left maxillary canine and one distal to the right maxillary canine, going about 4-5 mm in the alveolar mucosa. On the alveolar crest, a horizontal incision was done on the vestibular side. All the incisions were split-thickness. Deep split-thickness elevation was done 3-4 mm parallel to the bone. On the palatal side, "palatal island flap" was performed as described by Tinti et al. [14] and modified by Hürzeler et al. [15], in order to achieve primary intention closure. In brief, a horizontal incision was done in the palatal side, connecting the palatal sides of the right maxillary central incisor and the left maxillary lateral incisor, followed by two full thickness releasing vertical incisions that were then connected by a full-thickness horizontal incision, parallel to the first horizontal incision, about 10 mm more apically. At this point, a split-thickness incision was done from the coronal horizontal incision for about 5 mm into the apical direction, and another split-thickness incision was done from the apical horizontal incision for about 3 mm into the coronal

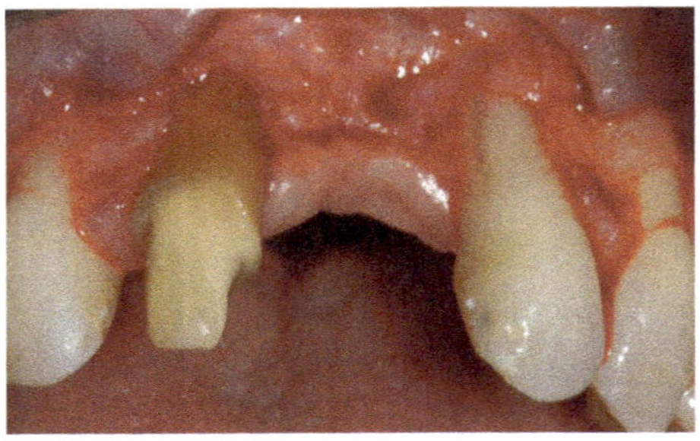

Figure 3: Flap is released (split-full-split) following coronally advanced flap design (as described by Zucchelli & De Sanctis).

direction, all done using a microblade. All root surfaces were dried and conditioned with EDTA for 2 minutes and then with Emdogain.

After the elevation of the flap, the occlusal surface between the two horizontal incisions in the edentulous area was deepithelialized, as it was the recipient site for the soft-tissue graft.

Afterwards, free gingival grafts (FGGs) were harvested from the right and left sides of the palate, from the second molar up to the lateral incisor, as described by Zucchelli et al. [16]. Both grafts were deepithelialized with a 15C blade, to obtain connective tissue grafts.

The first graft, harvested from the right palate, of about 20 mm in length (Figure 4(a)), was folded (Figure 4(b)), and then secured by two vertical mattress sutures, with 7/0 PGA sutures, to form a two-layered graft. The two-layered graft was sutured on the connective tissue of the occlusal side of the edentulous deepithelialized area, with a horizontal mattress suture and an interrupted suture, to secure the graft in place (Figure 5). Then, the second graft was harvested from the other side of the palate, which was of 20 mm length and 7 mm in width (Figure 6). This second graft was cut in two parts; the first part, which was about 13 mm in length, was sutured on the periosteum of the buccal side, with a horizontal mattress suture on the apical side and with a single interrupted suture on the first graft on the deepithelialized anatomical papillae (Figure 7).

After securing and stabilizing the first part of the second graft in place, the second part of the second graft, which was about 7 mm length (Figure 8), was then sutured occlusally with two sling sutures around the right maxillary central incisor and the left maxillary lateral incisor (Figures 9 and 10).

Coronal advancement of the buccal flap was obtained by means of two split-thickness incisions: a deep one, to cut the muscle insertions in the periosteum, and a superficial one, to detach the muscle inserting in the inner aspect of the mucosa lining the flap. This second incision allowed for the coronal advancement of the flap. The flap mobilization was considered appropriate when the buccal horizontal incision of the edentulous area reached the palatal horizontal incision without any tension. Sling sutures suspended around the palatal cingula of the involved teeth were used to anchor the surgical papillae to the corresponding deepithelialized anatomical papillae. Single interrupted sutures, with 6/0 prolene, were performed to have a complete closure between the horizontal incisions of the edentulous area and the palatal island flap (Figure 11).

3.2. Second Mucogingival Surgery. Due to incomplete soft-tissue augmentation, we performed a second mucogingival surgery, 6 months after the first one (Figure 12). There was a complete absence of pocketing around the area of the first surgery. The same flap design, which was applied in the first surgery, was utilized. After split-thickness flap elevation, probing depth around the anterior maxillary teeth was 2 mm (Figures 13 and 14), which could mean that we might have a connective tissue attachment to the root surface of the right maxillary central incisor and the left maxillary lateral incisor.

The first graft, which was harvested from the right palate and was about 20 mm in length, was folded and then secured by two vertical mattress sutures, with 6/0 PGA sutures, to form a two-layered graft. The two-layered graft was sutured on the connective tissue of the occlusal side of the edentulous deepithelialized area with a horizontal mattress suture and an interrupted suture to secure the graft in place.

A second graft was then harvested from the other side of the palate and was of 25 mm length and 7 mm in width. This second graft was cut in two parts; the first part (about 18 mm length) was sutured on the periosteum of the buccal side, with a horizontal mattress suture on the apical side and with a single interrupted suture on the first graft and on the deepithelialized anatomical papillae. This graft, which was 5 mm longer than the buccal one done in the first surgery, covered the buccal area from the right maxillary central incisor up to the left maxillary lateral incisor.

After the first part of the second graft was secured in place and was completely stable, the second part of the graft (which was about 7 mm length) was then sutured occlusally with two sling sutures around the right maxillary central incisor and the left maxillary lateral incisor (Figures 15 and 16). All the sutures used to stabilize the grafts in place were 6/0 PGA sutures. Flap closure was obtained in the same way as the first surgery by utilizing interrupted and sling sutures with 6/0 prolene (Figure 17). The palatal island flap facilitated primary intention closure of the flap as shown in Figure 18. In both surgeries, the palatal wound was protected with cyanoacrylate and collagen pack as previously described in literature [17], which helped limit the patient's postoperative discomfort, despite having multiple grafts harvested from both palatal sides.

3.3. Laser Frenectomy. We proposed the patient to undergo a strip technique [18, 19] to correct the amount of keratinized tissue and remove all muscular insertions. The patient was satisfied with the outcome and declined to undergo another graft harvesting surgery, so we performed a frenectomy with an apically positioned flap, using laser; six months after the second mucogingival surgery, the frenum was removed with a diode laser [20, 21] to relieve muscle attachment in the area.

3.4. Prosthetic Reconstruction. A temporary cantilever resin-bonded bridge was used during the surgical periods to allow for proper tissue healing. Sixteen months after the first

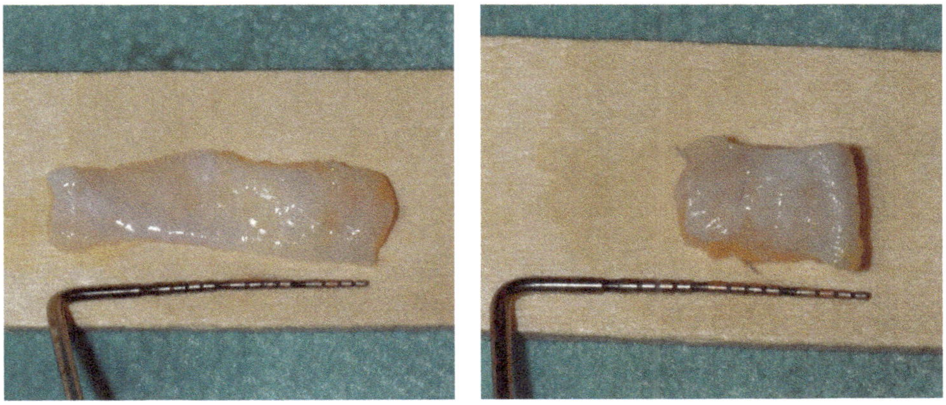

(a) (b)

FIGURE 4: (a) Deepithelialized free gingival graft. (b) Connective tissue graft folded in two layers and then sutured, to gain soft-tissue thickness in the vertical direction.

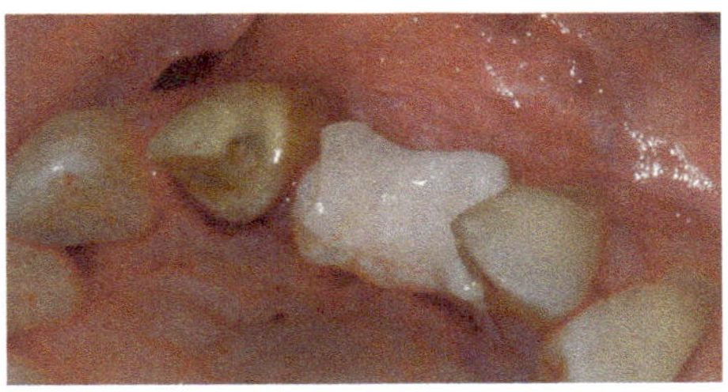

FIGURE 5: Folded connective tissue graft sutured at the defect site.

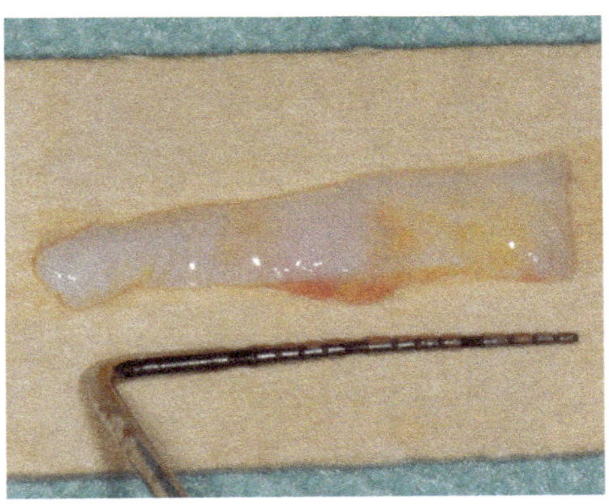

FIGURE 6: Second deepithelialized free gingival graft.

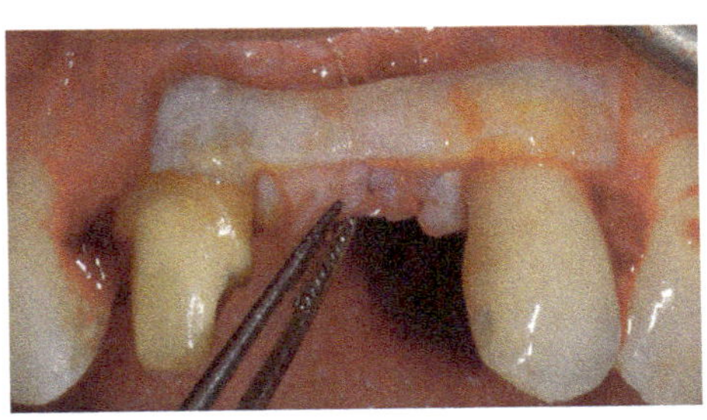

FIGURE 7: First part of the second deepithelialized free gingival graft sutured on the buccal side.

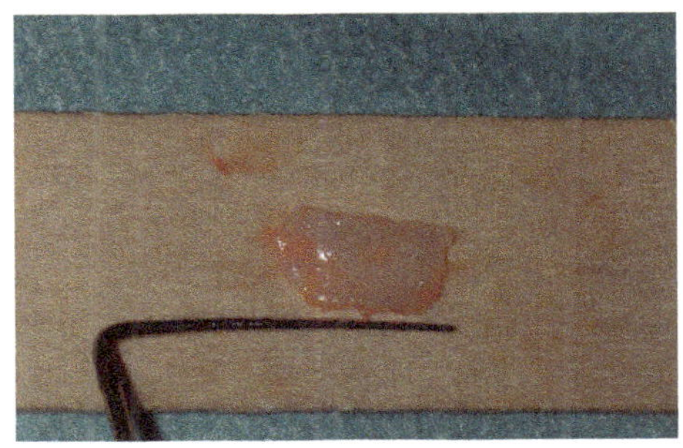

FIGURE 8: Second part of the second deepithelialized free gingival graft.

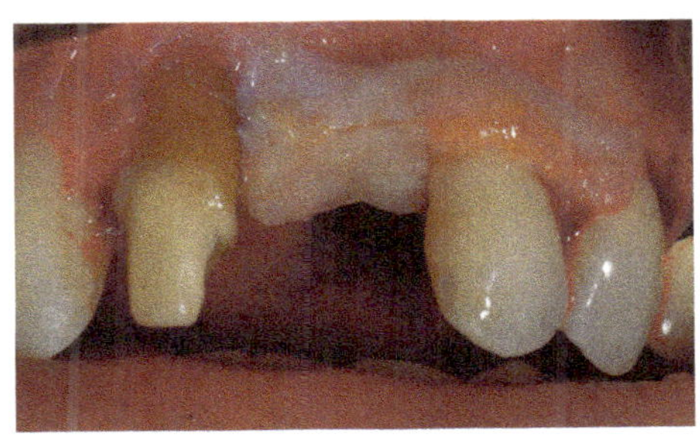

FIGURE 9: Sutured multilayered connective tissue graft (frontal view).

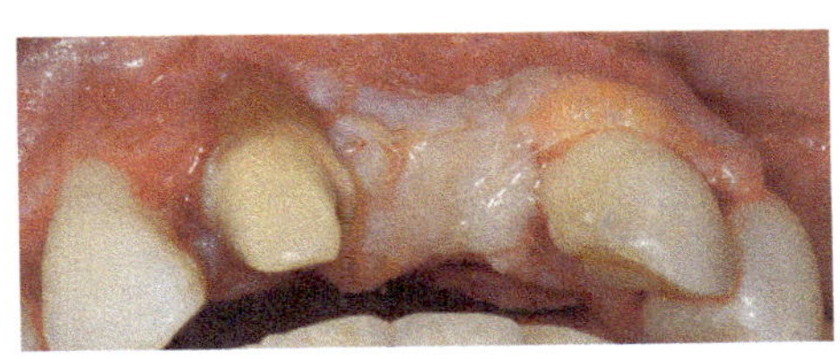

FIGURE 10: Sutured multilayered connective tissue graft (occlusal view).

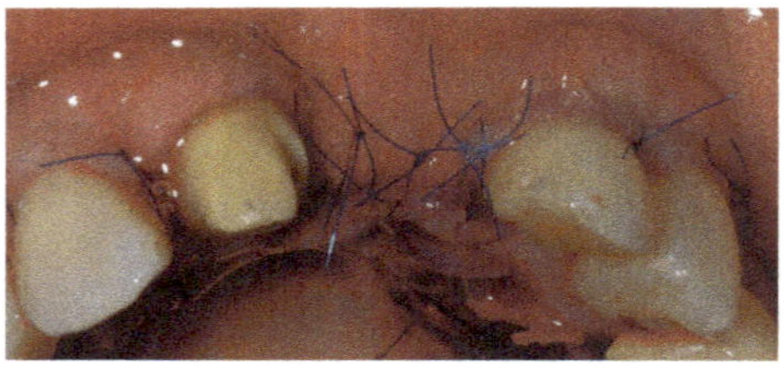

Figure 11: Suturing of the flap.

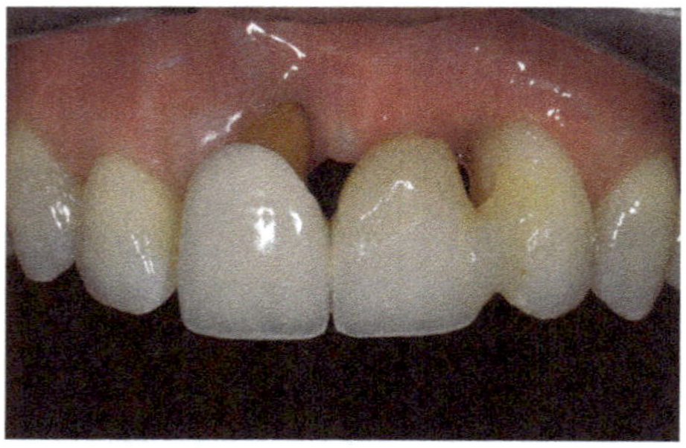

Figure 12: Healing after 6 months. Incomplete soft-tissue augmentation is evident.

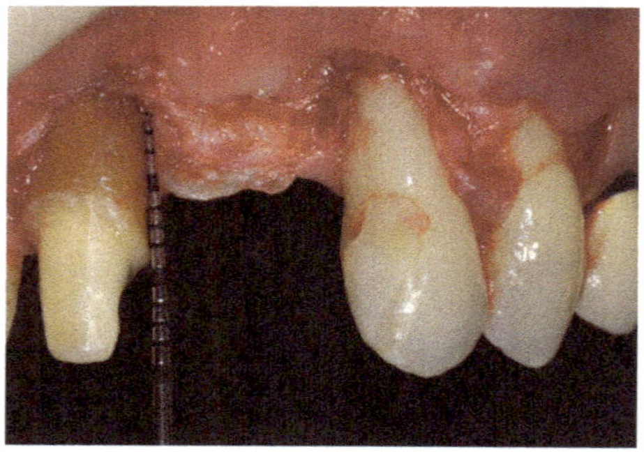

Figure 13: Probing depth after flap elevation.

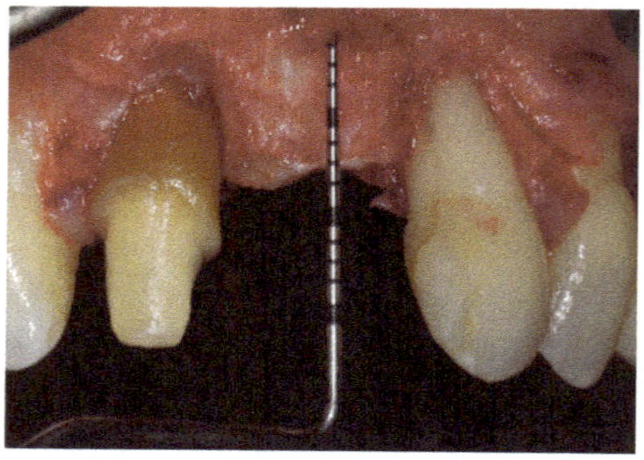

Figure 14: The previous connective tissue graft augmentation is evident after flap elevation.

mucogingival surgery, the definitive prosthesis, a Zirconia cantilever bridge, restored the right and left maxillary central incisors, supported by a rest on the left maxillary lateral incisor. Clinical and radiographic final results can be seen in

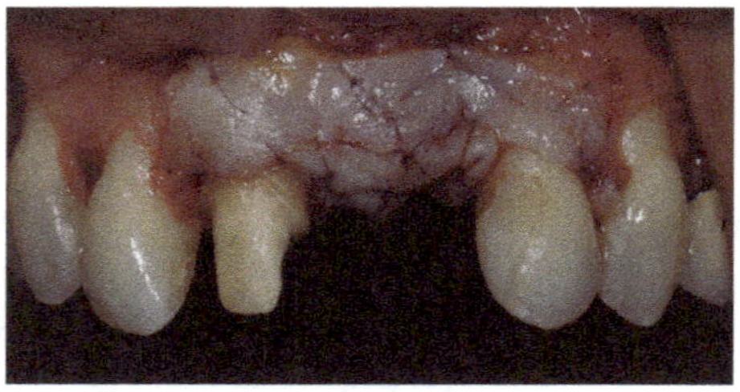

Figure 15: Sutured multilayered connective tissue graft (3 layers of occlusal connective tissue graft and one layer of buccal connective tissue graft).

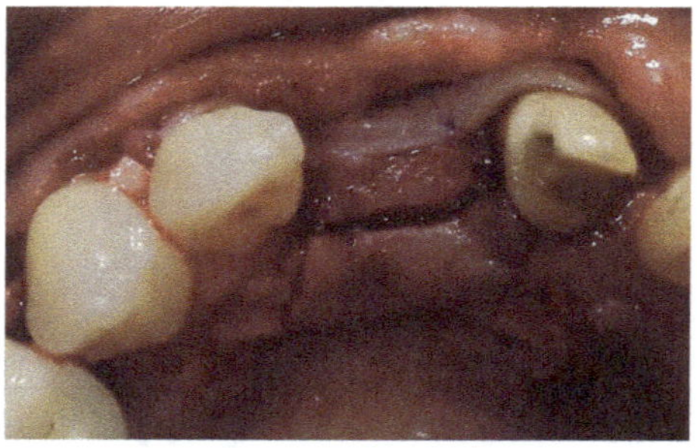

Figure 16: Connective tissue graft sutured on the buccal side. Coronal incision line of the palatal island flap is evident.

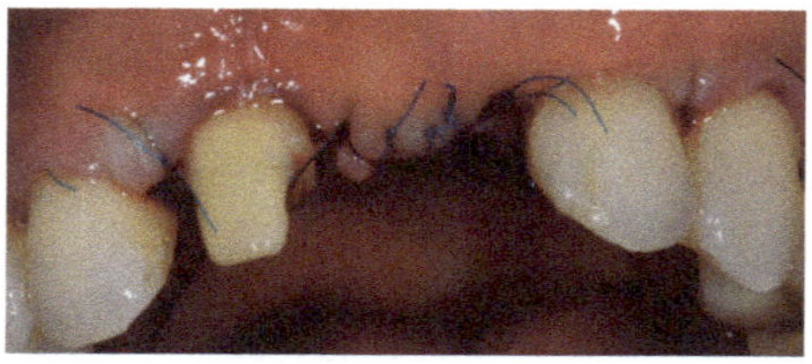

Figure 17: Final suturing of the flap with interrupted sutures.

Figures 19 and 20. The patient was satisfied with the final results and aesthetic outcomes.

3.5. Overall Results of Postsurgical Follow-Ups. Probing around tissues was done 4 months postfrenectomy, which was 16 months after the first mucogingival surgery. The probing depth was 3 mm around the right maxillary central incisor. Buccal and palatal probing depths around the left maxillary lateral incisor were 5 mm. There were no signs of bleeding on probing. Gingival recessions were fully covered. Ten months after the second mucogingival surgery, a soft-tissue augmentation of 9 mm in the vertical direction was achieved. After the definitive prosthesis was placed, a satisfactory aesthetic outcome was reached. The color and shape of the bridge were in harmony with the other teeth (Figure 19), and the emergence profile of the pontic was easy to clean. The left maxillary lateral incisor showed no signs of mobility, while the right maxillary central incisor showed a degree I mobility.

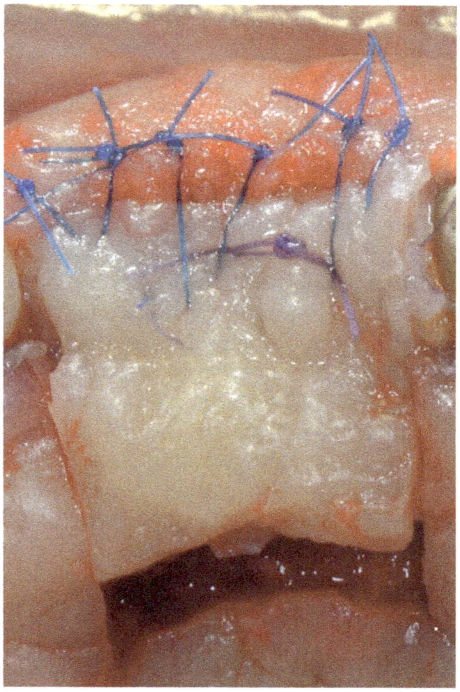

FIGURE 18: Primary intention closure with palatal island flap.

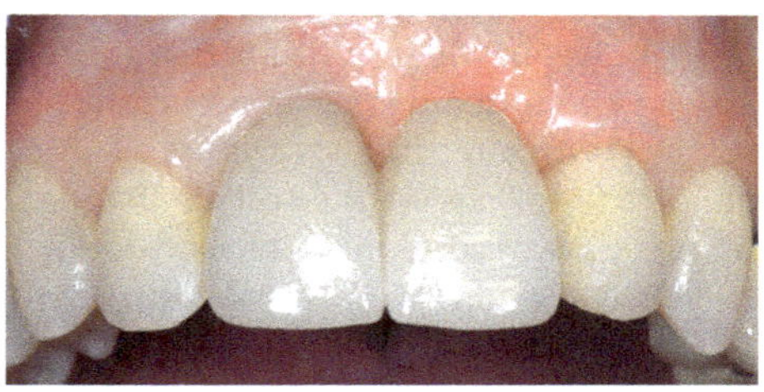

FIGURE 19: Final results, 16 months after the first mucogingival surgery.

4. Discussion

Vertical and horizontal bone augmentation procedures prior to dental implant placement employ different techniques to improve the overall bone volume and ensure final successful outcomes of dental implant therapy. Although vertical bone augmentation procedures, which include vertical GBR, onlay grafting, inlay grafting, and distraction osteogenesis [4, 5], are as technique sensitive as horizontal bone augmentation procedures, they are still more challenging. In fact, vertical bone augmentation procedures are associated with a high complication rate, mainly soft-tissue dehiscence and bone graft exposure [22], resulting in partial or complete loss of the bone-grafting material. In a systematic review on the use of nonresorbable membranes in vertical bone augmentation, the range of reported complications was 0%-45% [4].

In the present case, the patient previously underwent a vertical GBR procedure in the anterior maxilla, utilizing an e-PTFE membrane with an underlying autogenous/xenograft of a 1 : 1 ratio. In general, early or late exposure of membranes is considered as the main cause of GBR failure due to subsequent infection and contamination of the underlying bone grafting material [5, 23–25]. In a recent randomized controlled clinical trial, Cucchi et al. [26] reported a 15% healing complication rate in posterior mandibles treated with vertical bone augmentation utilizing nonresorbable e-PTFE membranes. Similarly, Simion et al. [27] experienced an 18% healing complication rate when the membrane technique was utilized with autogenous or allografts for vertical bone augmentation. The same research group reported similar findings when the e-PTFE membrane was utilized in combination with autograft/xenograft with a 1 : 1 ratio [28].

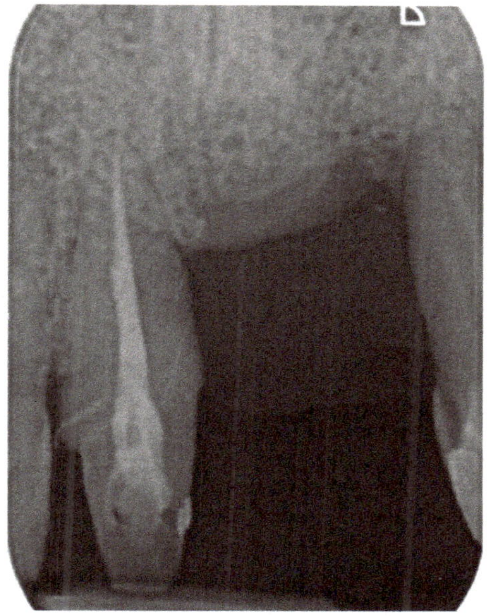

FIGURE 20: Final intraoral periapical radiograph.

In the present case, GBR failure in the anterior maxilla is classified as "complete failure," according to the classification proposed by Checchi et al. [29], which is strictly confined to the aesthetic consequences and treatment options of bone augmentation procedure failures in the atrophic anterior maxillae. In this classification, complete failure of bone augmentation procedures in the anterior maxilla is defined as "failure of the whole procedure which needs to be performed again, often with lower amount and poorer quality of hard and soft tissues than those present in the initial pre-surgical condition" [29]. However, since performing the same surgical procedure all over again might be unpredictable, a nonsurgical correction could be an alternative, which is usually influenced by the patient's decision [29]. In this scenario, the patient might not want to undergo a new bone augmentation procedure due to previous failure.

It must be noted that the correction of failed bone augmentation procedures in the anterior maxilla is more challenging than that in the mandible due to higher aesthetic demands [29]. Therefore, soft-tissue grafting is recommended in the reconstruction of a deficient alveolar ridge in the regions of high aesthetic demands [9]. In this context, different soft-tissue grafting techniques are applied in the correction of alveolar ridge defects for aesthetic purposes such as deepithelialized free gingival grafts [10], epithelial and subepithelial connective tissue grafts, roll pedicle graft, onlay graft, interpositional graft, and combined onlay interpositional graft [30–36], and the differences in the outcomes between different grafting procedures for deficient ridge reconstruction have been investigated. For example, Agarwal and Gupta [9] assessed the differences between subepithelial connective tissue graft in a pouch and combined onlay/connective tissue graft for the reconstruction of class III (Seibert) alveolar ridge defects. Findings of this study demonstrated that the combined onlay/connective tissue graft resulted in more significant gains in the horizontal and vertical ridge dimensions, after 3 and 6 months compared to baseline, due to better revascularization of the onlay graft and better control of the buccolingual and apicocoronal augmentation during the surgery [37].

In another randomized controlled clinical trial, vascularized interpositional periosteal-connective tissue graft (pediculated graft) and free subepithelial connective tissue graft were compared in correcting alveolar ridge deficiency of the anterior maxilla, however in Seibert class I [8]. The authors concluded that after 6 months, sites treated by the pediculated graft were superior in maintaining the initially augmented volume and showed less shrinkage of the graft, attributed to better perfusion of the pediculated graft [8].

Taking all the previous findings together, the GBR failure in the present case was corrected with soft-tissue grafting, taking into consideration the classification proposed by Checchi et al. [29] and also the patient's decision; the patient refused to undergo a new bone augmentation procedure because of the previous failure of the procedure. Due to the severe lack of soft-tissue volume in both the apicocoronal and buccolingual dimensions in the anterior edentulous maxillary area and the simultaneous gingival recession of adjacent teeth, GBR failure was corrected with "multiple soft tissue grafts" in two separate mucogingival surgeries, first to create an initial soft-tissue volume that would serve as a platform for successive soft-tissue augmentation to further increase soft-tissue volume in the edentulous area and second to cover the gingival recessions of adjacent teeth.

The surgical technique we used was similar to the subepithelial connective tissue graft (CTG) augmentation procedures, especially the one described by Zucchelli et al. [10], but with several modifications. In their novel subepithelial connective tissue graft technique for soft-tissue augmentation in a localized class III ridge defect (Seibert) in the anterior maxilla, Zucchelli et al. [10] utilized two folded subepithelial connective tissue grafts , obtained from depithelializing free gingival grafts, to create double thickness CTGs; one sutured buccolingually to create a platform and treat the horizontal component of the soft-tissue defect, and the second graft was sutured above the occlusal surface of the platform, to treat the vertical component of the soft-tissue defect. In the present case report, we have modified this technique.

First, we have reconstructed soft tissues in two separate mucogingival surgeries not only due to the larger defect area and the severely compromised soft-tissue quantity and quality following GBR failure but also due to the unpredictable shrinkage of augmented tissues [33]. Second, for the buccal flap design, we have adopted the one described for coronally advanced flap in the treatment of multiple gingival recessions [12, 13]; however, we have added two vertical releasing incisions, distal to the right and left maxillary canines, in order to better mobilize the flap because of the larger defect area, while Zucchelli et al. [10] avoided the incorporation of any vertical releasing incisions.

Third, we utilized the palatal island flap, as described by Tinti et al. [14] and modified by Hürzeler et al. [15], to move the palatal horizontal incision more coronally for about 3-4 mm to achieve primary intention closure.

Walter et al. [33] previously described a two-step approach for localized alveolar ridge augmentation of class III Seibert in the anterior maxilla, using different soft-tissue grafts: onlay-interpositional graft and subepithelial connective tissue graft. The first soft-tissue augmentation procedure was immediately followed by a separate frenulotomy; then three months later, a second soft-tissue surgical procedure was performed, with achieved satisfactory aesthetic outcomes. In the present case, we have also applied a two-step approach, but we have completed the two mucogingival surgeries first, with a 6-month interval between both surgeries, and then we performed frenectomy, 6 months after the second mucogingival surgery, keeping in mind that about 4-6 months are required for soft-tissue remodeling of the augmented tissues [33].

One of the main advantages of using soft-tissue grafting in correcting an alveolar ridge defect is that it is not as technique sensitive as bone augmentation procedures [38]. However, soft-tissue grafting techniques require a second surgical site, i.e., donor site to harvest the soft-tissue graft [38] and could be associated with unpredictable soft-tissue shrinkage over time, due to the long-term healing process [33], also around pontic areas.

Data on volumetric changes around pontic areas after soft-tissue augmentation procedures are available from retrospective 5-year [39] and 10-year [40] follow-up studies. Sanz-Martín et al. [39] reported that at 5 years, 24 patients receiving fixed dental prosthesis, with and without subepithelial CTGs, showed the same volumetric stability over the period of 5 years. In fact, the changes in soft-tissue pontic height amounted to a loss in the height of 0.34 mm in the group that received CTG and 0.35 mm in the group that did not receive any CTG, noting that there were no statistically significant differences in the baseline linear measurements between both groups [39]. Out of the 24 patients that were enrolled in the previous study, 17 were evaluated for a 10-year follow-up [40], with a calculation between the 5- and 10-year results being performed. Results showed that there were no statistically significant differences in pontic height between 5-year and 10-year results, suggesting a slight but continuous loss of tissue volume from baseline to 5 and 10 years, without any significant differences between sites with or without soft-tissue volume augmentation.

At the 16-month follow-up of the present case, no bleeding on probing was evident, gingival recessions were fully covered, and even levels of gingival margins were achieved. The soft tissues were stable. However, soft-tissue shrinkage, even if slight, is to be expected over time, also around pontics as confirmed by previous authors [39, 40].

5. Conclusions

The following conclusions can be inferred from the present case report:

(1) Multilayered connective tissue grafting technique might be successful in correcting soft tissues after failed bone augmentation procedures

(2) Vertical soft-tissue augmentation is possible with this technique

(3) Two mucogingival surgeries were needed due to the large defect area

(4) Palatal island flap is utilized with this technique to easily achieve a primary intention closure of the flap

(5) Slight soft-tissue shrinkage is still to be expected over time

Acknowledgments

FA is supported by the Osteology Research Scholarship (Osteology Foundation, Lucerne, Switzerland).

References

[1] T. Albrektsson, G. Zarb, P. Worthington, and A. R. Eriksson, "The long-term efficacy of currently used dental implants: a review and proposed criteria of success," *The International Journal of Oral & Maxillofacial Implants*, vol. 1, no. 1, pp. 11–25, 1986.

[2] I. A. Urban, E. Montero, A. Monje, and I. Sanz-Sánchez, "Effectiveness of vertical ridge augmentation interventions: a systematic review and meta-analysis," *Journal of Clinical Periodontology*, vol. 46, pp. 319–339, 2019.

[3] F. Khoury and T. Hanser, "Three-dimensional vertical alveolar ridge augmentation in the posterior maxilla: a 10-year clinical study," *The International Journal of Oral & Maxillofacial Implants*, vol. 34, no. 2, pp. 471–480, 2019.

[4] I. Rocchietta, F. Fontana, and M. Simion, "Clinical outcomes of vertical bone augmentation to enable dental implant placement: a systematic review," *Journal of Clinical Periodontology*, vol. 35, Supplement 8, pp. 203–215, 2008.

[5] M. Esposito, M. G. Grusovin, P. Felice et al., "Interventions for replacing missing teeth: horizontal and vertical bone augmentation techniques for dental implant treatment," *Cochrane Database of Systematic Reviews*, vol. 4, article CD003607, 2009.

[6] P. Gallo and D. Díaz-Báez, "Management of 80 complications in vertical and horizontal ridge augmentation with nonresorbable membrane (d-PTFE): a cross-sectional study," *The International Journal of Oral & Maxillofacial Implants*, vol. 34, no. 4, pp. 927–935, 2019.

[7] B. Langer and L. J. Calagna, "The subepithelial connective tissue graft. A new approach to the enhancement of anterior cosmetics," *The International Journal of Periodontics & Restorative Dentistry*, vol. 2, no. 2, pp. 22–33, 1982.

[8] A. Akcalı, D. Schneider, F. Ünlü, N. Bıcakcı, T. Köse, and C. H. F. Hämmerle, "Soft tissue augmentation of ridge defects in the maxillary anterior area using two different methods: a randomized controlled clinical trial," *Clinical Oral Implants Research*, vol. 26, no. 6, pp. 688–695, 2015.

[9] A. Agarwal and N. D. Gupta, "Alveolar ridge augmentation by connective tissue grafting using a pouch method and modified connective tissue technique: a prospective study," *Dental Research Journal*, vol. 12, no. 6, pp. 548–553, 2015.

[10] G. Zucchelli, C. Mazzotti, V. Bentivogli, I. Mounssif, M. Marzadori, and C. Monaco, "The connective tissue platform technique for soft tissue augmentation," *The International Journal of Periodontics & Restorative Dentistry*, vol. 32, no. 6, pp. 665–675, 2012.

[11] J. S. Seibert, "Reconstruction of deformed, partially edentulous ridges, using full thickness onlay grafts. Part I. Technique and wound healing," *The Compendium of Continuing Education in Dentistry*, vol. 4, pp. 437–453.2, 1983.

[12] G. Zucchelli and M. De Sanctis, "Treatment of multiple recession-type defects in patients with esthetic demands," *Journal of Periodontology*, vol. 71, no. 9, pp. 1506–1514, 2000.

[13] G. Zucchelli, M. Mele, C. Mazzotti, M. Marzadori, L. Montebugnoli, and M. de Sanctis, "Coronally advanced flap with and without vertical releasing incisions for the treatment of multiple gingival recessions: a comparative controlled randomized clinical trial," *Journal of Periodontology*, vol. 80, no. 7, pp. 1083–1094, 2009.

[14] C. Tinti and S. Parma-Benfenati, "Coronally positioned palatal sliding flap," *The International Journal of Periodontics & Restorative Dentistry*, vol. 15, no. 3, pp. 298–310, 1995.

[15] M. B. Hürzeler, S. von Mohrenschildt, and O. Zuhr, "Stage-two implant surgery in the esthetic zone: a new technique," *The International Journal of Periodontics & Restorative Dentistry*, vol. 30, no. 2, pp. 187–193, 2010.

[16] G. Zucchelli, M. Mele, M. Stefanini et al., "Patient morbidity and root coverage outcome after subepithelial connective tissue and de-epithelialized grafts: a comparative randomized-controlled clinical trial," *Journal of Clinical Periodontology*, vol. 37, no. 8, pp. 728–738, 2010.

[17] L. Tavelli, F. Asa'ad, R. Acunzo, G. Pagni, D. Consonni, and G. Rasperini, "Minimizing patient morbidity following palatal gingival harvesting: a randomized controlled clinical study," *The International Journal of Periodontics & Restorative Dentistry*, vol. 38, no. 6, pp. e127–e134, 2018.

[18] I. A. Urban, K. Nagy, S. Werner, and M. Meyer, "Evaluation of the combination of strip gingival grafts and a xenogeneic collagen matrix for the treatment of severe mucogingival defects: a human histologic study," *The International Journal of Periodontics & Restorative Dentistry*, vol. 39, no. 1, pp. 9–14, 2019.

[19] T. J. Han, P. R. Klokkevold, and H. H. Takei, "Strip gingival autograft used to correct mucogingival problems around implants," *The International journal of periodontics & restorative dentistry*, vol. 15, no. 4, pp. 404–411, 1995.

[20] A. Desiate, S. Cantore, D. Tullo, G. Profeta, F. R. Grassi, and A. Ballini, "980 nm diode lasers in oral and facial practice: current state of the science and art," *International Journal of Medical Sciences*, vol. 6, no. 6, pp. 358–364, 2009.

[21] D. De Santis, D. Bertossi, G. Zanotti et al., "Nd-YAP laser assisted frenulectomy: a case series on 23 patients," *Minerva stomatologica*, vol. 62, 8 Supplement 1, pp. 27–36, 2013.

[22] S. Lundgren, M. Sjöström, E. Nyström, and L. Sennerby,

"Strategies in reconstruction of the atrophic maxilla with autogenous bone grafts and endosseous implants," *Periodontol 2000*, vol. 47, no. 1, pp. 143–161, 2008.

[23] E. E. Machtei, "The effect of membrane exposure on the outcome of regenerative procedures in humans: a meta-analysis," *Journal of Periodontology*, vol. 72, no. 4, pp. 512–516, 2001.

[24] S. Verardi and M. Simion, "Management of the exposure of e-PTFE membranes in guided bone regeneration," *Practical Procedures & Aesthetic Dentistry*, vol. 19, no. 2, pp. 111–117, 2007.

[25] F. Fontana, E. Maschera, I. Rocchietta, and M. Simion, "Clinical classification of complications in guided bone regeneration procedures by means of a nonresorbable membrane," *The International Journal of Periodontics & Restorative Dentistry*, vol. 31, no. 3, pp. 265–273, 2011.

[26] A. Cucchi, E. Vignudelli, A. Napolitano, C. Marchetti, and G. Corinaldesi, "Evaluation of complication rates and vertical bone gain after guided bone regeneration with non-resorbable membranes versus titanium meshes and resorbable membranes. A randomized clinical trial," *Clinical Implant Dentistry and Related Research*, vol. 19, no. 5, pp. 821–832, 2017.

[27] M. Simion, S. A. Jovanovic, P. Trisi, A. Scarano, and A. Piattelli, "Vertical ridge augmentation around dental implants using a membrane technique and autogenous bone or allografts in humans," *The International Journal of Periodontics & Restorative Dentistry*, vol. 18, no. 1, pp. 8–23, 1998.

[28] M. Simion, F. Fontana, G. Rasperini, and C. Maiorana, "Vertical ridge augmentation by expanded-polytetrafluoroethylene membrane and a combination of intraoral autogenous bone graft and deproteinized anorganic bovine bone (Bio Oss)," *Clinical Oral Implants Research*, vol. 18, no. 5, pp. 620–629, 2007.

[29] V. Checchi, R. Gasparro, R. Pistilli, L. Canullo, and P. Felice, "Clinical classification of bone augmentation procedure failures in the atrophic anterior maxillae: esthetic consequences and treatment options," *BioMed Research International*, vol. 2019, Article ID 4386709, 16 pages, 2019.

[30] S. Studer, R. Naef, and P. Schärer, "Adjustment of localized alveolar ridge defects by soft tissue transplantation to improve mucogingival esthetics: a proposal for clinical classification and an evaluation of procedures," *Quintessence International*, vol. 28, no. 12, pp. 785–805, 1997.

[31] S. P. Studer, E. P. Allen, T. C. Rees, and A. Kouba, "The thickness of masticatory mucosa in the human hard palate and tuberosity as potential donor sites for ridge augmentation procedures," *Journal of Periodontology*, vol. 68, no. 2, pp. 145–151, 1997.

[32] J. S. Seibert and H. Salama, "Alveolar ridge preservation and reconstruction," *Periodontol 2000*, vol. 11, no. 1, pp. 69–84, 1996.

[33] C. Walter, L. Büttel, and R. Weiger, "Localized alveolar ridge augmentation using a two-step approach with different soft tissue grafts: a clinical report," *The Journal of Contemporary Dental Practice*, vol. 9, no. 4, pp. 99–106, 2008.

[34] D. R. Scharf and D. P. Tarnow, "Modified roll technique for localized alveolar ridge augmentation," *The International Journal of Periodontics & Restorative Dentistry*, vol. 12, no. 5, pp. 415–425, 1992.

[35] J. S. Seibert, "Reconstruction of deformed, partially edentulous ridges, using full thickness onlay grafts. Part II. Prosthetic/periodontal interrelationships," *The Compendium of Continuing Education in Dentistry*, vol. 4, no. 6, pp. 549–562, 1983.

[36] D. S. Thoma, G. I. Benić, M. Zwahlen, C. H. F. Hämmerle, and R. E. Jung, "A systematic review assessing soft tissue augmentation techniques," *Clinical Oral Implants Research*, vol. 20, Supplement 4, pp. 146–165, 2009.

[37] J. S. Seibert and J. V. Louis, "Soft tissue ridge augmentation utilizing a combination onlay-interpositional graft procedure: a case report," *The International Journal of Periodontics & Restorative Dentistry*, vol. 16, no. 4, pp. 310–321, 1996.

[38] P. Y. Lai and S. W. Yip, "Alveolar ridge augmentation using subepithelial connective tissue grafts: a case report," *Journal of Prosthodontics and Implantology*, vol. 1, no. 2, pp. 60–65, 2012.

[39] I. Sanz-Martín, I. Sailer, C. H. F. Hämmerle, and D. S. Thoma, "Soft tissue stability and volumetric changes after 5 years in pontic sites with or without soft tissue grafting: a retrospective cohort study," *Clinical Oral Implants Research*, vol. 27, no. 8, pp. 969–974, 2016.

[40] S. P. Bienz, I. Sailer, I. Sanz-Martín, R. E. Jung, C. H. F. Hämmerle, and D. S. Thoma, "Volumetric changes at pontic sites with or without soft tissue grafting: a controlled clinical study with a 10-year follow-up," *Journal of Clinical Periodontology*, vol. 44, no. 2, pp. 178–184, 2017.

6

Impacted Palatal Canines and Diode Laser Surgery: A Case Report

Marina Consuelo Vitale,[1] Maria Gloria Nardi,[2] Matteo Pellegrini,[2] Francesco Spadari,[3,4] Federica Pulicari,[3,4] Roberto Alcozer,[1] Martina Minardi,[1] Maria Francesca Sfondrini,[1] Karin Bertino,[1] and Andrea Scribante[1]

[1]*Unit of Orthodontics and Pediatric Dentistry, Section of Dentistry, Department of Clinical, Surgical, Diagnostic and Pediatric Sciences, University of Pavia, Pavia 27100, Italy*
[2]*Section of Dentistry, Department of Clinical, Surgical, Diagnostic and Pediatric Sciences, University of Pavia, Pavia 27100, Italy*
[3]*Maxillo-Facial and Odontostomatology Unit, Fondazione IRCCS Cà Granda Ospedale Maggiore Policlinico, Milan 20122, Italy*
[4]*Department of Biomedical, Surgical and Dental Sciences, University of Milan, Via Della Commenda 10, Milan 20122, Italy*

Correspondence should be addressed to Andrea Scribante; andrea.scribante@unipv.it

Academic Editor: Giuseppe Alessandro Scardina

Introduction. Maxillary canine is the most frequent dental element that could likely remain impacted in the bone structure, with a percentage between 1 and 5%. This study presents a case report using a diode laser for surgical-orthodontics disinclusion of a palatal mucosal impacted permanent left upper canine (2.3) and the simultaneous application of an orthodontic bracket. *Methods.* After cementation of the trans-palatal bar to the upper first molars with a hook for orthodontic traction, local anaesthesia with articaine was performed, followed by surgical operculectomy using a diode laser (810 nm wavelength, continuous wave mode with a power output of 3 W, and a 0.4 mm diameter optical fiber), and the orthodontic bracket with a passive metal looped ligature was applied. Subsequently, active elastic traction was applied on 2.3 and the upper arch was bonded for the application of a series of orthodontic wires, lace-back, and metal ligatures. A progressive reactivation of the elastic traction and extraction of 6.3 was necessary to translate the canine into the correct arch position. *Results.* Diode laser surgical-orthodontic disinclusion of impacted upper canine was performed successively, resulting in a dry surgical field ideal for orthodontic bracket adhesion. No pain and no swelling have been reported from the patient. The orthodontic treatment allowed the canine to be moved to the correct position in the arch. *Conclusions.* This case showed that the diode laser is a valid alternative for the surgical-orthodontic disinclusion of an included tooth element.

1. Introduction

After the third molar, maxillary canine is the most frequent dental element that could likely remain impacted in the bone structure, with a percentage between 1 and 5%, depending on the patient. It is more common in females than in males, with a ratio of 2 : 1, and only 8% of patients are bilateral [1]. Impaction of the maxillary canine has a ratio of 10 : 1 to mandibular canine and 85% of the upper impaction are palatal [2].

Numerous etiological factors are associated with impacted canines and, according to the literature, they can be classified as localized, systemic, and genetic (Table 1) [3–9].

It is essential to make an early diagnosis of the impacted canine to plan the treatment of this dental anomaly in advance and to properly replace this tooth in the arch as soon as possible, considering the importance of canine guidance role in the occlusion and consequently in the correct body posture. [10]. Early diagnosis of canine displacement in relation to the surrounding structures is mainly based on radiographic examination: in Panoramic X-ray more mesial is located in the canine crown, further likelihood of canine eruption is reduced [11].

Table 1: Etiologic factors associated with impacted canines.

Localized [3, 4]				
Loss of arch space	Trauma	Ankylosis	Root dilacerations	Supernumerary teeth
Cyst or neoplasm	Reconstructive surgery for cleft lip/ palate repair	Thickened overlying bone or soft tissue	Missing adjacent lateral incisor	Variation in root size of the lateral incisor
Variation in timing of lateral incisor root formation		Over-retained primary canine or early loss of the primary canine		Idiopathic factors
Systemic [5]				
Endocrine disorders		Febrile illness		Irradiation
Genetic [5–9]				
Gardner syndrome	Cleidocranial dysostosis	Yunis–Varon syndrome	Malposed tooth germ	Presence of an alveolar cleft

The choice of treatment in the patient with an impacted canine changes with the age, oral health, and etiologic factors [3, 12]: monitoring of the impacted element, in the absence of clinical problems [13], extraction of the deciduous element, if the impacted permanent canine is close to eruption [3], extraction of the deciduous tooth and simultaneous uncovering of the permanent tooth with the application of an orthodontic appliance to increase the space in the arch, and allowing the physiological eruption of the canine [13]. In some cases, it is possible to perform dental reimplantation, when the orthodontic treatment turns out to be too complex, unsuccessful, or not accepted by the patient [13].

At the end of growth, surgical-orthodontic treatment is the only choice to align teeth in the dental arch; alternatively, it is possible to extract the impacted element with subsequent prosthetic or implant-prosthetic treatment [3].

Laser is the acronym of light amplification by stimulated emission of radiation, and it represents a new technology introduced in Dentistry by Theodore Harold Maiman in 1960, but only in 1989, Nd:YAG laser and CO_2 laser were commercially available in the dental market [14]. The light emitted is monochromatic, collimated, and coherent [15]. The essential elements of a laser device are a sounding box in which an active medium is stimulated by a pumping process in a population inversion and in a suitable geometry of the optical feedback elements. Depending on the active medium (gas, liquid, or solid), laser radiation could be in the ultraviolet, visible, or in infrared section of the electrophotometer spectrum [16].

Different authors described laser efficacy in the treatment of oral pathologies, carrying out studies on photodynamic therapy [17, 18] and surgical procedures [19, 20]. Laser provides an excellent alternative to conventional surgical techniques for soft tissue [21]. Many authors described the use of laser in surgical treatments, such as gingivectomy, labial, lingual frenectomies, and fiberotomy [22]. Furthermore, laser can prevent aphthae and cold sores, ablate benign and irritant tissue excess, correct lip, and tongue bands [23]. Laser can also be used in endodontics to remove bacteria from infected teeth [24]. Laser plays an important role in the treatment of periodontal disease: it can modulate many inflammatory pathways, improves wound healing by stimulating fibroblast proliferation, it has a positive biomodulatory effect on bone healing, it performs an antimicrobial activity, and could be a reliable adjunctive agent to mechanical debridement in the non-surgical treatment of periodontal disease [25]. Additionally, it is also used to treat dentin hypersensitivity [26]. Laser can also be useful in dental bleaching: studies have shown how it can accelerate the release of free radicals within the bleaching gel to decrease the duration of the treatment [27]. Some authors described how low-level laser therapy and photodynamic therapy after scaling and root planning can improve the therapeutic outcomes in patients affected by chronic periodontitis [28]. In the literature the role of laser in cavity preparation, carious removal, and pulp therapy is also discussed [29]. Meanwhile, laser, safe and effective technology, has become widely used in dentistry. The potential advantages include less or no bleeding during the surgical procedure, reduction, or elimination of the need for local anaesthesia, reduced postoperative pain, and less patient anxiety [30].

Finally, laser can be applied in orthodontics to etch enamel prior to adhesive application and orthodontic brackets [31] and can reduce pain following band application on maxillary first molars for orthodontic treatment [32]. Photobiomodulation (or low-level laser therapy) with laser or LED can also be used to reduce pain intensity during and following lower third molar extraction and to improve symptoms related to Burning Mouth Syndrome through a reduction of the capillary diameter [33, 34].

Since there are few studies assessing laser application's advantages in surgical-orthodontics disinclusion of an impacted canine, the aim of the present study is to present a case report using a diode laser for the disinclusion of an impacted permanent left upper canine (2.3) and the simultaneous application of an orthodontic bracket.

2. Case Report

2.1. Diagnosis and Etiology. A 17.5-year-old female patient was referred to the Unit of Orthodontics and Paediatric Dentistry from the Unit of Oral Surgery of the Department of Clinical, Surgical, Diagnostic, and Paediatric Sciences of the University of Pavia. In the past, she had a root canal treatment on upper central incisors after dental trauma.

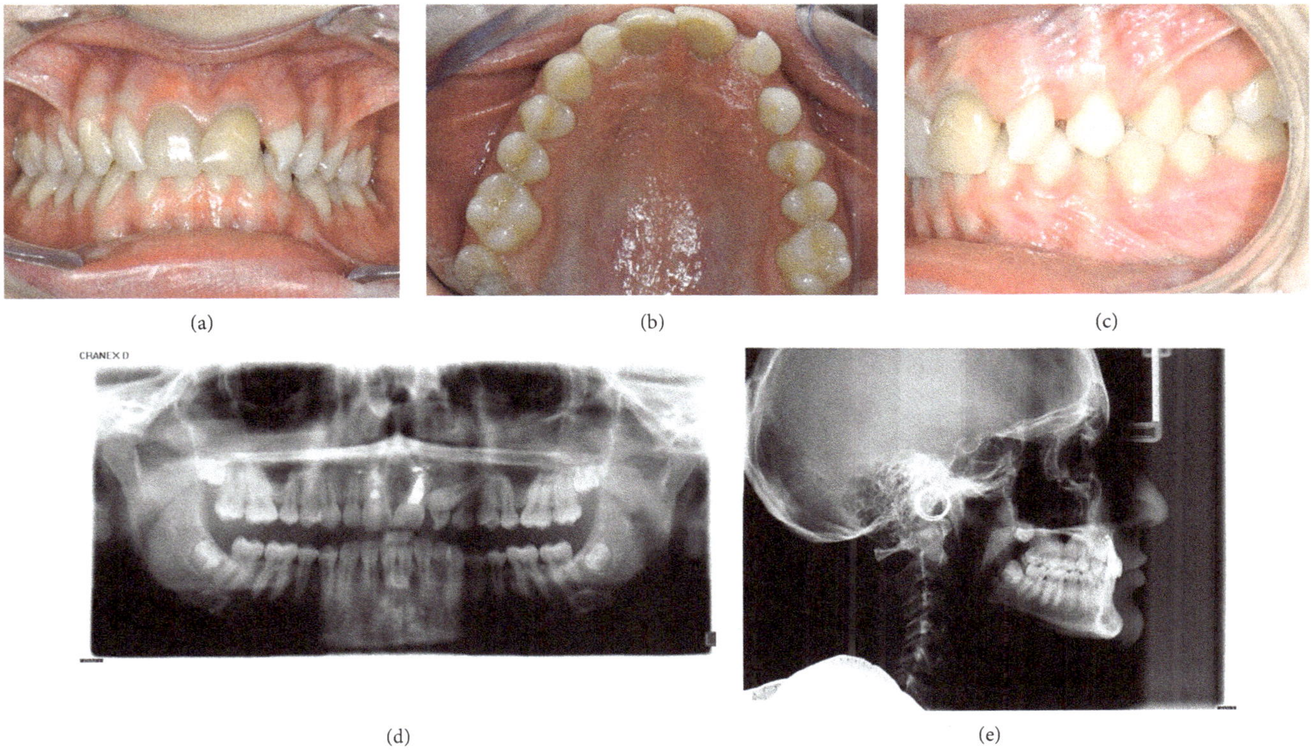

Figure 1: (a–c) Pretreatment intraoral and (d and e) radiographical recordings.

The patient showed facial symmetry, competent lips, and normal facial height. Upper and lower dental midlines coincided. Fox plane was not completely parallel to the interpupillary line. Panoramic and lateral cephalometric radiographs were taken (Figures 1(d) and 1(e); Cranex® D, Soredex®, Tuusula, Finland): the panoramic radiograph showed the presence of third molars' germs, lower deciduous canines' persistence, and upper left canine's impaction without apparent left maxillary incisors' radicular resorption.

Cephalometric analysis was performed (DeltaDent, version 2.3, Outside Format, Paullo, Italy): class I skeletal with bimaxillary protrusion (ANB 1.2°, SNA 87°, SNB 85.8°, and Wits index—1.4 mm), hypodivergency, and anterior remaining growth were shown.

The facial profile was normal, the facial angle was slightly increased (171.3°), while the nasolabial angle was slightly decreased (93.3°). Upper incisors were correctly inclined, in fact, the angle formed by the upper incisor's longitudinal axis and bispinal plane (Sna-Snp) measured 107.9°, whereas lower incisors were retroclined, considering that the angle formed by the lower incisor's longitudinal axis and mandibular plane (Go-Gn) measured 87.8°. Intraoral pictures (Figures 1(a)–1(c); taken with Nikon Digital Camera D3500, Nikon Corporation, Tokyo, Japan) showed coincident dental midlines, deep bite, conservative treatments on upper central incisors, and upper lateral incisors' malposition. Overjet measured 0 mm, while overbite measured 4 mm. The patient presented class I molar and class I canine on the right with upper central incisors discolouration. On the left, the patient showed class I molar, while canine classification was not possible. Lower deciduous canines were still present, left maxillary lateral incisors were rotated and many diastemas could be found. The morphology of the upper arch was correct, the retroincisive papilla was hypertrophic, and the first upper maxillary molars were rotated. The lower arch showed a correct morphology as well, lower left canine was lingually inclined. There was no dentoalveolar discrepancy. Bolton's analysis was appropriate, considering that the impacted canine was the same size as the contralateral teeth and excluding the lower left canine. Furthermore, clinical recordings highlighted normal Periodontal Screening and Recording and slight mobility on upper central incisors, multiple gingival recessions in the upper and lower posterior jaws and good oral hygiene.

Clinical and radiological recordings led to the diagnosis of the upper left canine's palatal impaction and surgical exposure of the impacted tooth was planned for subsequent orthodontic traction. The impacted canine provided a "sector 2" position with an α angle, formed by the tooth's midline and long axis, of approximately 80° and a short distance from the alveolar ridge [35].

2.2. Treatment Objectives. The aim of the treatment is surgical operculectomy of the mucosal tissue overlying the left upper permanent canine (2.3) in palatal mucosal impaction, with good surgical haemostasis, allowing intra-operative adhesion of the orthodontic bracket, thus exerting a more rapid onset of orthodontic traction. The extraction of the deciduous canine (6.3) is necessary to allow the permanent canine to be moved into the dental arch after the disinclusion has been completed.

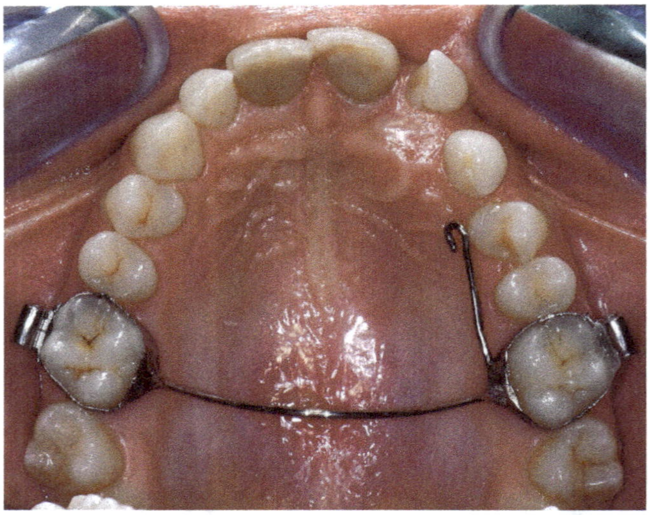

FIGURE 2: Intraoral photo with the TPB cemented to the first molars and the orthodontic traction hook welded.

2.3. Treatment Alternatives. The first possible alternative is a surgical treatment with lasers of various wavelengths: 10,600 nm (CO_2 laser), 2940 nm (Er:YAG laser), and 1064 nm (Nd:YAG laser).

Another possible alternative is the use of the electric scalpel, which presents different risks associated with its use, including burns due to the use of high-frequency current, fire risks due to the presence of combustible liquids or gases in the room where it is used, and electrical risks due to the radiated power, which may disturb any equipment applied to the patient [36].

The last alternative is a conventional surgical approach using a cold-blade scalpel, with the consequent risks of intra- and post-operative bleeding and the impossibility of maintaining a dry surgical field, essential to ensure proper adhesion of the orthodontic bracket, the need to apply sutures, potential difficulties in wound healing, and increased post-operative pain [37].

2.4. Treatment Progress. Written informed consent was obtained from the patient's parents to proceed with the surgical-orthodontic procedure of canine disinclusion. An upper silicone impression (Elite HD+ Putty Soft, Zhermack S.p.A., Badia Polesine, Italy) was made and sent to the dental technician for fabrication of a trans-palatal bar (TPB) with a hook for orthodontic traction of 2.3 impacted. After the use of orthodontic separators (Loose S Modules S2, 3M Company, St. Paul, MN, USA), the TPB was cemented to the upper first permanent molars (3M™ Unitek™ Multi-Cure Glass Ionomer Band Cement, 3M Company, St. Paul, MN, USA) and cement was light-cured (Starlight Pro, Power Output 1400 mW/cm^2, Mectron S.p.A., Carasco, Italy; Figure 2). The patient and all staff wore protective glasses to prevent eye damage [38]. After local anaesthesia (Septanest, articaine hydrochloride 4% with adrenaline 1/100,000), a diode laser (Fotona XD-2, Fotona d.o.o., Ljubljana, Slovenia) was used to perform surgical operculectomy, being an element in superficial palatal impaction, with the following parameters [39]: 810 nm wavelength, continuous wave mode with a power output of 3 W and a 0.4 mm diameter optical fiber (Figures 3(a) and 3(b)). Figure 4 shows how the surgical incision did not cause intra-operative bleeding, thus creating an ideal condition for the adhesion of the orthodontic bracket. No pain and no swelling have been reported from the patient.

The bonding protocol used is as follows [40]: etching of the enamel with 35% phosphoric acid applied for 20–30 seconds and rinsing for an equivalent time. Drying using aspiration to obtain the chalky white appearance of the enamel. Application of light cure adhesive (3M™ Transbond™ PLUS Color Change Adhesive, 3M Company, St. Paul, MN, USA) on the enamel and on the intrados of the orthodontic bracket using a Microbrush® (Microbrush International, Algonquin, IL, USA). Positioning of the orthodontic bracket (3M Unitek APC™ II Victory Series™, 3M Company, St. Paul, MN, USA) and application of continuous pressure for a light curing time of twice 20 seconds under constant suction (Starlight Pro, Power Output 1400 mW/cm^2, Mectron S.p.A.). Immediate traction with an elastic connection to the wire: if an error has been made in the bonding protocol, the orthodontic bracket is immediately taken off and a new bonding procedure is begun.

The orthodontic bracket was placed with a passive metal looped ligature, secured with composite (Figure 5). No sutures and no additional analgesic or antibiotic were recommended, thanks to the photo-bio-stimulating effect (LLLT) of laser [41]. The patient was discharged with necessary postoperative instructions for maintenance of good oral hygiene and keeping the area clean.

The patient was visited with a follow-up of 2 weeks, twice, and monthly thereafter. After 2 weeks, active elastic traction on 2.3 has been applied and one month after surgery the upper arch was bonded through Straight-Wire MBT™ technique with a 0.14″ NiTi arch-wire (3M™ Unitek™ Nitinol Classic Archwire, 3M Company, St. Paul, MN, USA), performing a mesial lace-back 1.2–2.2 and metal ligation on 2.2 with preformed ligature wire 0.10″ (K4210-25, Leone S.p.A. Ortodonzia e Implantologia, Sesto Fiorentino, Italy; Figure 6).

Subsequently, the canine was gradually translated into the correct position in the dental arch by progressive reactivations of elastic traction with elastic cotton threads (Leone, Sesto Fiorentino, Italy), lace-back 1.2–2.2, and metal ligatures on 2.2 and 2.4 with preformed ligature wire 0.10″ (K4210-25, Leone); in addition, a super elastic NiTi arch-wire (0.12″) upper arch has been used (3M™ Unitek™ Nitinol Classic Archwire, 3M Company).

Table 2 shows the procedures checklist of surgical-orthodontic disinclusion of the left upper canine (2.3) in palatal mucosal impaction and its orthodontic translation in the upper arch.

The patient is still undergoing orthodontic treatment to finalize therapy for closing diastema between 2.2 and 2.3.

2.5. Treatment Results. After excision, the patient had no signs of respiratory distress, and no feeding difficulty was reported from the parents. After 2 weeks and 1 month

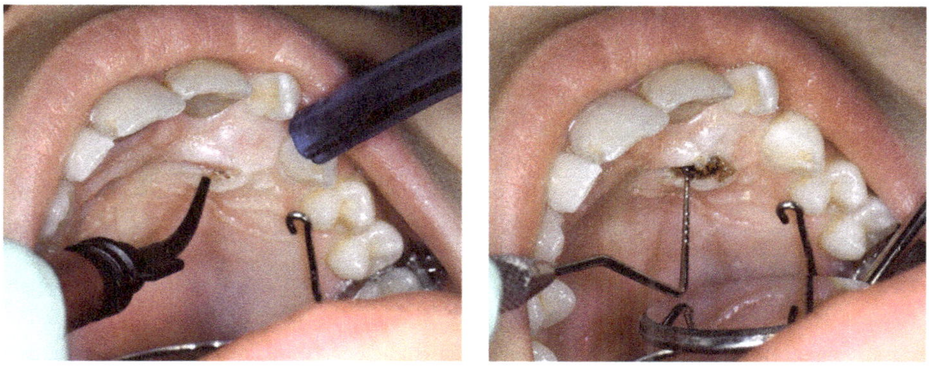

(a) (b)

Figure 3: (a and b) Intraoral photo during surgical procedure.

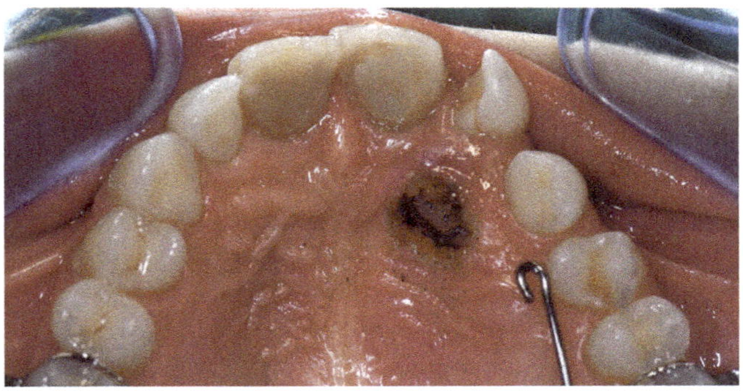

Figure 4: Surgical incision after laser surgery.

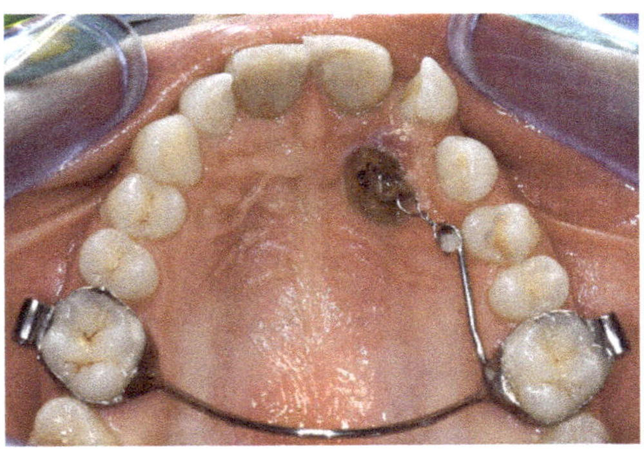

Figure 5: Orthodontic bracket positioned after surgical operculectomy, with a passive metal looped ligature and secured with composite.

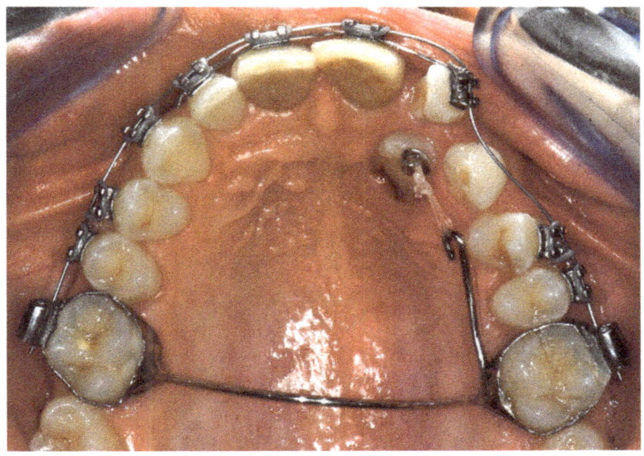

Figure 6: Intraoral photo 1 month after surgery with active elastic traction on 2.3 and upper arch bonded.

follow-up, the intraoral wound healed without complications and no signs of infection (Figure 6); 3 months after surgery, the position of the upper canine can be appreciated and thanks to the orthodontic traction applied (Figure 7); 12 months after surgery, the upper canine 2.3, once included, is positioned at the level of the dental arch but a diastema remains between 2.2 and 2.3, for which orthodontic finalization is necessary to close it (Figures 8(a)–8(d)).

2.6. Discussion. This case report described surgical disinclusion of a left upper canine using a diode laser, followed by orthodontic treatment to translate the impacted canine into the dental arch, highlighting some advantages, such as no intra-operative bleeding, thus providing orthodontic bracket adhesion, no sutures, and no post-operative pain or swelling.

In the literature, there are several articles in which laser technology has been used in the surgical management of impacted teeth; however, to our knowledge, no case reports have not yet been presented in literature where an 810 nm wavelength diode laser has been used to perform surgical operculectomy of the palatal impacted canines with a subsequent intra-operative application of the orthodontic bracket. A previous clinical study showed the application of a 980 nm wavelength diode laser for surgical operculectomy of a palatal included left upper canine, preventing bleeding and need for sutures, reducing pain, and allowing placement of orthodontic brackets [42]. A recent case report showed a surgical operculectomy of both impacted upper permanent canines through a CO_2 laser, postponing orthodontic bracket placement to a later date and highlighting many advantages, such as no bleeding, no need for sutures, relative ease, and speed of the procedure, reduced or no postoperative symptoms, antimicrobial activity, and rapid wound healing [43]. A case series study showed a combination of two laser (Nd:YAG and Er:YAG) for the surgical treatment of a left upper canine in osteo-mucosal impaction. Er:YAG was used for hard

Table 2: Procedures checklist of surgical-orthodontic disinclusion of the left upper canine (2.3) in palatal mucosal impaction and its orthodontic translation in the upper arch.

1. Diagnosis of palatal mucosal impaction of the left upper canine (2.3) by clinical and radiological recordings.
2. Definition of treatment objectives: surgical-orthodontic disinclusion of impacted 2.3 by diode laser and its orthodontic translation in the arch after extraction of 6.3.
3. Obtaining informed consent from the patient's parents to proceed with surgical-orthodontic disinclusion.
4. Performing an upper silicone impression for the fabrication of a trans-palatal bar (TPB) with a hook for orthodontic traction of 2.3 impacted.
5. After application of the orthodontic separators, cementing and light-curing the TPB on the upper first permanent molars.
6. Wearing safety glasses and performing local anaesthesia.
7. Performing a diode laser surgical operculectomy with the following parameters: 810 nm wavelength, continuous wave mode with a power output of 3 W, and a 0.4 mm diameter optical fiber.
8. Adhesion of the orthodontic bracket to achieve orthodontic traction.
9. Etching of the enamel with 35% phosphoric acid applied for 20–30 seconds and rinsing for an equivalent time.
10. Drying using aspiration to obtain the chalky white appearance of the enamel.
11. Application of light cure adhesive on the enamel and on orthodontic bracket baseplate using a Microbrush®.
12. Positioning of the orthodontic bracket and application of continuous pressure for a light curing time of twice 20 seconds under constant suction.
13. Immediate traction with an elastic connected to the wire: if an error has been made in the bonding protocol, the orthodontic bracket is immediately taken off and a new bonding procedure is begun.
14. Placement of the orthodontic bracket with a passive metal looped ligature, secured with composite.
15. Discharge the patient with necessary postoperative instructions for maintenance of good oral hygiene and keeping the area clean.
16. See the patient 2 weeks after surgery, twice, and monthly thereafter. Application of active elastic traction on 2.3 after 2 weeks and upper arch bonding one month after surgery through Straight-Wire MBT™ technique with a 0.14″ NiTi arch-wire, performing a mesial lace-back 1.2–2.2 and metal ligation on 2.2.
17. Progressive translation of the canine into the correct position in the dental arch through reactivations of elastic traction with elastic cotton threads, lace-back 1.2–2.2, metal ligatures on 2.2 and 2.4 and super elastic NiTi (0.12) upper arch.

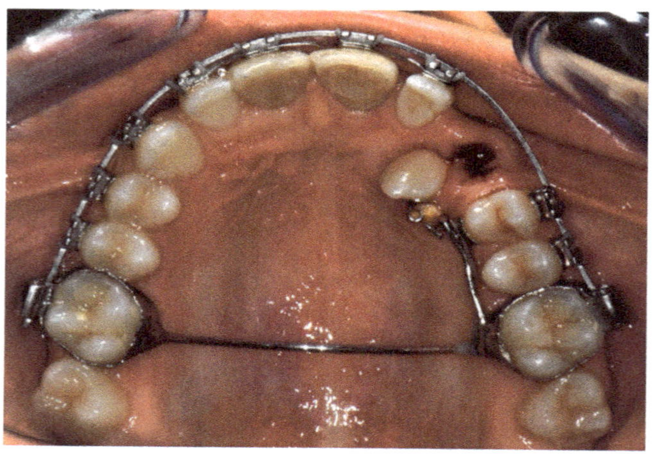

Figure 7: Position of 2.3 after 3 months of orthodontic traction and the extraction of deciduous 6.3.

tissue while Nd:YAG for soft tissue. Er:YAG does not show a haemostatic effect, therefore the surgical field was coagulated with Nd:YAG, ensuring bracket adhesion to enamel, and also reducing or avoiding the need for anaesthesia and reducing post-operative pain [44].

In addition, numerous studies in the literature showed the positive effect of the laser on soft tissue, leading to no post-operative pain, no discomfort, no post-operative bleeding, and optimal healing by second intention through the formation of a thin, aesthetically excellent scar. In fact, patients rate the procedure as well tolerable and acceptable [45–47].

A brief review of the dosimetry and techniques used in previous clinical studies is reported in Table 3.

Studies in the literature point to some important disadvantages in the use of the other surgical alternatives, which contributed to the choice of using the diode laser. Specifically, the use of the CO_2 laser results in thermal damage and a stress effect on soft tissue cells, evident through the presence of elongated cells with fusiform nuclei devoid of nucleoli (therefore inactive), depletion of glycogen, and a reduction in the expression of immunocytochemical markers of intracellular proteins, nuclear cell cycle proliferation, and apoptosis [49]. This cellular damage is also determined following the use of the Er:YAG laser; however, it is significantly reduced, highlighting the possibility of faster healing [49, 50]. An important disadvantage of this laser, considering the importance of having a dry operating field to be able to apply the orthodontic bracket, is the absence of a coagulating effect [49, 50]. Obviously, the same disadvantage is represented using a cold-blade scalpel [37]. The Nd:YAG laser has an unsatisfactory analgesic effect and, consequently, local anaesthesia is required and the fibrous tissue is not easily removed [51]. Finally, the electrosurgical scalpel presents numerous disadvantages and risks associated with its use, from risk of burns, due to the use of

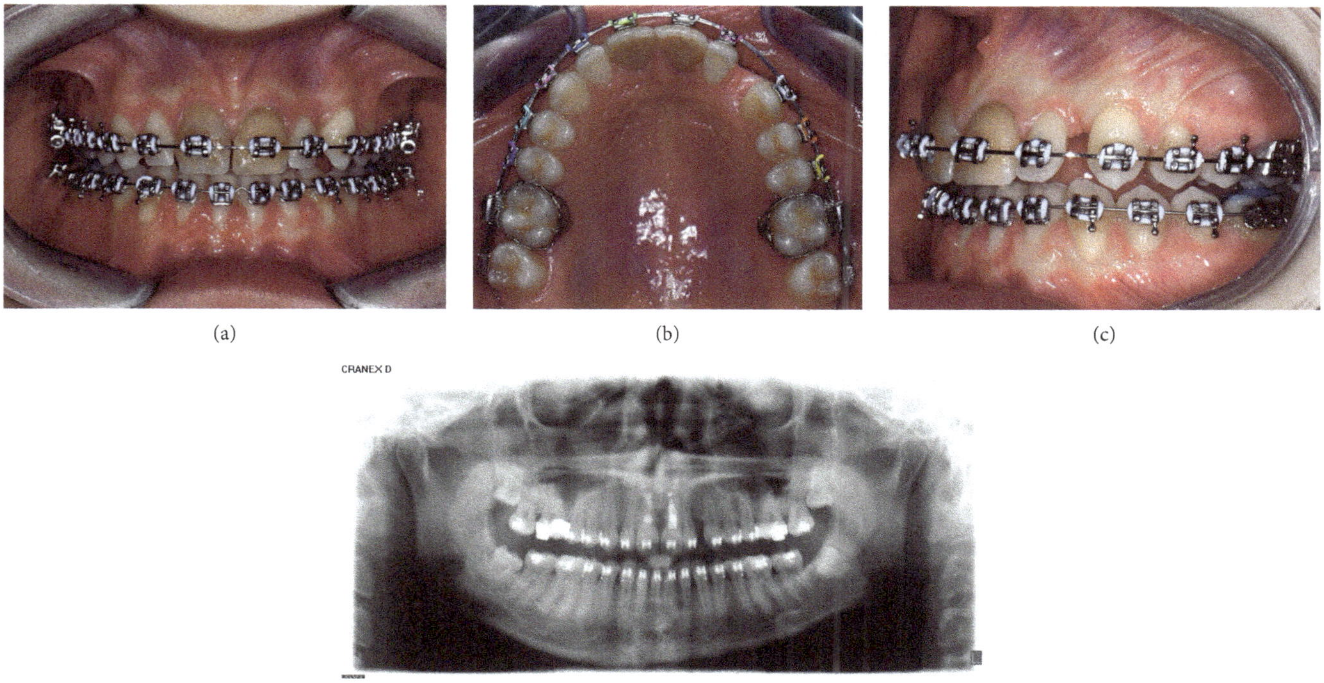

(a) (b) (c) (d)

Figure 8: (a–c) Intraoral photo and (d) panoramic radiograph 12 month after surgical-orthodontics disinclusion. Upper canine 2.3, once included, is positioned in the dental arch.

Table 3: Brief review of the dosimetry and techniques used in previous clinical reports.

Authors	Laser	Mode	Power setting	Wavelength (nm)
Migliario et al. [42, 48]	Diode	Pulsed (20 s)	1.5 W	980
Impellizzeri et al. [43]	CO_2	Superpulsed (80 Hz)	4.5 W	10,600
Fornaini et al. [44]	Nd:YAG	Superpulsed (40 Hz)	4 W	1064
	Er:YAG	Medium-short pulse (10 Hz)	300 mJ	2940
Olivi et al. [45]	Er:YAG	Superpulsed (300 μs)	2.25–3 W	2940
Kato and Wijeyeweera [46]	CO_2	Continuous	3 W or 4 W	10,600
Ramkumar et al. [47]	Diode	Continuous	1.5 W	940

high-frequency current, to a fire risk, due to the presence of combustible liquids or gases in the room where it is used, in an electrical risk, due to the radiated power that can disturb various medical devices applied to the patient. Furthermore, it has been shown, from a histological, histochemical, and immunocytochemical point of view, that the epithelial damage due to the use of electrocautery is higher than the epithelial damage induced using the CO_2 laser, delaying the healing of the surgical wound more [36, 52].

This study has some limitations. First, this is a case report with a short-term follow-up. More cases with long-term follow-up are needed to prove the success of this technique. Finally, we can also consider a limitation: laser equipment can involve a high investment and require a learning curve to achieve an optimal result. Based on these observations, several clinical trials are needed to evaluate the advantages and disadvantages of different laser and electrosurgery in surgical disinclusion of impacted teeth.

3. Conclusion

This case report shows how an 810 nm diode laser can be used during orthodontic treatment for dental exposure without causing post-operative pain and swelling and how it allows maintaining a dry field in order to apply an orthodontic bracket during the operation.

Consent

A written informed consent was obtained from all patients before the commencement of the study.

Authors' Contributions

MCV: conceptualization, supervision, data curation, formal analysis, investigation, methodology, and project administration. MFS: conceptualization, project administration, and supervision. MGN writing—original draft. MP: writing—original draft. SF: methodology. FP: methodology. RA: investigation. MM: investigation. KB: investigation. AS: conceptualization, supervision, and writing—review and editing.

References

[1] A. R. Chapokas, K. Almas, and G. P. Schincaglia, "The impacted maxillary canine: a proposed classification for surgical exposure," *Oral Surgery, Oral Medicine, Oral Pathology and Oral Radiology*, vol. 113, no. 2, pp. 222–228, 2012.

[2] Y. Brorsson and J. Naoumova, "Delayed diagnosis of displaced and impacted canines—a prospective longitudinal study," *Acta Odontologica Scandinavica*, vol. 78, no. 3, pp. 165–172, 2020.

[3] M. M. Bedoya and J. H. Park, "A review of the diagnosis and management of impacted maxillary canines," *The Journal of the American Dental Association*, vol. 140, no. 12, pp. 1485–1493, 2009.

[4] A. K. Sajnani, "Permanent maxillary canines - review of eruption pattern and local etiological factors leading to impaction," *Journal of Investigative and Clinical Dentistry*, vol. 6, no. 1, pp. 1–7, 2015.

[5] A. Becker and S. Chaushu, "Etiology of maxillary canine impaction: a review," *American Journal of Orthodontics and Dentofacial Orthopedics*, vol. 148, no. 4, pp. 557–567, 2015.

[6] M. de Oliveira Ribas, W. D. Martins, M. H. de Sousa et al., "Oral and maxillofacial manifestations of familial adenomatous polyposis (Gardner's syndrome): a report of two cases," *The Journal of Contemporary Dental Practice*, vol. 10, no. 1, pp. 82–90, 2009.

[7] G. R. Bayar, K. Ortakoglu, and M. Sencimen, "Multiple impacted teeth: report of 3 cases," *European Journal of Dentistry*, vol. 2, no. 1, pp. 73–78, 2008.

[8] P. M. Campeau, G. M. Lenk, J. T. Lu et al., "Yunis–Varon syndrome is caused by mutations in FIG4, encoding a phosphoinositide phosphatase," *American Journal of Human Genetics*, vol. 92, no. 5, pp. 781–791, 2013.

[9] C. L. Antunes, A. M. Aranha, M. C. Bandeca et al., "Eruption of impacted teeth in cleft lip and palate patients following alveolar bone graft," *The Journal of Contemporary Dental Practice*, vol. 19, no. 9, pp. 1072–1075, 2018.

[10] S. Sambataro, S. Bocchieri, G. Cervino et al., "Correlations between malocclusion and postural anomalies in children with mixed dentition," *Journal of Functional Morphology Kinesiology*, vol. 4, no. 3, p. 45, 2019.

[11] A. Alqerban, A. S. Storms, M. Voet, S. Fieuws, and G. Willems, "Early prediction of maxillary canine impaction," *Dentomaxillofacial Radiology*, vol. 45, no. 3, p. 20150232, 2016.

[12] R. M. Cruz, "Orthodontic traction of impacted canines: concepts and clinical application," *Dental Press Journal of Orthodontics*, vol. 24, no. 1, pp. 74–87, 2019.

[13] I. Izadikhah, D. Cao, Z. Zhao, and B. Yan, "Different management approaches in impacted maxillary canines: an overview on current trends and literature," *The Journal of Contemporary Dental Practice*, vol. 21, no. 3, pp. 326–336, 2020.

[14] J. Hecht, "A short history of laser development," *Applied Optics*, vol. 49, no. 25, pp. F99–F122, 2010.

[15] V. Heiskanen and M. R. Hamblin, "Correction: photobiomodulation: lasersvs.light emitting diodes?," *Photochemical & Photobiological Sciences*, vol. 18, no. 1, p. 259, 2019.

[16] L. C. Martens, "Laser physics and a review of laser applications in dentistry for children," *European Archives of Paediatric Dentistry*, vol. 12, no. 2, pp. 61–67, 2011.

[17] A. Romano, D. di Stasio, D. Lauritano et al., "Topical photodynamic therapy in the treatment of benign oral mucosal lesions: a systematic review," *Journal of Oral Pathology & Medicine*, vol. 50, no. 7, pp. 639–648, 2021.

[18] A. Romano, D. di Stasio, E. Gentile, M. Petruzzi, R. Serpico, and A. Lucchese, "The potential role of photodynamic therapy in oral premalignant and malignant lesions: a systematic review," *Journal of Oral Pathology & Medicine*, vol. 50, no. 4, pp. 333–344, 2021.

[19] R. Hanna and S. Parker, "The advantages of carbon dioxide laser applications in paediatric oral surgery. A prospective cohort study," *Lasers in Medical Science*, vol. 31, no. 8, pp. 1527–1536, 2016.

[20] J. H. Ahn, S. Power, and E. Thickett, "Application of the diode laser for soft-tissue surgery in orthodontics: case series," *Journal of Orthodontics*, vol. 48, no. 1, pp. 82–87, 2021.

[21] S. Nammour, "Laser dentistry, current advantages, and limits," *Photomedicine and Laser Surgery*, vol. 30, no. 1, pp. 1–4, 2012.

[22] E. F. Sant'Anna, M. T. Araújo, L. I. Nojima, A. C. Cunha, B. L. Silveira, and M. Marquezan, "High-intensity laser application in *Orthodontics*," *Journal of Orthodontics*, vol. 22, no. 6, pp. 99–109, 2017.

[23] E. Sutter, B. Giacomelli-Hiestand, M. Rücker, and S. Valdec, "CO_2 laser application in stomatology," *Swiss Dental journal*, vol. 129, no. 3, pp. 214-215, 2019.

[24] Y. Saydjari, T. Kuypers, and N. Gutknecht, "Laser application in dentistry: irradiation effects of Nd:YAG 1064 nm and diode 810 nm and 980 nm in infected root canals—a literature overview," *BioMed Research International*, vol. 2016, 10 pages, 2016.

[25] A. Scribante, S. Gallo, M. Pascadopoli et al., "Management of periodontal disease with adjunctive therapy with ozone and photobiomodulation (PBM): a randomized clinical trial," *Photonics*, vol. 9, no. 3, p. 138, 2022.

[26] C. de Paula Eduardo, P. M. de Freitas, M. Esteves-Oliveira et al., "Laser phototherapy in the treatment of periodontal disease. A review," *Lasers in Medical Science*, vol. 25, no. 6, pp. 781–792, 2010.

[27] R. Fekrazad, S. Alimazandarani, K. A. Kalhori, H. Assadian, and S. M. Mirmohammadi, "Comparison of laser and power bleaching techniques in tooth color change," *Journal of Clinical and Experimental Dentistry*, vol. 9, no. 4, pp. e511–e515, 2017.

[28] K. K. Gandhi, R. Pavaskar, E. G. Cappetta, and H. J. Drew, "Effectiveness of adjunctive use of low-level laser therapy and photodynamic therapy after scaling and root planing in patients with chronic periodontitis," *The International Journal of Periodontics & Restorative Dentistry*, vol. 39, no. 6, pp. 837–843, 2019.

[29] G. Olivi, M. D. Genovese, and C. Caprioglio, "Evidence-based dentistry on laser paediatric dentistry: review and outlook," *European Journal of Paediatric Dentistry*, vol. 10, no. 1, pp. 29–40, 2009.

[30] D. Ortega-Concepcion, J. Cano-Duran, J. Peña-Cardelles, V. Paredes-Rodriguez, J. Gonzalez-Serrano, and J. Lopez-Quiles, "The application of diode laser in the treatment of oral soft tissues lesions. A literature *review*," *Dentistry*, vol. 9, no. 7, pp. e925–e928, 2017.

[31] M. F. Sfondrini, G. Calderoni, M. C. Vitale, P. Gandini, and A. Scribante, "Is laser conditioning a valid alternative to conventional etching for aesthetic brackets?," *European Journal of Paediatric Dentistry*, vol. 19, no. 1, pp. 61–66, 2018.

[32] M. F. Sfondrini, M. C. Vitale, A. L. B. Pinheiro et al., "Photobiomodulation and pain reduction in patients requiring orthodontic band application: randomized clinical trial," *BioMed Research International*, vol. 2020, 2020.

[33] S. Tortorici, P. Messina, and G. A. Scardina, "Effectiveness of low-level laser therapy on pain intensity after lower third molar extraction," *International Journal of Clinical Dentistry*, vol. 12, no. 4, pp. 357–367, 2019.

[34] G. A. Scardina, S. Casella, G. Bilello, and P. Messina, "Photobiomodulation therapy in the management of burning mouth syndrome: morphological variations in the capillary bed," *Dentistry Journal*, vol. 8, no. 3, p. 99, 2020.

[35] D. E. S. Malik, M. Fida, and R. H. Sukhia, "Correlation between radiographic parameters for the prediction of palatally impacted maxillary canines," *Journal of Orthodontics*, vol. 46, no. 1, pp. 6–13, 2019.

[36] S. L. Soon and C. V. Washington, "Electrosurgery, electrocoagulation, electrofulguration, electrodesiccation, electrosection, electrocautery," in *Surgery of the Skin*, J. K. Robinson, C. W. Hanke, and D. M. Siegel, Eds., vol. 9pp. 177–190, Elsevier, New York, 2nd edition edition, 2010.

[37] D. O. Eyarefe, D. I. Kuforiji, T. A. Jarikre, and B. O. Emikpe, "Enhanced electroscalpel incisional wound healing potential of honey in Wistar rats," *International Journal of Veterinary Science and Medicine*, vol. 5, no. 2, pp. 128–134, 2017.

[38] C. Sweeney, "Laser safety in dentistry," *General Dentistry*, vol. 56, no. 7, pp. 653–659, 2008.

[39] N. Akbulut, E. S. Kursun, M. K. Tumer, K. Kamburoglu, and U. Gulsen, "Is the 810-nm diode laser the best choice in oral soft tissue therapy?," *European Journal of Dentistry*, vol. 7, no. 2, pp. 207–211, 2013.

[40] M. F. Sfondrini, V. Cacciafesta, A. Scribante, M. De Angelis, and C. Klersy, "Effect of blood contamination on shear bond strength of brackets bonded with conventional and self-etching primers," *American Journal of Orthodontics and Dentofacial Orthopedics*, vol. 125, no. 3, pp. 357–360, 2004.

[41] R. A. Mussttaf, D. F. L. Jenkins, and A. N. Jha, "Assessing the impact of low level laser therapy (LLLT) on biological systems: a review," *International Journal of Radiation Biology*, vol. 95, no. 2, pp. 120–143, 2019.

[42] M. Migliario, M. Rizzi, A. G. Lucchina, and F. Renò, "Diode laser clinical efficacy and mini-invasivity in surgical exposure of impacted teeth," *Journal of Craniofacial Surgery*, vol. 27, no. 8, pp. e779–e784, 2016.

[43] A. Impellizzeri, M. Horodynski, E. Serritella et al., "Uncovering and autonomous eruption of palatally impacted canines—a case report," *Dentistry Journal*, vol. 9, no. 6, p. 66, 2021.

[44] C. Fornaini, E. Merigo, P. Vescovi, G. Lagori, and J. Rocca, "Use of laser in orthodontics: applications and perspectives," *Laser Therapy*, vol. 22, no. 2, pp. 115–124, 2013.

[45] M. Olivi, M. D. Genovese, and G. Olivi, "Laser labial frenectomy: a simplified and predictable technique. Retrospective clinical study," *European Journal of Paediatric Dentistry*, vol. 19, no. 1, pp. 56–60, 2018.

[46] J. Kato and R. L. Wijeyeweera, "The effect of CO_2 laser irradiation on oral soft tissue problems in children in Sri Lanka," *Photomedicine and Laser Surgery*, vol. 25, no. 4, pp. 264–268, 2007.

[47] S. Ramkumar, L. Ramkumar, N. Malathi, and R. Suganya, "Excision of mucocele using diode laser in lower lip," *Case Reports in Dentistry*, vol. 2016, 4 pages, 2016.

[48] M. Migliario, L. A. Greco, V. Rocchetti, and F. Renò, "Laser surgical approach to impacted maxillary incisors: case series and brief review," *European Review for Medical and Pharmacological Sciences*, vol. 23, no. 22, pp. 9691–9696, 2019.

[49] D. Zaffe, M. C. Vitale, A. Martignone, F. Scarpelli, and A. R. Botticelli, "Morphological, histochemical, and immunocytochemical study of CO2 and Er:YAG laser effect on oral soft tissues," *Photomedicine and Laser Surgery*, vol. 22, no. 3, pp. 185–189, 2004.

[50] G. L. Sfasciotti, F. Zara, L Vozza, V. Carocci, G. Ierardo, and A. Polimeni, "Diode versus CO_2 laser therapy in the treatment of high labial frenulum attachment: a pilot randomized, double-blinded clinical trial," *International Journal of Environmental Research and Public Health*, vol. 17, no. 21, p. 7708, 2020.

[51] I. Giovannacci, G. Mergoni, M. Meleti et al., "Postoperative discomfort in oral soft tissue surgery: a comparative perspective evaluation of Nd:YAG laser, quantic molecular resonance scalpel and cold blade," *Minerva Stomatologica*, vol. 64, no. 1, pp. 9–20, 2015.

[52] M. C. Vitale, A. R. Botticelli, D. Zaffe et al., "CO_2 laser biopsies of oral mucosa: an immunocytological and histological comparative study," *Lasers in Dentistry VII*, vol. 4249, pp. 139–144, 2001.

7

A Rare Case of Nonsyndromic Generalized Radiculomegaly with a Literature Review

Mohammad Al-Obaida

Department of Restorative Dental Sciences, King Saud University, Riyadh, Saudi Arabia

Correspondence should be addressed to Mohammad Al-Obaida; malobaida@ksu.edu.sa

Academic Editor: Kevin Seymour

Radiculomegaly is a rare condition involving elongated tooth roots. This condition has significant clinical implications and has been associated with syndromes such as oculofaciocardiodental syndrome. However, only a few nonsyndromic cases of radiculomegaly have been reported. Here, we report a case of nonsyndromic radiculomegaly in a Saudi individual. A subsequent review of the literature suggests endodontic management modalities for individuals with the dental findings demonstrated in the present case.

1. Introduction

Tooth development is a complex physiological process which involves bud, cap, and bell stages, as well as tooth root development and tooth eruption. After a crown is nearly completed, the root begins to develop according to guidance provided by the double layer of the epithelial sheath referred to as "Hertwig's epithelial root sheath" [1]. The most common root malformations in humans arise from either developmental disorders of the root alone or disorders of radicular development as part of general tooth dysplasia [2]. However, there is limited information regarding mechanisms of root morphogenesis and elongation [3].

Abnormal tooth morphology and number, including hyperdontia, hypodontia, oligodontia, multiple roots, and taurodontia, are obvious dental anomalies [4]. Among these anomalies is a rare congenital condition called, "radiculomegaly," which involves a pronounced elongation of dental roots (either in isolation or affecting multiple teeth). This rare condition has seldom been reported in the literature. The first reports of radiculomegaly [5–7] described it as a characteristic of the X-linked rare congenital syndrome, oculofaciocardiodental syndrome (OFCD), which only affects females. However, radiculomegaly was later reported as a characteristic feature of males affected by Klinefelter syndrome [3, 8]. To date, only a few nonsyndromic cases of radiculomegaly have been reported [9, 10]. Here, we report a case of nonsyndromic radiculomegaly in a Saudi individual and then discuss the aspects of this case in relation to previous studies (Table 1).

2. Case Report

2.1. Patient History. A 31-year-old Saudi male patient presented to a restorative clinic at the College of Dentistry, King Saud University, Saudi Arabia. The patient was seeking permanent restoration of an endodontically treated tooth on the left side of his lower jaw which had undergone significant decay many years prior.

The dental history of the patient included extraction of a mandibular left molar, multiple restorations, and a root canal treatment. The patient stated that he underwent a surgical procedure to the gingiva to help his anterior permanent teeth erupt during childhood. Medical history revealed no significant reports. The family history for the patient also revealed no evidence of any medical condition.

2.2. Physical Examination. Height and weight recorded for the patient were 185 cm and 114 kg, respectively. A head and neck extraoral examination revealed a mandibular protrusion leading to a straight facial profile (Figure 1) and tight lips upon closure with a thick lower lip. An

Table 1: Published cases of nonsyndromic radiculomegaly.

Title of publication	Authors	Year of publication	Journal
Cuspid gigantism	Hayward JR	1980	Oral Surgery, Oral Medicine, Oral Pathology
A very long cuspid	Weine FS	1986	Journal of Endodontics
Radiculomegaly of canines and congenital cataracts - a syndrome?	Marashi and Gorlin	1990	Oral Surgery, Oral Medicine, Oral Pathology
A very large maxillary cuspid	Wilkie and Chambers	1990	Oral Surgery, Oral Medicine, Oral Pathology
Long root of deciduous anterior teeth	Fujmura et al.	2008	Odontology
Bilateral second premolars agenesia together with a unilateral canine radiculomegaly	Kemoli and Junior	2017	Contemporary Clinical Dentistry
Radiculomegaly: a case report of this rare dental finding with review of the associated oculofacio-cardio-dental syndrome	Smith et al.	2018	Oral and Maxillofacial Pathology

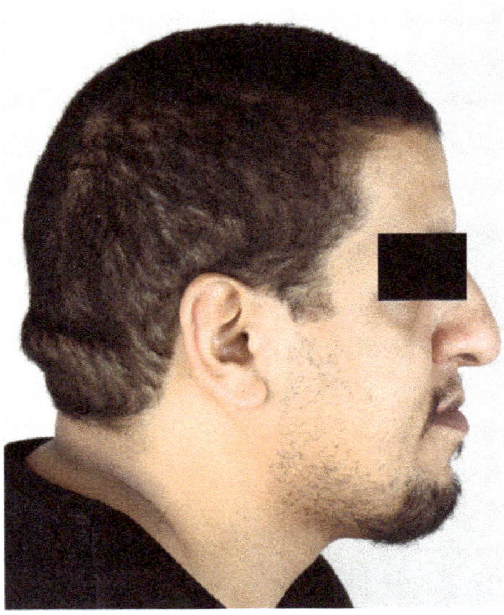

Figure 1: A profile view of the patient's mandibular protrusion.

intraoral examination showed racial melanin pigmentation, especially on attached gingiva, with anterior and bilateral cross bites (Figures 2 and 3). Generalized gingivitis with bad oral hygiene and heavy plaque accumulation were observed in the crowded anterior segments. Areas of deep pockets and bleeding were also noted. Tooth #32 presented hypomineralization, while a very deep vault in the hard palate and bony enlargement of the posterior areas of the maxillary arch were also observed (Figure 4). Crowded teeth characterize both of the patient's arches since the patient has a full set of teeth and narrow upper and lower arches.

2.3. Radiographic Examination. A panoramic view of the patient's teeth show long roots (radiculomegaly) for most of the teeth, especially for the molar teeth (Figure 5). Periapical radiographs also show unusually long roots (Figure 6). Cone beam computed tomography (CBCT) software was used to measure the length of the patient's entire set of teeth. Measurements were made from the apex to the tip of the cusps in a slice orientation manner (Figure 7).

3. Discussion

Radiculomegaly, a condition which manifests as elongated dental roots (whether isolated or generalized), is rare. Radiculomegaly was first mentioned as an entity in 1980 [5], and then subsequently in 1986 and 1990 [6, 7]. In 1990, Marashi and Gorlin further observed a potential association between radiculomegaly and cataracts. Based on their observations, they proposed the likelihood of a syndrome [11]. In 1993, Wilkie et al. hypothesized that a combination of eye, facial, heart, and teeth abnormalities represent characteristics of OFCD. Support for this hypothesis was subsequently provided by Gorlin et al. in 1996.

In the present case, an association between radiculomegaly and OFCD was excluded since OFCD is an X-chromosome linked disease and is fatal in males [4, 10, 12]. Our patient also did not exhibit any eye or heart problems. Similarly, Klinefelter syndrome was excluded since males with Klinefelter syndrome often manifest clinical signs and symptoms which affect their physical and intellectual development (e.g., infertility, primary testicular insufficiency, breast enlargement (gynecomastia)). Other manifestations can include abnormal fusion of certain bones in the forearm (radioulnar synostosis), curved pinky fingers (fifth finger clinodactyly), and flat feet (pes planus). Furthermore, individuals affected by Klinefelter syndrome tend to experience anxiety, depression, impaired social skills, behavioral problems (e.g., emotional immaturity, impulsivity, attention-deficit/hyperactivity disorder), and limited problem-solving skills (executive functioning). Approximately 10% of boys and men with Klinefelter syndrome exhibit autism spectrum disorder. Therefore, Klinefelter syndrome was also excluded since our patient exhibited no clinical or social problems [8]. Finally, Cockayne syndrome (CS) is a rare, autosomal recessive disorder which was first described in 1936 by Edward Cockayne. Early descriptions of CS identified microcephaly and growth failure as cardinal clinical features. Other recognized features include hearing loss,

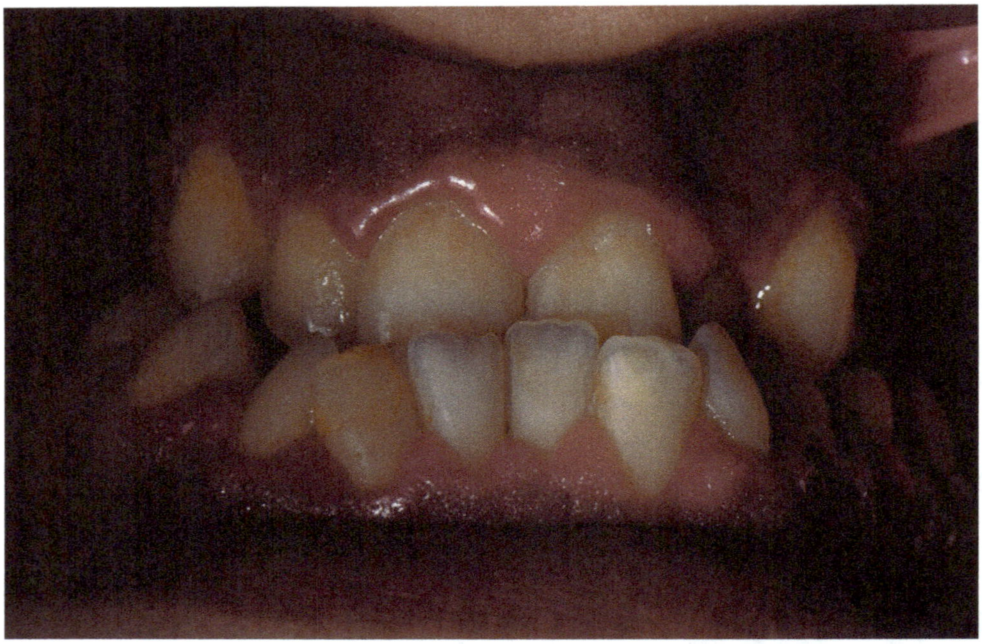

FIGURE 2: An intraoral anterior view of the patient's anterior cross bite.

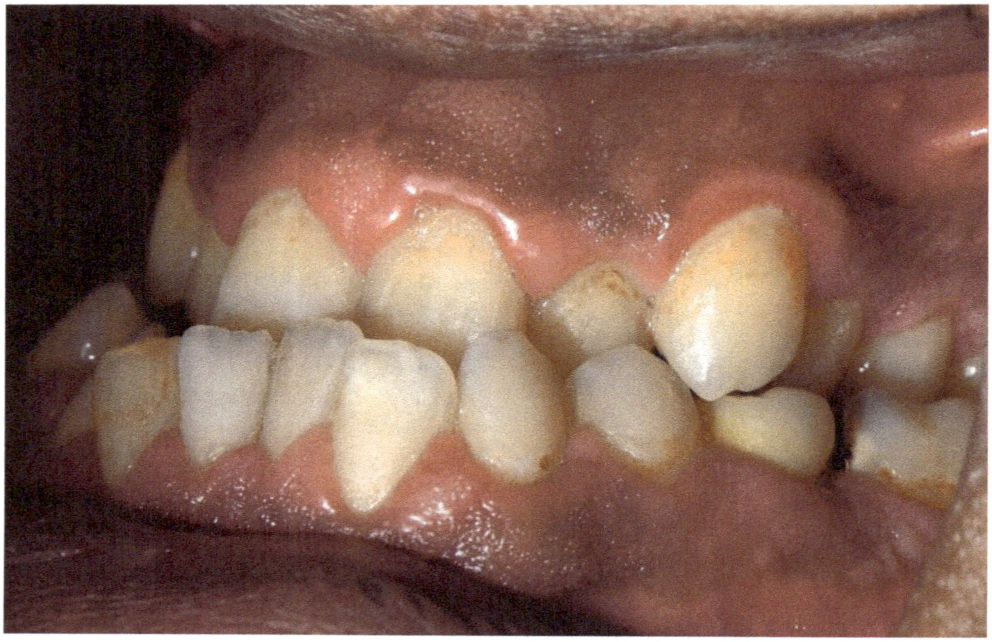

FIGURE 3: An intraoral lateral view of the patient's posterior cross bite.

cataracts, retinal dystrophy, and developmental delays [13, 14]. In the present case, CS was excluded since none of the patient's clinical features were consistent with this diagnosis. Thus, the present case was excluded from any associations with reported syndromes which are characterized by similar features.

The morphology of permanent premolars and molars has been reviewed extensively.

Descriptive data regarding morphological or anatomical landmarks for various types of teeth have been used to identify average variations among different populations [15, 16]. These studies provide basic knowledge for clinicians to recognize potential issues or aspects during treatment or case management. One of the anatomical landmarks which could be used as a reference for all teeth is vertical length. Despite small variations among the findings of different

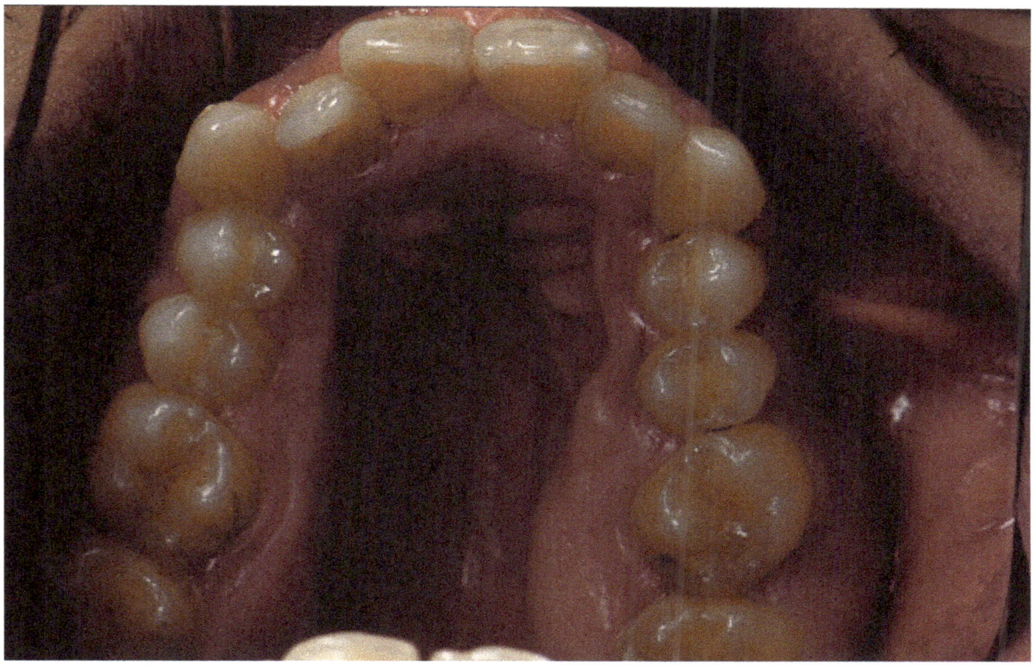

FIGURE 4: A view of the deep V-shaped maxillary vault of the patient. Bone enlargement in the molar area is also observed.

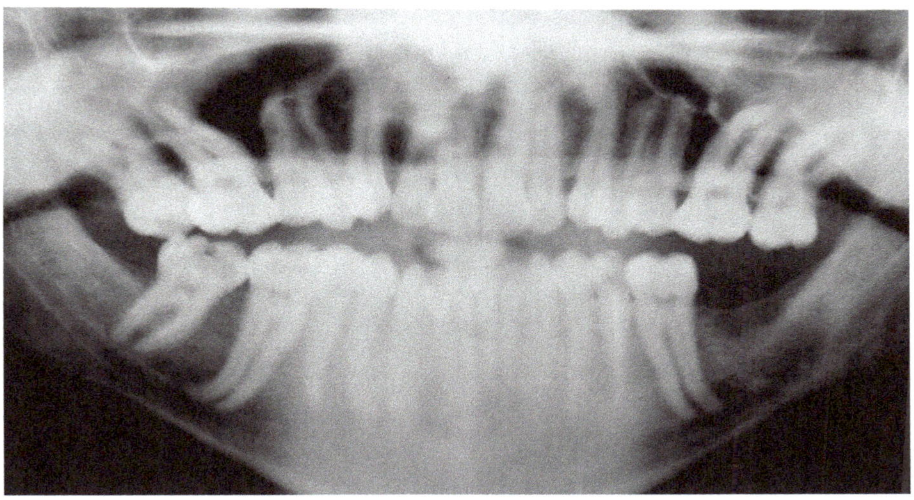

FIGURE 5: A panoramic radiograph showing the elongated roots of the teeth.

studies [15–19], it has generally been reported that the vertical lengths of teeth share similar averages. In the present case, an extreme variation in root length was detected in periapical radiographs (PAs) and with CBCT. Among published reports of radiculomegaly, canine teeth are most commonly affected [4, 9, 10, 20, 21]. Being able to obtain accurate root canal length measurements after treatment is also essential for determining the success of a treatment. Conventional methods for measurement involve tools such as an electronic apex locator (EAL) and PAs [22]. However, a limitation of obtaining measurements from two-dimensional PAs is that root canal length is frequently overestimated [23]. Similarly, when measuring tooth length from PAs, the likelihood of distortion relative to the projection angle of the X-ray unit must be considered. CBCT-based data can be used as a reference for evaluating root length and resorption of teeth without metal restorations in patients with malocclusions [24]. In addition, CBCT is a validated tool for exploring root canal morphology in three dimensions [25]. However, when dealing with ionizing radiation, the indication for each new image has to be critically evaluated. Particularly with regard to endodontic treatments, it must be determined whether spatial imaging is really needed or whether conventional two-dimensional PAs are sufficient, according to the ALARA principle in medical radiology [26].

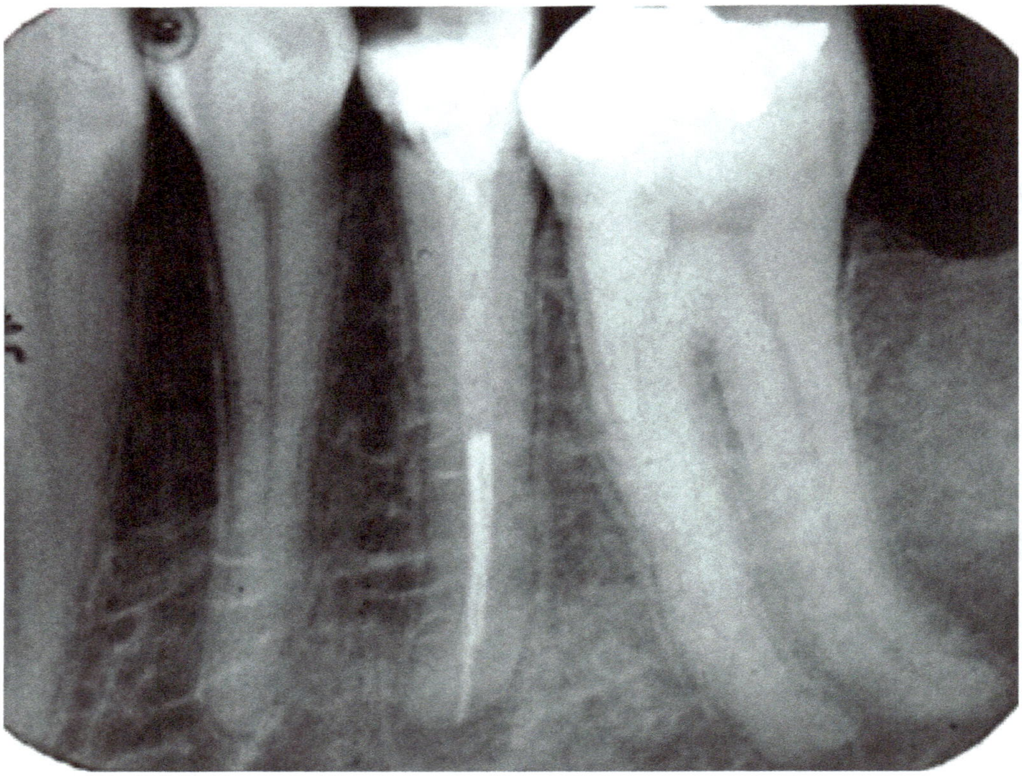

Figure 6: PA X-ray of the long root of the teeth.

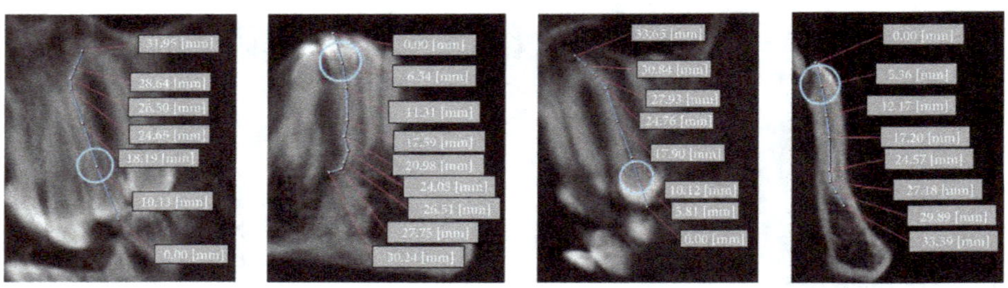

Figure 7: CBCT view of some teeth.

For endodontic treatment of elongated roots, longer manual and rotary files are needed. Due to concerns raised nearly 40 years ago, efforts were made to standardize endodontic files and root canal filling materials. As a result, an international organization for standardization of endodontic files (ISO) was established. Currently, there are three standard lengths available for endodontic files: 21 mm, 25 mm, and 31 mm. In addition, various studies have been conducted to improve the intraoral accessibility of instruments for endodontic treatment [27]. Thus, modified endodontic files and obturation techniques have been developed (Pace et al., 2011). In some cases, KReamer veterinary instruments have been used (Vetinox; Dentsply Maillefer, Ballaigues, Switzerland). To perform obturation, a Thermafil-modified technique has been developed. Briefly, the plastic handle of a Thermafil obturator is removed and a Thermafil stem is inserted into a stainless-steel straight wire to complete the obturation. Mehran et al. described another modified technique for fabricating long files. Their technique involves cutting and removing the plastic handle of a 31-mm K-file and the handle of another file at the initiation of the flutes (thereby keeping the handle). The two parts are then attached with soldering [28]. A technique to fabricate long Gutta-Percha cones has also been described by Maden et al. Briefly, an artificial canal is created in a plastic mold by using veterinary files. Thermoplastized gutta-percha is subsequently injected into the mold to create a cone [21].

Another treatment option to consider for patients with radiculomegaly involves use of Mineral Trioxide Aggregate (MTA). The introduction of bioceramics has showed promising results in the treatment of mature permanent teeth with carious exposures [29]. For example, Taha et al. reported that a full pulpotomy performed with biodentine was successful up to a year after mature permanent teeth with carious-exposed pulps, and clinical signs and symptoms indicative of irreversible pulpitis were treated [30]. In 2017, Linu et al. also reported a technique using a biometric material which exhibited better biocompatibility and sealing properties. As a result, application of this technique provided more predictable outcomes for direct pulp capping of mature permanent teeth with carious exposure [31]. Given the hypomineralization which was noted for tooth #32 in the present case, it is possible that this represents Molar-Incisor Hypomineralization (MIH), a condition which affects the enamel of permanent teeth. First permanent (adult) molars and incisors (front teeth) are most commonly affected by MIH. Normally, enamel appears white and is very hard. However, in cases of MIH, the enamel has a creamy or yellow/brown color [32]. There was no caries detected in tooth #32 in our patient.

A bony expansion was observed in the palatal sides of the patient's maxilla. This expansion was characterized as hard, bony, and painless, and it did not exhibit any signs of growth. Therefore, this expansion was considered clinically to represent a palatal exostosis. The latter is a benign lesion which can be left alone, or can be surgically removed to obtain functional benefits [33].

4. Conclusion

Radiculomegaly has been associated with many syndromes in the literature, while only a few reports of nonsyndromic cases have been published. Here, we report a nonsyndromic case of generalized radiculomegaly in a Saudi individual. Initially, patients with radiculomegaly should receive counseling regarding caries prevention since extensive caries can lead to pulpal involvement. Furthermore, the latter may require root canal treatment or dental extractions, and these have adverse treatment complications to consider. If it is decided that endodontic treatment is needed, special management protocols and tools should then be considered.

Consent

The patient signed a written consent to allow his information and images to be published in this paper.

Acknowledgments

The author extends his appreciation to the College of Dentistry at King Saud University for supporting this research and publishing the case.

References

[1] X.-F. Huang and Y. Chai, "Molecular regulatory mechanism of tooth root development," *International Journal of Oral Science*, vol. 4, no. 4, pp. 177–181, 2012.

[2] H. U. Luder, "Malformations of the tooth root in humans," *Frontiers in Physiology*, vol. 6, p. 307, 2015.

[3] N. Suda and K. Moriyama, "Human diseases associated with abnormal tooth roots," *Journal of Oral Biosciences*, vol. 51, no. 4, pp. 199–204, 2009.

[4] J. Kato, K. Kushima, and F. Kushima, "New radiological findings and radiculomegaly in oculofaciocardiodental syndrome with a novel BCOR mutation: a case report," *Medicine*, vol. 97, no. 49, article e13444, 2018.

[5] J. R. Hayward, "Cuspid gigantism," *Oral Surgery, Oral Medicine, and Oral Pathology*, vol. 49, no. 6, pp. 500-501, 1980.

[6] F. S. Weine, "A very long cuspid!," *Journal of Endodontia*, vol. 12, no. 2, pp. 80-81, 1986.

[7] G. J. Wilkie and I. G. Chambers, "A very large maxillary cuspid," *Oral Surgery, Oral Medicine, and Oral Pathology*, vol. 70, no. 2, pp. 159-160, 1990.

[8] R. Lähdesmäki and L. Alvesalo, "Root lengths in the permanent teeth of Klinefelter (47,XXY) men," *Archives of Oral Biology*, vol. 52, no. 9, pp. 822–827, 2007.

[9] A. M. Kemoli and T. M. Junior, "Bilateral second premolars agenesia together with a unilateral canine radiculomegaly," *Contemporary Clinical Dentistry*, vol. 8, no. 1, pp. 151–154, 2017.

[10] M. H. Smith, D. M. Cohen, I. Bhattacharyya, N. M. Islam, and D. Kashtwari, "Radiculomegaly: a case report of this rare dental finding with review of the associated oculo-facio-cardio-dental syndrome," *Oral Surgery, Oral Medicine, Oral Pathology, Oral Radiology*, vol. 126, no. 4, pp. e220–e227, 2018.

[11] A. H. Marashi and R. J. Gorlin, "Radiculomegaly of canine teeth and congenital cataracts: confirmation of a syndrome," *American Journal of Medical Genetics*, vol. 42, no. 1, p. 143, 1992.

[12] A. Davoody, I.-P. Chen, R. Nanda, F. Uribe, and E. J. Reichenberger, "Oculofaciocardiodental syndrome: a rare case and review of the literature," *The Cleft Palate-Craniofacial Journal*, vol. 49, no. 5, pp. e55–e60, 2012.

[13] A. Bloch-Zupan, M. Rousseaux, V. Laugel et al., "A possible cranio-oro-facial phenotype in Cockayne syndrome," *Orphanet Journal of Rare Diseases*, vol. 8, no. 1, p. 9, 2013.

[14] B. T. Wilson, Z. Stark, R. E. Sutton et al., "The Cockayne Syndrome Natural History (CoSyNH) study: clinical findings in 102 individuals and recommendations for care," *Genetics in Medicine*, vol. 18, no. 5, pp. 483–493, 2016.

[15] P. Carrotte, "Endodontics: Part 4 Morphology of the root canal system," *British Dental Journal*, vol. 197, no. 7, pp. 379–383, 2004.

[16] S. J. Nelson, M. M. Ash, and M. M. Ash, *Wheeler's Dental Anatomy, Physiology, and Occlusion*, Saunders/Elsevier, St. Louis, MO, 9th ed edition, 2010.

[17] A. Jain and R. Bahuguna, "Root canal morphology of mandibular first premolar in a gujarati population - an in vitro study," *Dental Research Journal*, vol. 8, no. 3, pp. 118–122, 2011.

[18] J. D. Pécora, P. C. Saquy, M. D. Sousa Neto, and J. B. Woelfel, "Root form and canal anatomy of maxillary first premolars," *Brazilian Dental Journal*, vol. 2, no. 2, pp. 87–94, 1992.

[19] J. D. Pécora, J. B. Woelfel, and M. D. Sousa Neto, "Morphologic study of the maxillary molars. 1. External anatomy," *Brazilian Dental Journal*, vol. 2, no. 1, pp. 45–50, 1991.

[20] M. Iwase, H. Nishijima, G. Kondo, and M. Ito, "Radiculomegaly of permanent canines and first premolars: report of two cases in conjunction with oculo-facio-cardio-dental syndrome," *International Journal of Case Reports and Images*, vol. 6, no. 3, p. 189, 2015.

[21] M. Maden, A. Savgat, and G. Görgül, "Radiculomegaly of permanent canines: report of endodontic treatment in OFCD syndrome," *International Endodontic Journal*, vol. 43, no. 12, pp. 1152–1161, 2010.

[22] F. B. Jeger, S. F. M. Janner, M. M. Bornstein, and A. Lussi, "Endodontic working length measurement with preexisting cone-beam computed tomography scanning: a prospective, controlled clinical study," *Journal of Endodontia*, vol. 38, no. 7, pp. 884–888, 2012.

[23] C. B. Williams, A. P. Joyce, and S. Roberts, "A comparison between in vivo radiographic working length determination and measurement after extraction," *Journal of Endodontia*, vol. 32, no. 7, pp. 624–627, 2006.

[24] S.-Y. Kim, S.-H. Lim, S.-N. Gang, and H.-J. Kim, "Crown and root lengths of incisors, canines, and premolars measured by cone-beam computed tomography in patients with malocclusions," *The Korean Journal of Orthodontics*, vol. 43, no. 6, pp. 271–278, 2013.

[25] J. Michetti, D. Maret, J.-P. Mallet, and F. Diemer, "Validation of cone beam computed tomography as a tool to explore root canal anatomy," *Journal of Endodontics*, vol. 36, no. 7, pp. 1187–1190, 2010.

[26] R. Pauwels, J. Beinsberger, B. Collaert et al., "Effective dose range for dental cone beam computed tomography scanners," *European Journal of Radiology*, vol. 81, no. 2, pp. 267–271, 2012.

[27] J.-Y. Kim, S.-H. Lee, G.-H. Lee, and S.-H. Park, "Study of endodontic working length of Korean posterior teeth," *Journal of Korean Academy of Conservative Dentistry*, vol. 35, no. 6, p. 429, 2010.

[28] M. Taramsari, Z. Dalili Kajan, and L. Atash Biz Yeganeh, "Case report: an oculofaciocardiodental syndrome: challenges in endodontic treatment," *Journal of Dentomaxillofacial*, vol. 6, no. 3, pp. 77–82, 2017.

[29] N. A. Taha, M. B. Ahmad, and A. Ghanim, "Assessment of mineral trioxide aggregate pulpotomy in mature permanent teeth with carious exposures," *International Endodontic Journal*, vol. 50, no. 2, pp. 117–125, 2017.

[30] N. A. Taha and S. Z. Abdelkhader, "Outcome of full pulpotomy using Biodentine in adult patients with symptoms indicative of irreversible pulpitis," *International Endodontic Journal*, vol. 51, no. 8, pp. 819–828, 2018.

[31] S. Linu, M. S. Lekshmi, V. S. Varunkumar, and V. G. Sam Joseph, "Treatment outcome following direct pulp capping using bioceramic materials in mature permanent teeth with carious exposure: a pilot retrospective study," *Journal of Endodontics*, vol. 43, no. 10, pp. 1635–1639, 2017.

[32] Z. Almuallem and A. Busuttil-Naudi, "Molar incisor hypomineralisation (MIH) - an overview," *British Dental Journal*, vol. 225, no. 7, pp. 601–609, 2018.

[33] M. Isha, B. Nimma Vijayalaxmi, E. Ramaswami, and J. Desai Jimit, "Bony exostoses: case series and review of literature," *Acta Scientific Dental Sciences*, vol. 2, 2018.

8

Clinical Steps for Restoration of Fractured Anterior Teeth: Color Protocol with Non-VITA Scale

Ubiracy Gaião, Leonardo Fernandes da Cunha, Cibele de Almeida Kintopp, André Vivan Garcia, Carla Castiglia Gonzaga, Alexandre Moro, and Gisele Maria Correr

School of Health Sciences, Graduate Program in Dentistry, Universidade Positivo, Curitiba, PR, Brazil

Correspondence should be addressed to Leonardo Fernandes da Cunha; cunha_leo@yahoo.com.br

Academic Editor: Michelle A. Chinelatti

Direct composite resin restorations are commonly provided because of their satisfactory esthetics and minimal wear of opposing tooth structure. Recent restorative systems may not follow the nomenclature of the classical VITA shade guide, using instead a simplified resin color system. A better understanding of these systems and their behavior regarding the incidence of light is an excellent approach to anterior restorations, especially for fractured anterior teeth. This paper demonstrates the color selection and clinical sequence for the natural reproduction of tooth structure using a resin system that does not follow the VITA classical scale.

1. Introduction

Natural tooth is polychromatic, presenting a great variety of colors. Artificially reproducing these intrinsic characteristics of the tooth always demands time and often excessive adjustments. Dentists should use their artistic sense to identify details and define the different hues of each tooth [1–3]. For the professional to achieve this result, the restorative system must present a series of characteristics.

Changes in direct restorative systems have addressed the growing demand of patients and professionals for esthetics and optical characteristics that match those of natural teeth. Composite resins are available in a wide variety of colors and effects that allow combinations of translucency and opacity of dental structures [3].

Recently, direct restorative systems have tended not to use the VITA shade guide scale for their available colors. Their kits feature simplified enamel and dentin color options that are selected separately. Dentin confers the basic color, or hue, of the tooth, while the enamel does not change the hue but provides increased or reduced saturation, or chroma, according to its thickness [4]. The lightness or value will result from the placement of correct thicknesses of the resin layers. Thus, the technique is simplified and the clinical time reduced.

In addition, light-polymerized stains, which are flowable composite resins with low filler content, can be used to characterize occlusal cracks and grooves, darken teeth, or mimic the chromatic characteristics of the tooth as with an incisal opaque halo. They are available in various pigments, including brown, black, blue, and white ocher, to provide a direct restoration with a more natural appearance that is harmonious to the adjacent teeth [5].

The objective of this report was to present a predictable protocol for restoring an anterior tooth using a restorative system that does not use the VITA shade guide scale.

2. Case Report

A 21-year-old woman sought care to replace the resin restoration of her fractured anterior tooth. The existing restoration had a poor color match and excess material (Figure 1).

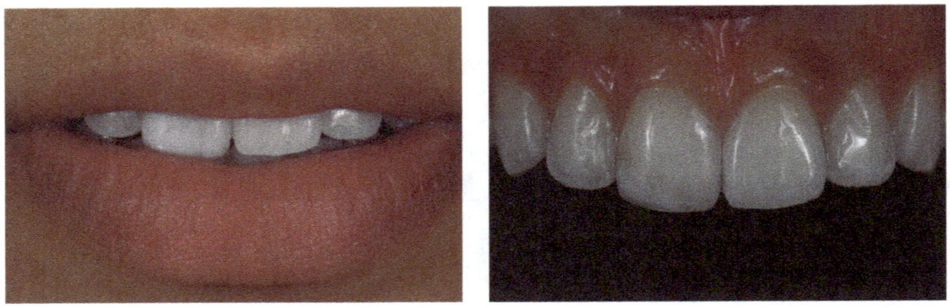

(a) (b)

Figure 1: Restored right maxillary central incisor showing poor color match. The restoration of the fractured tooth extended to the middle third.

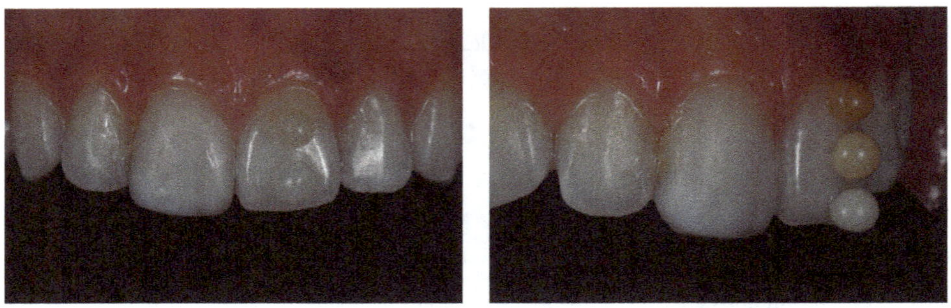

(a) (b)

Figure 2: Selection of color before tooth dehydration. The two enamel colors of the system were initially tested (LE and DE) (a). Then, the three dentin colors were tested (LD, MD, and DD) (b).

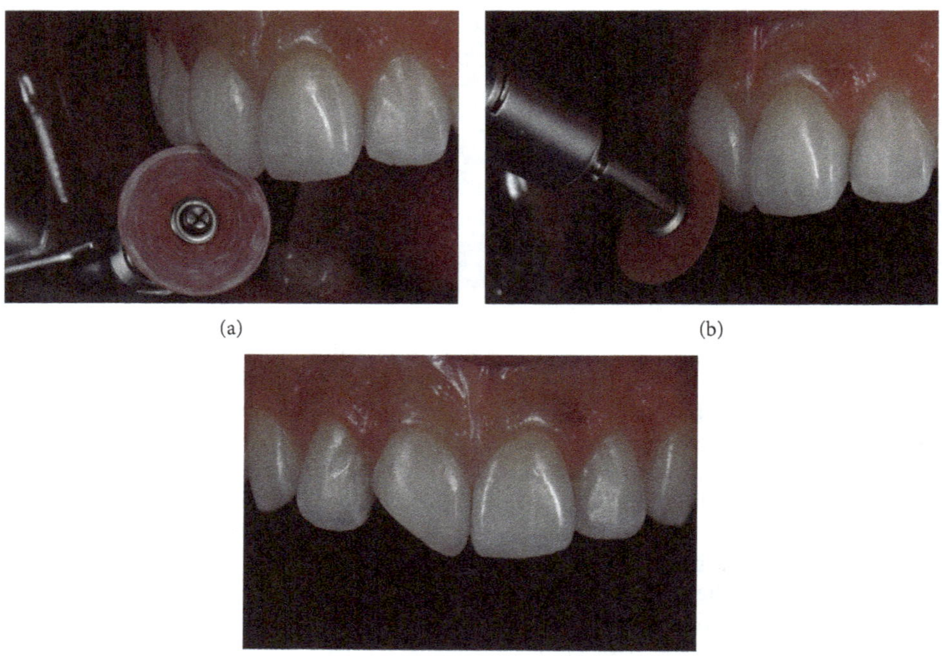

(a) (b)

(c)

Figure 3: Removing the existing restoration with abrasive disks. A beveled margin was made with coarse grit disks to remove the unsupported enamel.

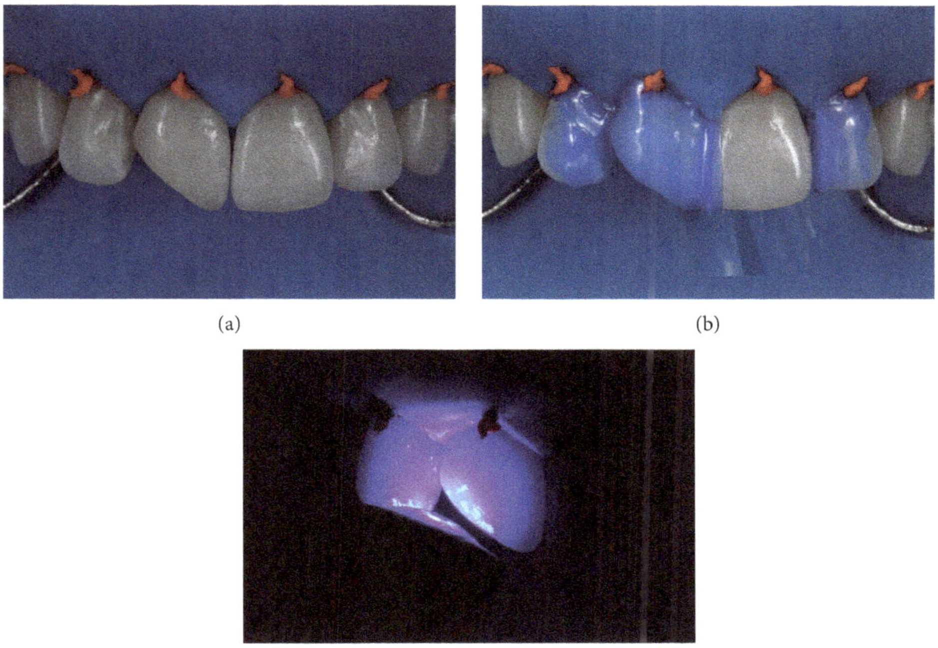

(a) (b) (c)

Figure 4: Rubber dam isolation of the operative field (a) and application of the adhesive system and polymerization according to the manufacturer's instructions (b, c).

Considering the age of the patient, the possibility of reversibility of the procedure, the time, and the cost, a direct adhesive restorative system was planned to restore the tooth.

After prophylaxis, the dentin and enamel color were selected using the Essentia, GC, resin system. For enamel color selection, each of the two enamel colors (light enamel and dark enamel) were placed on the tooth and polymerized (Figure 2(a)). The light enamel replicated the patient's tooth best. The dentin color was selected by applying the three dentin colors (light dentin, medium dentin, and dark dentin) on the patient's tooth and polymerizing. Light dentin was selected (Figure 2(b)).

After making a silicone putty matrix, the existing restoration was removed with abrasive disks (Sof-Lex, dark red, 3M; thick granulation). A beveled margin was made with the same disk (Figure 3). The operative field was isolated and the gingiva displaced with ligated rubber dam (Figure 4(a)). The adjacent teeth were protected with polyester tape. The enamel surface was conditioned with 37% phosphoric acid (Figure 4(b)), and the adhesive (G-BOND, GC) was then applied on the facial and lingual surfaces (Figure 4(c)) and polymerized according to the manufacturer's instructions.

The silicone matrix was positioned lingually to provide a well-contoured restoration (Figure 5(a)). Resin matching the lingual enamel was applied with the matrix in position (LE). After polymerization of this increment with the matrix in position, the lingual and incisal contour was established (Figure 6). Dentin resin was then applied to the middle third (LD), leaving room for the creation of a dentinal lobe in the incisal region (Figure 7). The incisal halo was made by using the opalescent translucent resin of the OM system (Figure 8),

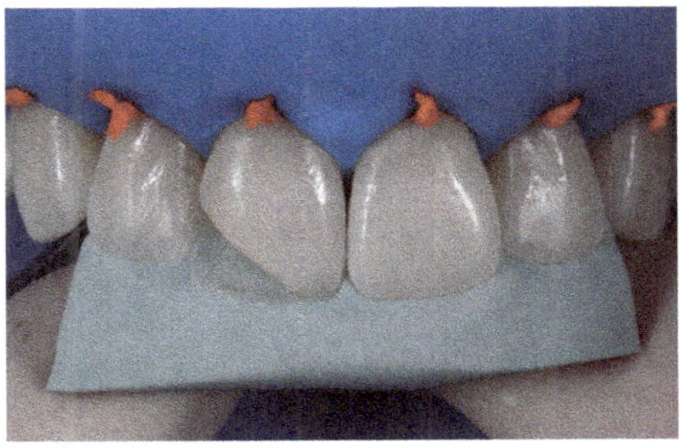

Figure 5: A silicone guide was used to assist the restoration of the lingual surface with the light enamel composite resin (LE: light enamel, Essentia, GC).

followed by a layer of white stain on that halo to simulate the opacity of this region (Figure 9). The dentin mamelons were made with clear resin (Figure 10), and opalescent resin was applied between the mamelons (Figure 11(a)). The enamel layer was applied to the facial surface and spread with the aid of a polyester strip and brush (Kota 4A) (Figure 11(b)).

Each increment was polymerized with an LED unit (Radii-cal, SDI) for the time recommended by the manufacturer. After removal of the rubber dam, any excess was removed, and the incisal edge adjusted.

In the following appointment, the restoration was finished and polished with sequential grit abrasive disks (Sof-Lex Pop-on, 3M). Rubber points and composite polishing paste applied with a felt disk were used to obtain the final gloss (Figure 12). The final restoration can be seen in

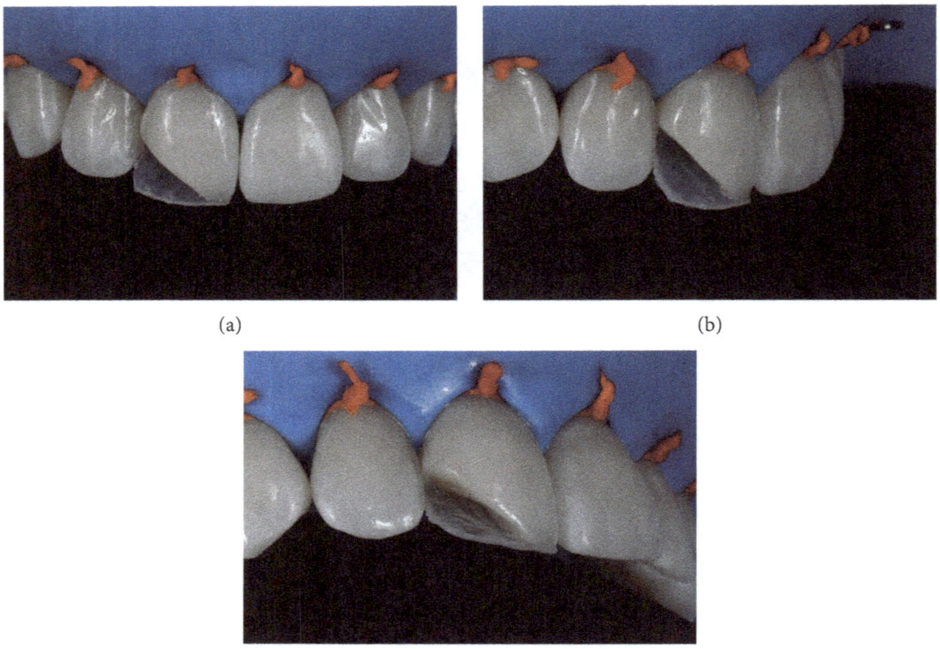

(a) (b)

(c)

FIGURE 6: Facial (a), lateral (b), and incisal (c) views immediately after application and polymerization of the resin to form the lingual "shell" with enamel resin.

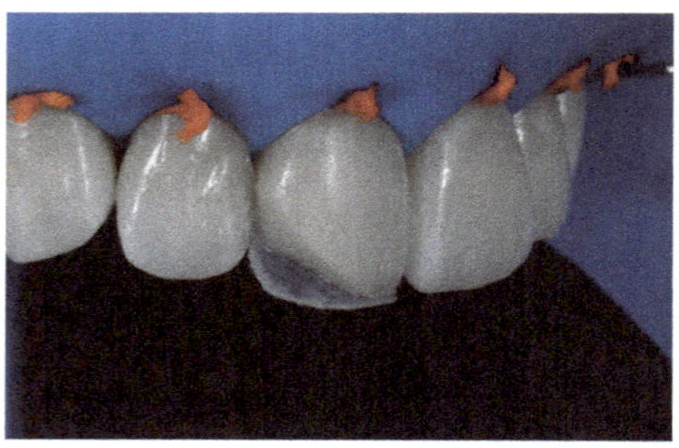

FIGURE 7: LD (light dentin; Essentia, GC) resin, corresponding to the dentin region, was then applied.

Figures 13(a) and 13(b). The definitive appearance of the restored smile can be seen in Figure 14.

3. Discussion

Current direct adhesive restorative systems have numerous advantages such as reversibility, durability, low cost, and speed of treatment. In the patient presented, the restoration was placed in a single appointment and finished and polished in a subsequent appointment. Maximum tooth structure was conserved when the existing restoration was removed, thus preserving enamel at the margins of the preparation and favoring the adhesion and longevity of the adhesive procedure [1]. The dentist should choose the restorative system according to each situation. The system used for the present patient was recently introduced and has not been tested in many studies. However, results appear to be comparable with those of other available systems [6].

Natural teeth possess translucency, opalescence, and fluorescence, all of which must be replicated by the restorative material to achieve clinical success. Enamel translucency varies from tooth to tooth and from individual to individual. The presence or absence of color, enamel thickness, degree of translucency, and surface texture is an essential component in determining translucency [7]. The system used provides variable shades and opacities that allow the reproduction of the chromaticity and translucency/opacity of enamel and dentin. The manipulation of the thickness of the enamel and dentin increments selected without using the VITA shade guide system allows the correct characteristics of the dental structures to be reproduced in a simplified way, as demonstrated in the present treatment.

The technique of intrinsic characterization of composite resin restorations with stains is routinely used in dental offices. Several manufacturers offer stains that enable individualized and customized composite resin restorations [5]. In the treatment presented, the white stain was used. These stains should be applied carefully with a fine brush as demonstrated in this treatment to avoid excess material that can lead to an unsightly appearance or decrease in cohesive strength between the resin increments [5, 8].

The dentin resins in the restorative system used have a microhybrid composition, while the enamel resins are nanohybrid, providing increased polishability for the external layer of the restoration. The color of the composite resin is not influenced by when the restoration is polished (immediately or later). Thus, the final polishing time can be scheduled according to the preferences of the clinician [9]. In the

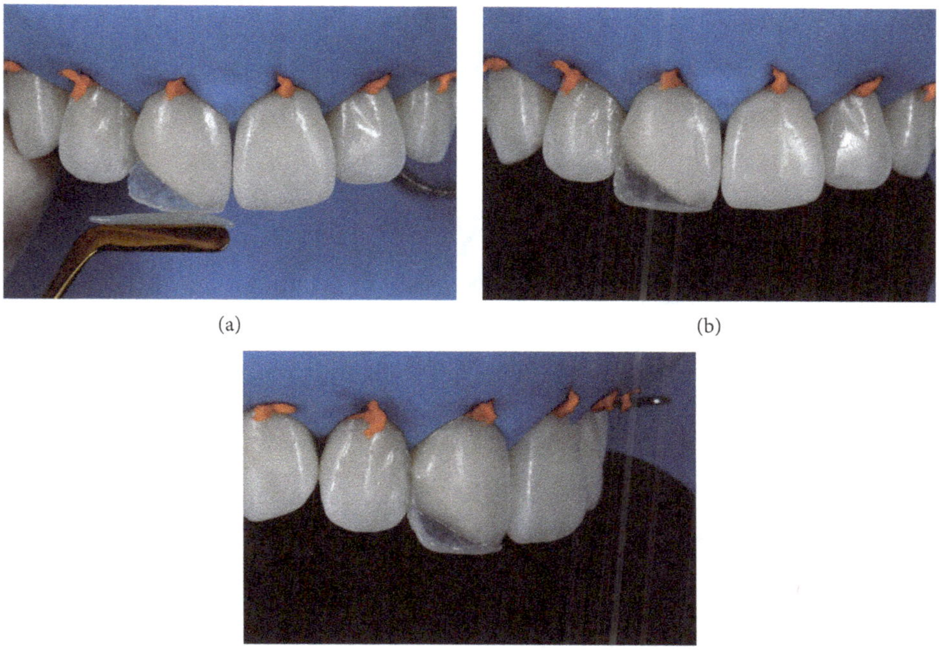

(a) (b) (c)

FIGURE 8: A resin with greater OM opalescence was placed to characterize the incisal area (a–c).

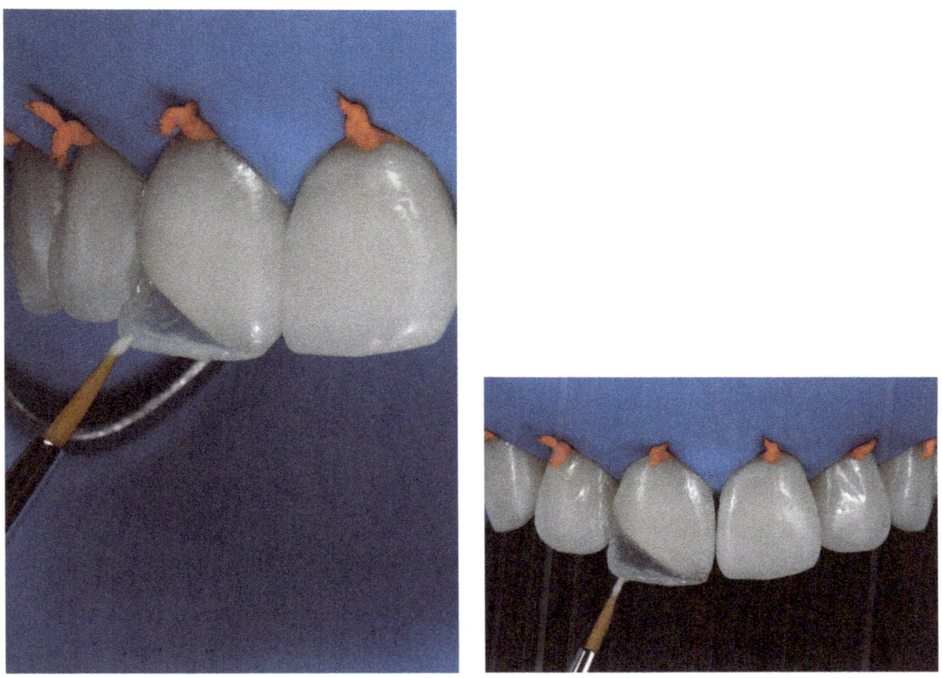

(a) (b)

FIGURE 9: Brush application of the white stain (Essentia, white modifier) to characterize the opaque incisal halo (a, b).

presented patient, the definitive finishing and polishing were performed in the next session to allow rehydration of the tooth and time for the clinician to determine the need for additional resin increments.

4. Conclusion

The use of resins that do not use the VITA shade guide scale is easy to understand and allows a simplified application of

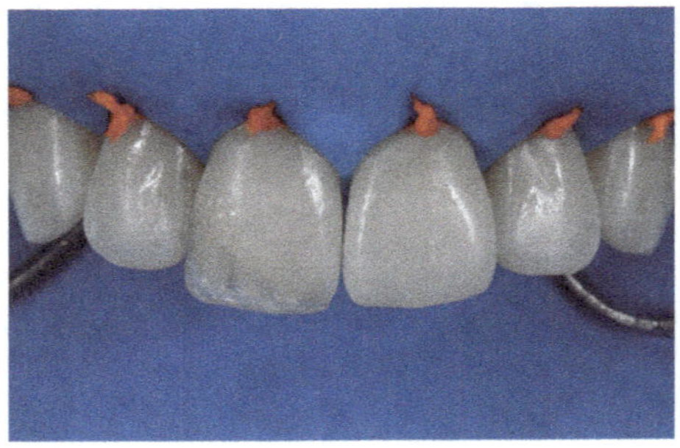

FIGURE 10: Application of LD dentin resin up to approximately half the width of the bevel. Observe the spaces between the developmental lobes, left when applying the opaque resin, in which the translucent incisal resin (OM) will be placed.

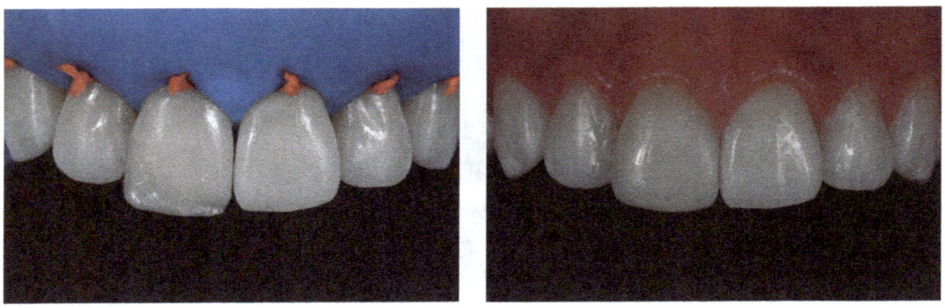

(a) (b)

FIGURE 11: Insertion of translucent incisal resin (OM) between dentin mamelons (a). Then, the resin was applied in the LE color over the entire facial surface of the restoration to simulate the enamel (b).

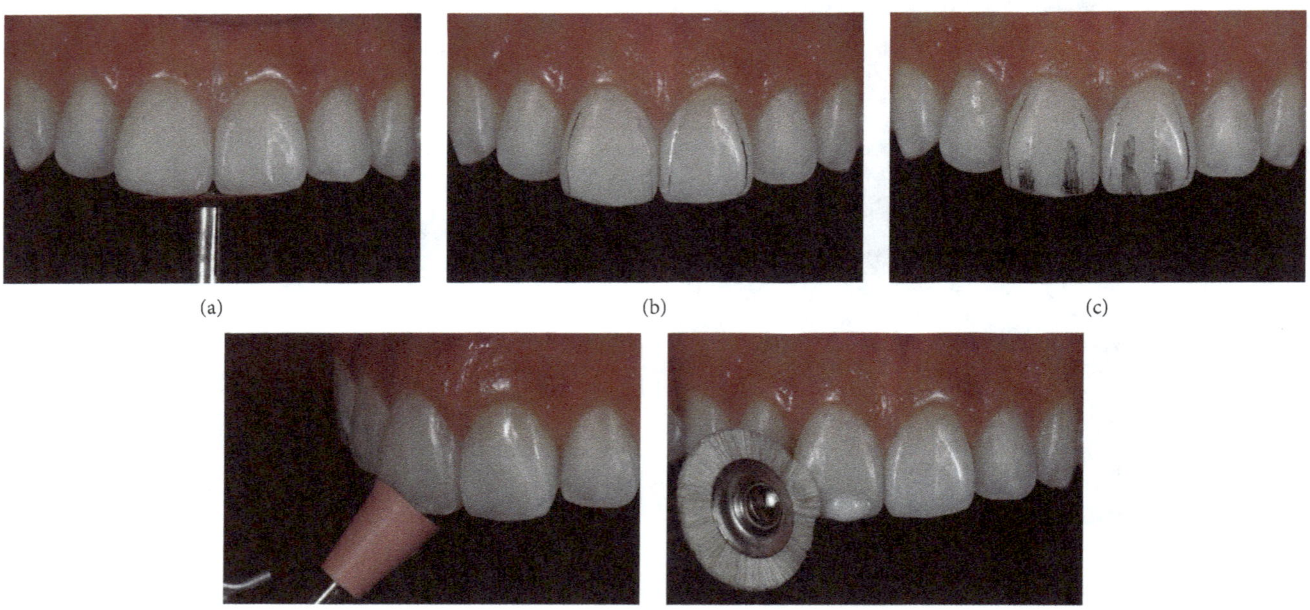

(a) (b) (c)

(d) (e)

FIGURE 12: Finishing and polishing of the restoration with abrasive disks (a), fine diamond rotary instruments (b, c), rubber points (d), and a felt disk with polishing paste (e).

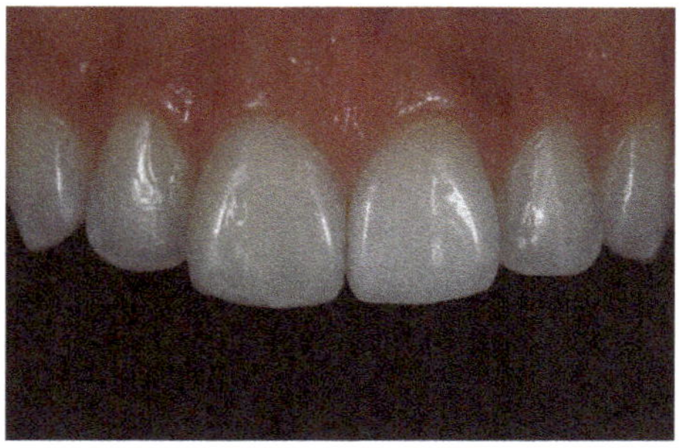

(a)

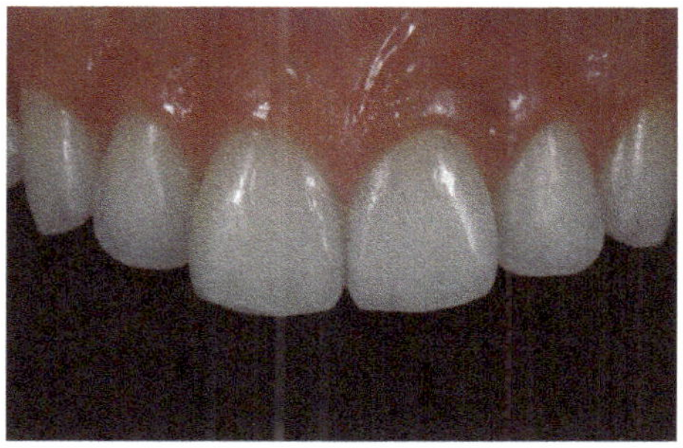

(b)

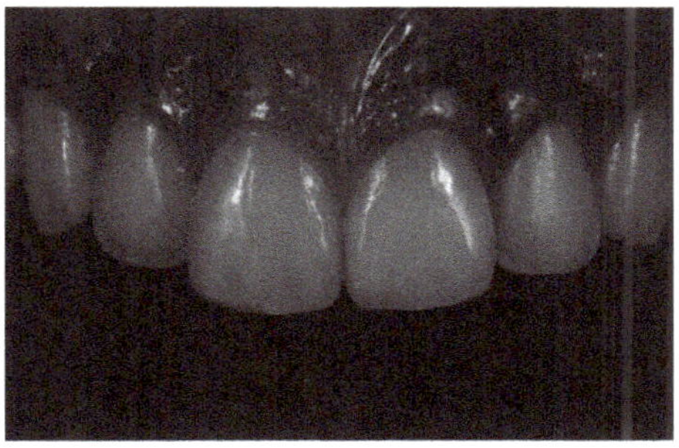

(c)

FIGURE 13: Detail of restorations after finishing and polishing procedures (a–c).

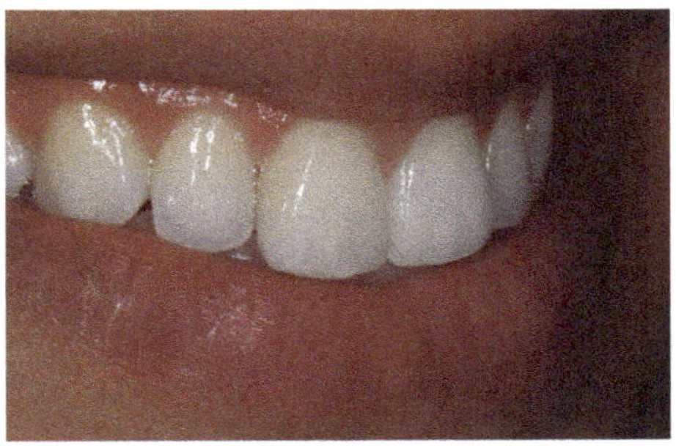

(a)

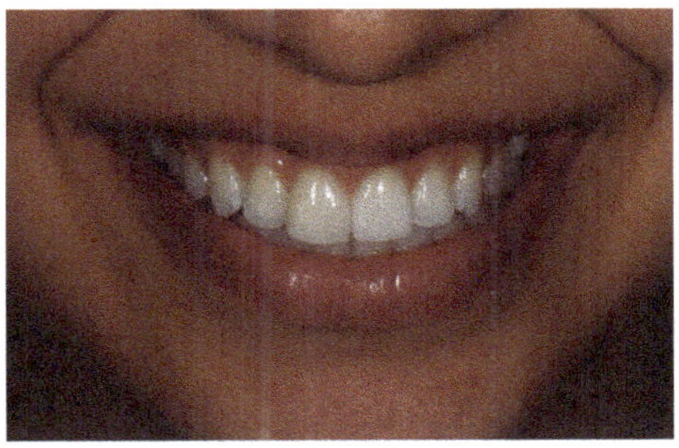

(b)

FIGURE 14: Smile view, harmony of shape, color, and function of the tooth have been restored (a, b).

the restorative system in a predictable, fast, and efficient way to reestablish the esthetics of anterior teeth.

References

[1] L. Vanini, "Light and color in previous composite restorations," *Practical Periodontics and Aesthetic Dentistry*, vol. 8, pp. 673–682, 1996.

[2] P. Magne and J. Holz, "Stratification of composite restorations: systematic and durable replication of natural aesthetics," *Practical Periodontics and Aesthetic Dentistry*, vol. 8, pp. 61–68, 1996.

[3] B. Zimmerli, M. Strub, F. Jeger, O. Stadler, and A. Lussi, "Composite materials: composition, properties and clinical applications. A literature review," *Schweizer Monatsschrift fur Zahnmedizin*, vol. 120, no. 11, pp. 972–986, 2010.

[4] D. Dietschi, "Optimising aesthetics and facilitating clinical application of free-hand bonding using the 'natural layering concept'," *British Dental Journal*, vol. 204, no. 4, pp. 181–185, 2008.

[5] D. C. Barcellos, M. T. Palazon, C. R. Pucci, L. H. Aizawa, and S. E. Gonçalves, "Influence of different surface treatments on bond strength of resin composite using the intrinsic characterization technique," *Operative Dentistry*, vol. 38, no. 6, pp. 635–643, 2013.

[6] H. Kermanshah, E. Yasini, and R. Hoseinifar, "Effect of cyclic loading on microleakage of silorane based composite compared with low shrinkage methacrylate-based composites," *Dental Research Journal*, vol. 13, no. 3, pp. 264–271, 2016.

[7] M. Villarroel, N. Fahl, A. M. de Sousa, and O. B. de Oliveira, "Direct esthetic restorations based on translucency and opacity of composite resins," *Journal of Esthetic and Restorative Dentistry*, vol. 23, no. 2, pp. 73–87, 2011.

[٤] C. R. Pucci, D. C. Barcellos, M. T. Palazon, A. B. Borges, M. A. da Silva, and S. E. de Paiva Gonçalves, "Evaluation of the cohesive strength between resin composite and light-curing characterizing materials," *The Journal of Adhesive Dentistry*, vol. 14, no. 1, pp. 69–73, 2012.

[٥] R. T. Pozzobon, T. C. Bohrer, P. E. Fontana, L. B. Durand, and M. Marquezan, "The effect of immediate and delayed polishing on the color stability of a composite resin," *General Dentistry*, vol. 65, no. 6, pp. e9–e12, 2017.

9

Multiple Nonsyndromic Unerupted Supernumerary Teeth: A Report of a Rare Case

Mehrnaz Moradinejad,[1] **Alireza Hashemi Ashtiani**,[2] **and Vahid Rakhshan**[3]

[1]*Department of Orthodontics, Dental School, Ahvaz Jundishapur University of Medical Sciences, Ahvaz, Iran*
[2]*Department of Prosthodontics, Dental School, Ahvaz Jundishapur University of Medical Sciences, Ahvaz, Iran*
[3]*Department of Anatomy, Dental School, Azad University of Medical Sciences, Tehran, Iran*

Correspondence should be addressed to Alireza Hashemi Ashtiani; arhashemee@gmail.com

Academic Editor: Husamettin Oktay

Introduction. The prevalence of nonsyndromic multiple supernumerary teeth is less than 1% of all hyperdontia cases which themselves have a rather small prevalence. Cases with 10 impacted nonsyndromic supernumerary teeth are extremely rare. This report presents such a case of nonsyndromic multiple impacted supernumerary teeth. *Case.* A 17-year-old boy with a completely orthodontic chief complaint attended our center. He had no systemic complaints and no signs or symptoms. Oral examination showed no abnormalities. On routine pretreatment panoramic radiography, numerous impacted supernumerary teeth appeared. A CBCT showed 10 impacted vertically aligned supplementary supernumerary teeth with incomplete roots: In the maxilla, the bilateral canine-premolar areas were involved, each having 2 supernumerary teeth palatal to the permanent teeth. In the mandible, the right premolar area included 2 supernumerary teeth. The left premolar-molar area contained 3 supernumerary teeth lingual to the permanent teeth. And in the right mandibular molar area, there was a distomolar tooth distal to the third molar. No bony ankyloses, root resorptions, or fusions were observed. The surrounding bone had become thinner and the mandibular alveolar canal was involved. *Interventions.* All supernumerary teeth except a mandibular distomolar were extracted carefully before beginning the orthodontic treatment. No complications were seen after the extraction, after orthodontic treatment, and 2 years after treatment. *Conclusions.* The possibility of completely hidden unerupted supernumerary teeth without any signs and symptoms might highlight the value of some radiographic screenings.

1. Introduction

Hyperdontia (also called supernumerary teeth) is a 'number' developmental dental anomaly, referring to any excess dental or odontological structure that is not a part of the normal dentition [1–5]. It has a prevalence ranging between 0.1% and 3.9% in permanent dentition and between 0.3 and 1.8% in primary dentition [1–5]. Hyperdontia can cause numerous esthetic and functional complications such as crowding, midline diastema, root resorption, ectopic eruption, cystic lesions, displacement of the crowns of the neighboring teeth, intraoral infections, and delayed or failed eruption [1–7], whereas, in some cases, supernumerary teeth might not disrupt occlusion or other clinical parameters and will be discerned only incidentally [7].

The etiology of hyperdontia is not known, perhaps multifactorial involving both genetic and environmental factors, with the most widely accepted hypothesis being the localized hyperactivity of the dental lamina [1, 2, 4–6, 8]. The cooccurrence of hyperdontia with numerous syndromes can indicate the genetic role; it can be seen in syndromes such as Marfan, Nance Horan, amelogenesis imperfecta, Crouzon, Franceschetti, Hallerman-Streiff, Down, Noonan, Rubenstein-Taybi, Zimmermann-Laband, Fabry, Ellis-Van Creveld, Ehlers-Danlos types III and IV, Rothmund–Thomson, Robinow, Hallermann-Streiff, Goldenhar, Gardner, incontinentia pigmenti, tricho-rhino-phalangeal syndrome, cleidocranial dysplasia, anophthalmia syndrome, craniosynostosis, orofaciodigital syndrome type I, and cleft lip and palate [1, 4, 9].

Hyperdontia usually involves few teeth: about 76-86% of patients have only 1 supernumerary tooth, while about 12-23% of patients will have only 2 supernumerary teeth [6]. Patients with more than 2 supernumerary teeth are quite rare, merely seen in about 2-8% of cases, with those having 5 or more supernumerary teeth being extremely rare and seen in less than 1% of all hyperdontia cases [5–7, 9] (perhaps about 1 in up to every 100,000 individuals, taking into account the prevalence of hyperdontia itself) [1–4, 6].

Such rare cases of multiple hyperdontia are usually a feature of syndromes and may not typically happen in nonsyndromic patients [5–7, 9]. Actually, nonsyndromic cases of multiple hyperdontia are even rarer, especially when the number of supernumerary teeth is greater than 6, and especially when all of them are impacted. We incidentally observed such an extremely rare case of 10 unerupted nonsyndromic supernumerary teeth in an orthodontic patient.

2. Case Presentation

The patient was a 17-year-old boy who had been referred to an orthodontic office. His chief complaint was that the canine teeth were protruding. His medical and family history did not indicate anything noteworthy. The person was healthy (although obese (height: 178 cm, weight: 135 kg, BMI = 42.6)) and had no complaints other than the said need for orthodontic treatment. No abnormalities were observed in his oral examination (Figure 1). No supernumerary teeth or any other anomalies were found on oral examination. For the sake of orthodontic diagnosis and treatment planning, first, a routine panoramic radiograph was prescribed. The examination of the panoramic radiograph showed evidence of supernumerary teeth (Figure 2).

To assess the condition of the supernumerary teeth more accurately, a cone-beam computed tomography (CBCT) was taken from all bimaxillary quadrants (NewTom VGI (Quantitative Radiology, Verona, Italy), FOV = 8 × 11 cm, high resolution), which indicated the presence of 10 supernumerary teeth in different areas (Figures 3–10). The patient was also referred to a physician for the assessment of any syndromes. The physician ruled out any syndrome in the patient.

2.1. CBCT Assessments. CBCT imaging was conducted. Cross-sectional, axial, coronal, and 3D images were reconstructed (Figures 4–11). The patient had all 32 normal permanent teeth. The locations of the found supernumerary teeth were as follows: In the maxilla, the bilateral canine-premolar areas were involved, each having 2 supernumerary teeth palatal to the permanent teeth. In the mandible, the right premolar area included 2 supernumerary teeth. The left premolar-molar area contained 3 supernumerary teeth lingual to the permanent teeth. And in the right mandibular molar area, there was a distomolar tooth distal to the third molar. The impaction type of all extra teeth was vertical. Anatomical features are as follows: All teeth show uncompleted roots; maxillary mesial ones had more developed roots. No bony ankylosis was detected (i.e., the periodontal ligament (PDL) space was visible around all the supernumerary teeth). Effects of supernumerary teeth on the normal teeth are as follows: No resorption and no fusion were detected at any sites. Effects of supernumerary teeth on the bone are as follows: Thinning of the palatal and lingual cortical bones were observed. Effects of supernumerary teeth on vital structures are as follows: Bilateral contacts of the roots of the supernumerary teeth with the inferior alveolar canals were observed. The supernumerary teeth had short roots, indicating that they had been developed lately. All of them were impacted, and none was erupted. All of them resembled normal teeth and hence were supplementary supernumerary teeth (there was no rudimentary hyperdontia).

2.2. Familial History. The patient, his parents, and his grandparents (who all were also patients attending the same dental clinic) were asked about any known cases of supernumerary teeth in any of their close or distant relatives. According to them, there was no person known for having any extra teeth among the close or distant relatives of them.

2.3. Orthodontic Diagnosis. The orthodontic assessments revealed that on the right side, the relationship was full-cusp molar and canine class II. On the left side, it was molar and canine class I. The lower midline was shifted to the right. Maxillary teeth were retruded.

2.4. Management and Any Complications. Fortunately, none of the supernumerary teeth had caused damage or root resorption to adjacent teeth, and there was no evidence of cystic or pathological changes in the extra teeth. Before starting orthodontic treatment, in order to prevent the supernumerary teeth from interfering with orthodontic movements of the teeth, all the supernumerary teeth (except the distomolar one) were extracted with the utmost care by an oral and maxillofacial surgeon under local anesthesia (Figure 11). The mandibular distomolar was not extracted because it did not interfere with orthodontic treatment or occlusion and also because its extraction might damage the surrounding tissues. After the extraction of supernumerary teeth, there were no complications on the adjacent bones and teeth.

2.5. Follow-Up. The orthodontic treatment was successful. No complication was seen after orthodontic treatment. The patient was followed up until two years (the present day), and he showed no problems.

3. Discussion

In the present case, most supernumerary teeth were located in the premolar areas. Our finding was in line with previous reports. In the case of sporadic supernumerary teeth, they usually happen in the premaxilla [2, 4, 10]. However, in the case of multiple supernumerary teeth, there might be a predominance of the hyperdontia occurrence in the premolar region (especially the mandibular premolar area), followed by the molar and the anterior areas, respectively; overall, about 60.9% of multiple supernumerary teeth may appear in the mandible, of which about 44.8% may appear in the premolar area [4, 8, 11, 12]. It is thought that supernumerary premolars might belong to a third (postpermanent) series, developing from extensions of the dental lamina [6, 13].

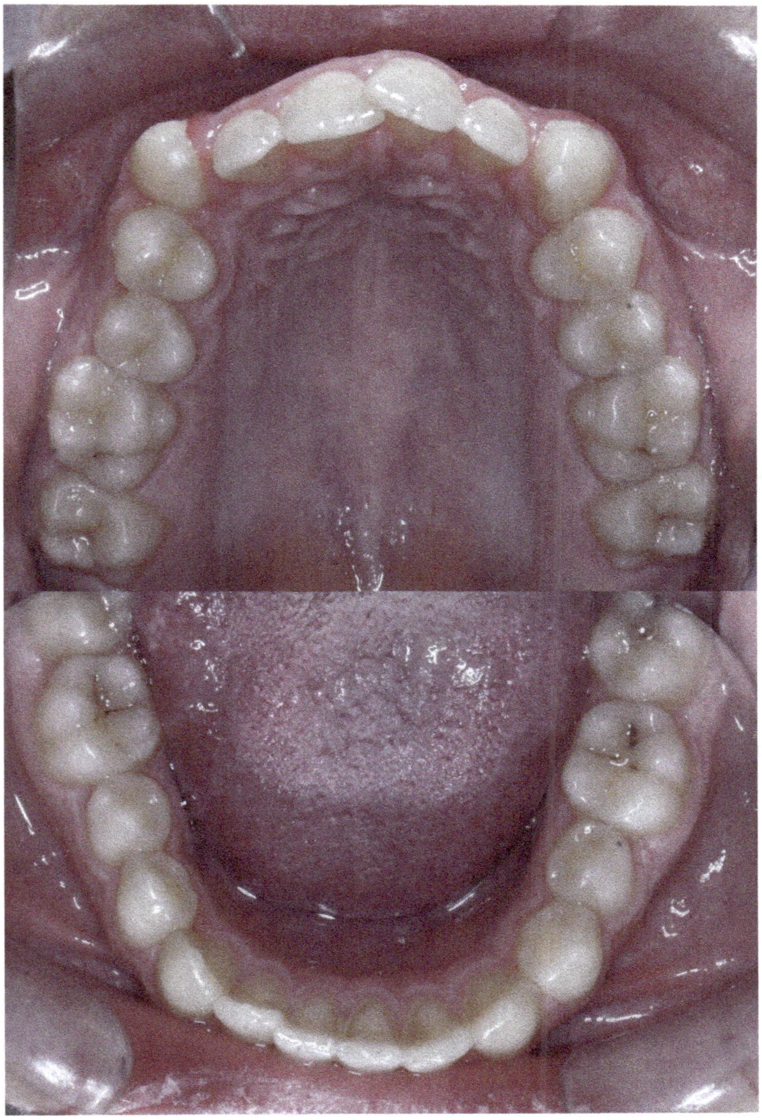

FIGURE 1: The lingual view of all teeth, showing no signs of any abnormalities.

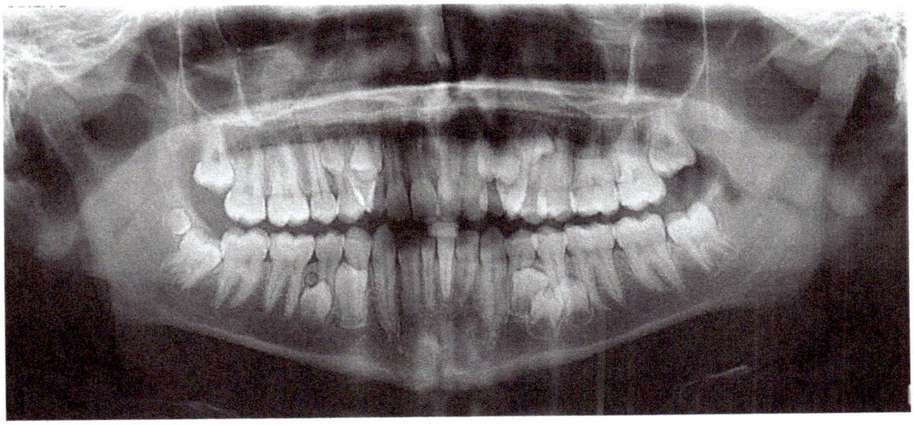

FIGURE 2: The original routine panoramic radiograph, showing supernumerary teeth.

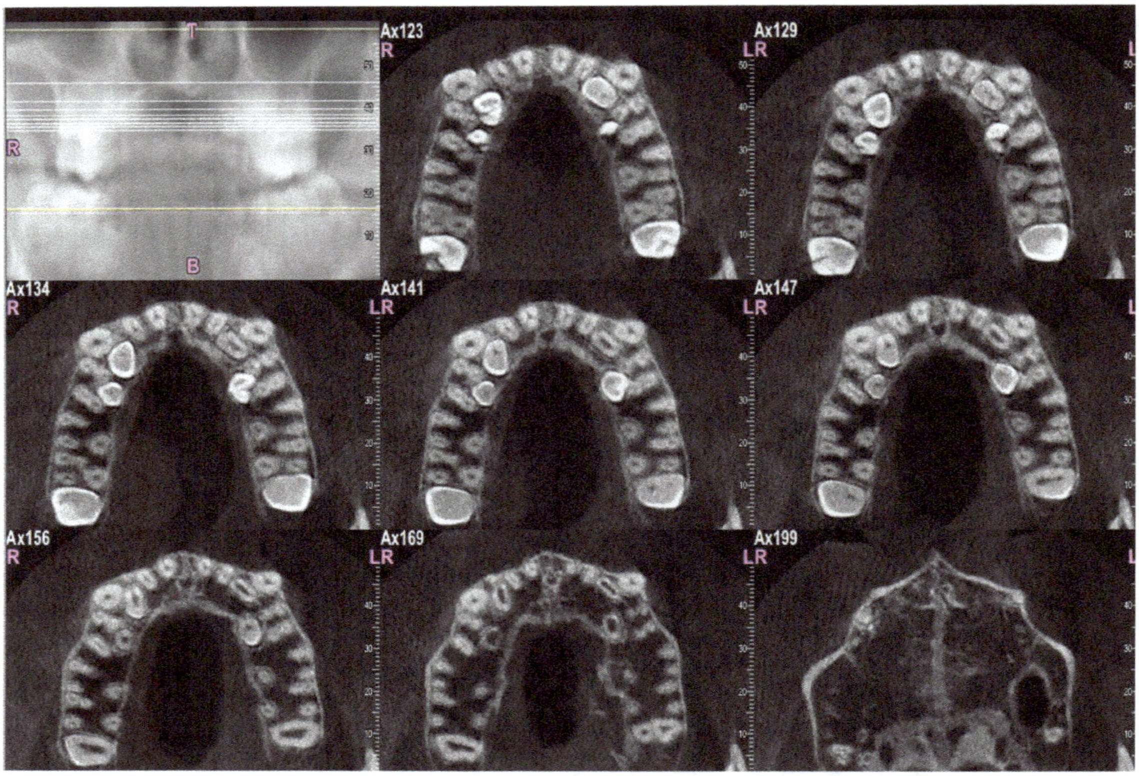

FIGURE 3: Transverse sections of the maxilla, showing sections of the maxillary supernumerary teeth.

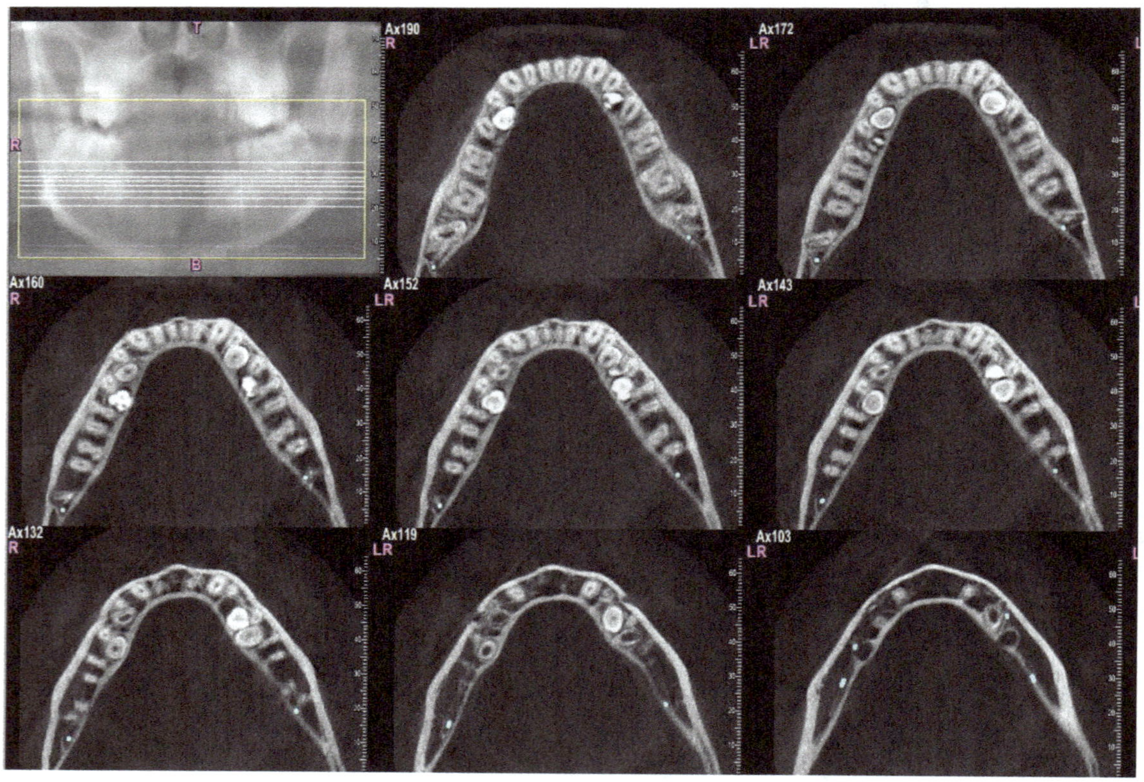

FIGURE 4: Transverse sections of the mandible, showing transverse sections of the mandibular supernumerary teeth.

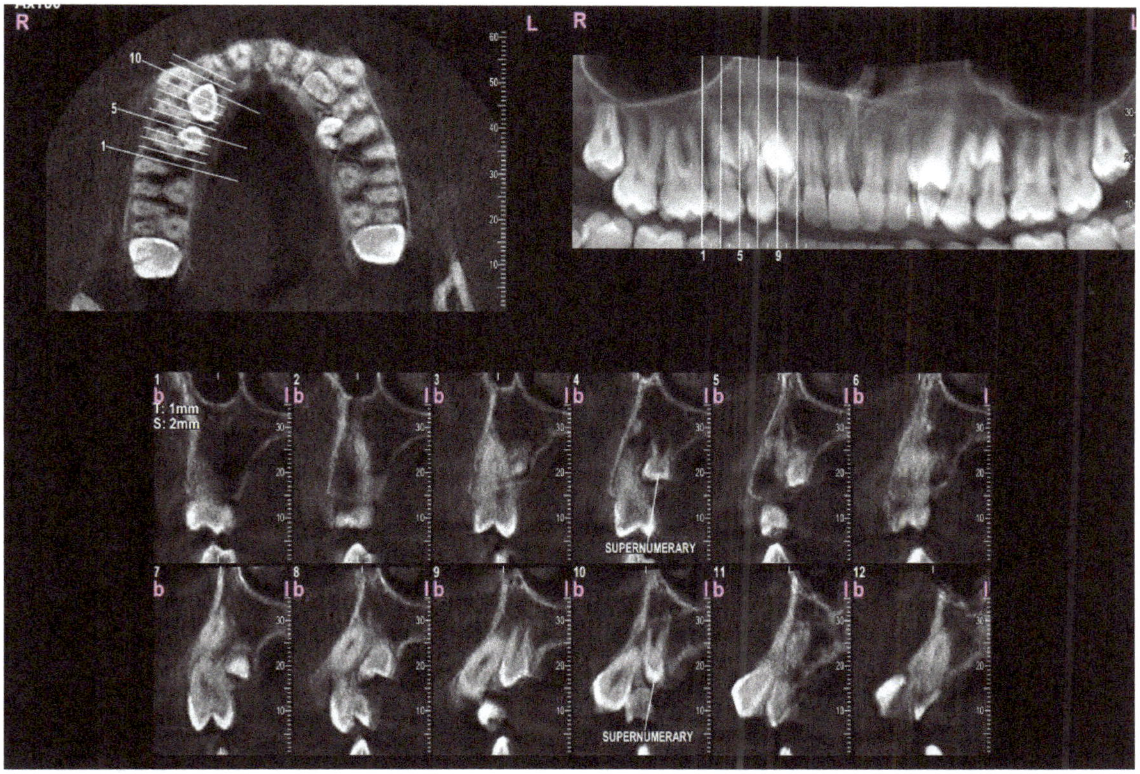

FIGURE 5: Vertical sections perpendicular to the alveolar ridge, showing the position and morphology of supernumerary teeth in the maxillary right quadrant.

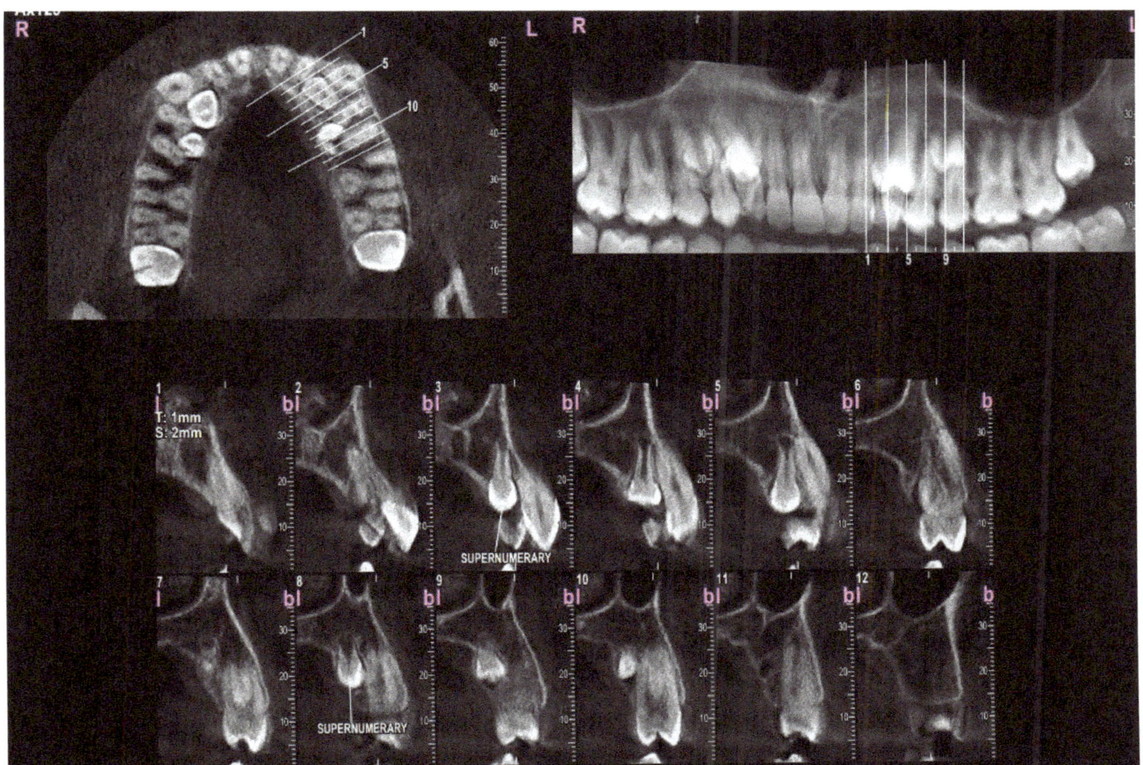

FIGURE 6: Vertical sections perpendicular to the alveolar ridge, showing the position and morphology of supernumerary teeth in the maxillary left quadrant.

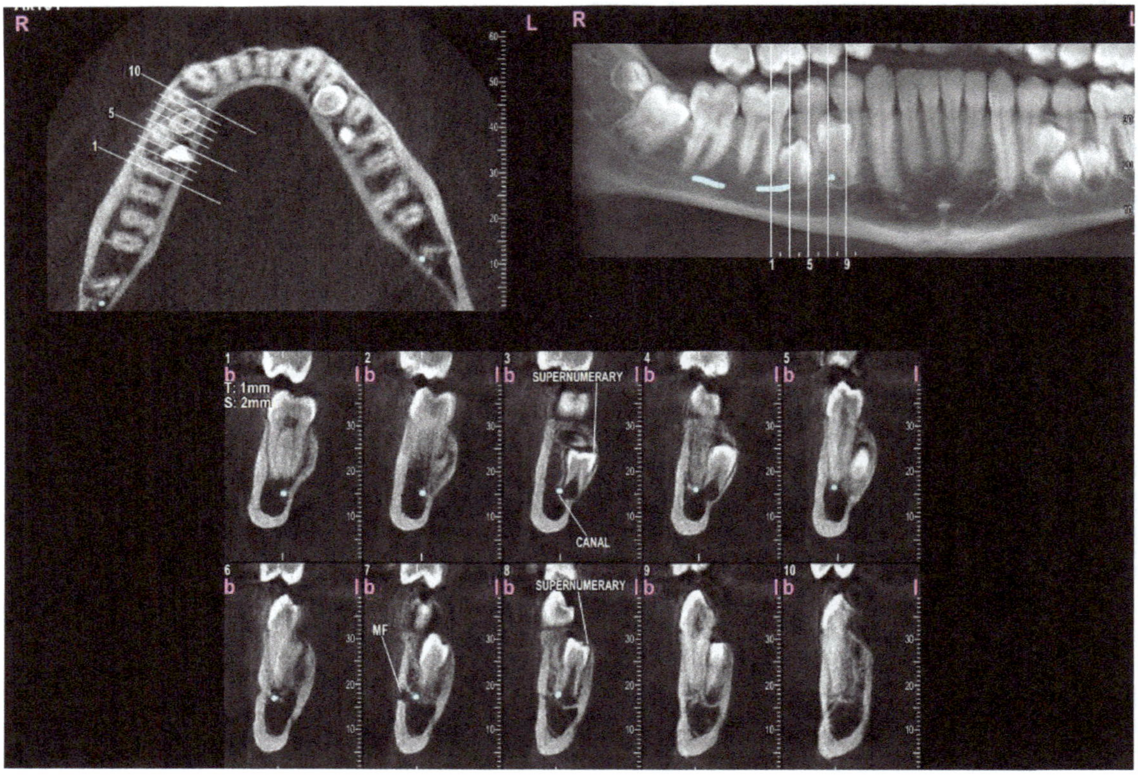

FIGURE 7: Vertical sections perpendicular to the alveolar ridge, showing the position and morphology of supernumerary teeth in the mandibular right quadrant.

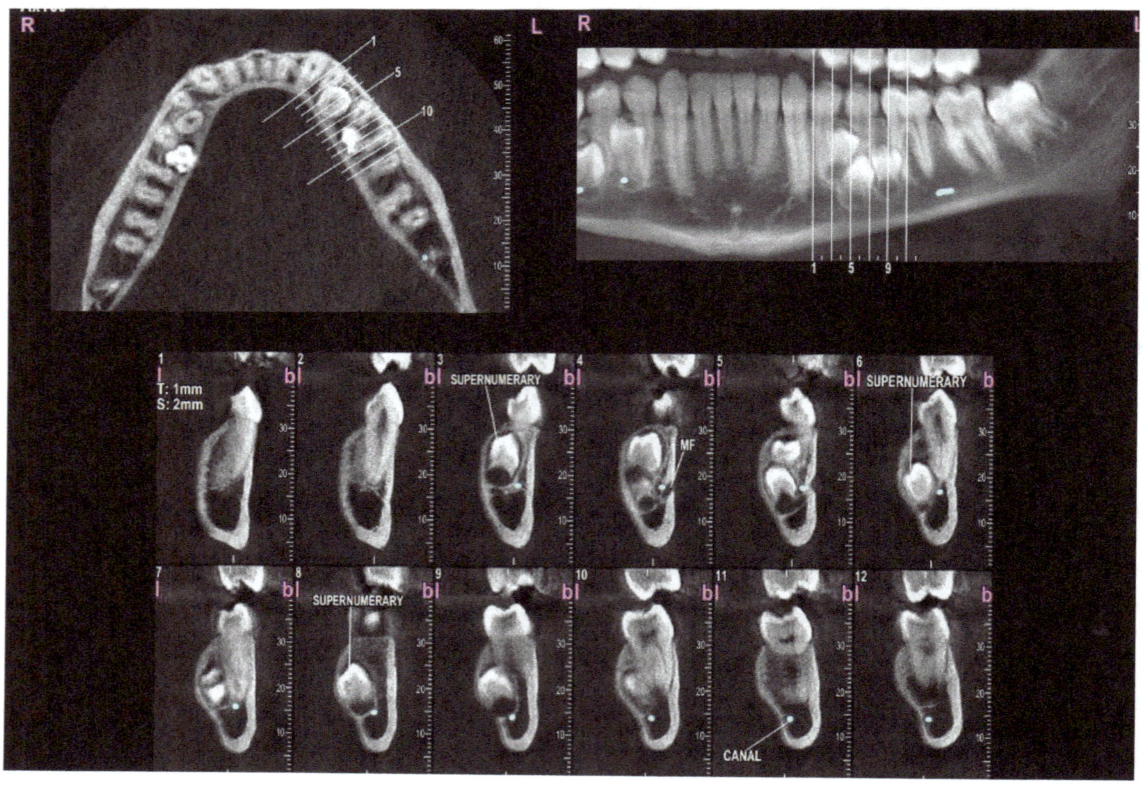

FIGURE 8: Vertical sections perpendicular to the alveolar ridge, showing the position and morphology of supernumerary teeth in the mandibular left quadrant.

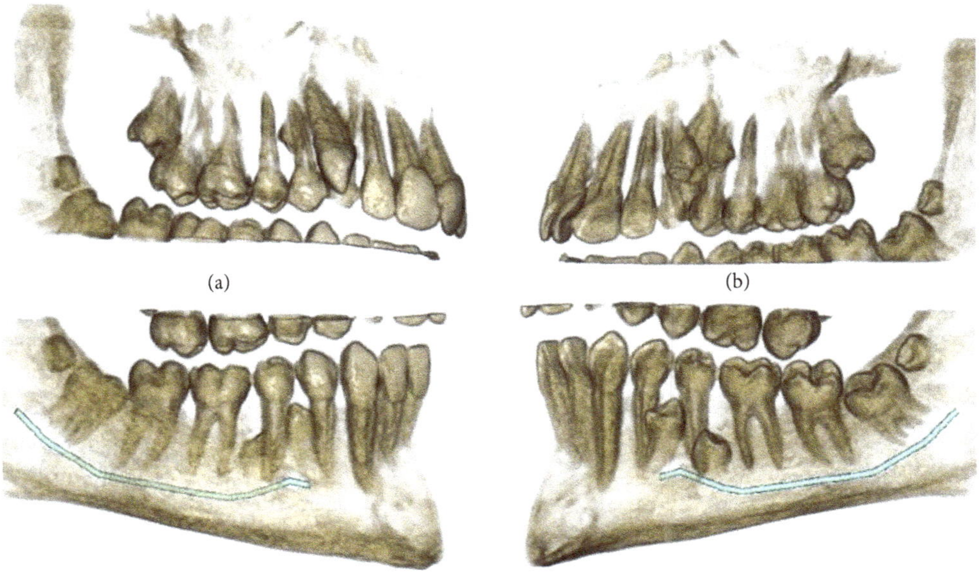

FIGURE 9: 3D reconstructions of the right upper and lower quadrants. (a, c) The buccal view (with slight adjustments in the point of view). (b, d) The palatal view. The mandibular nerve canal is highlighted.

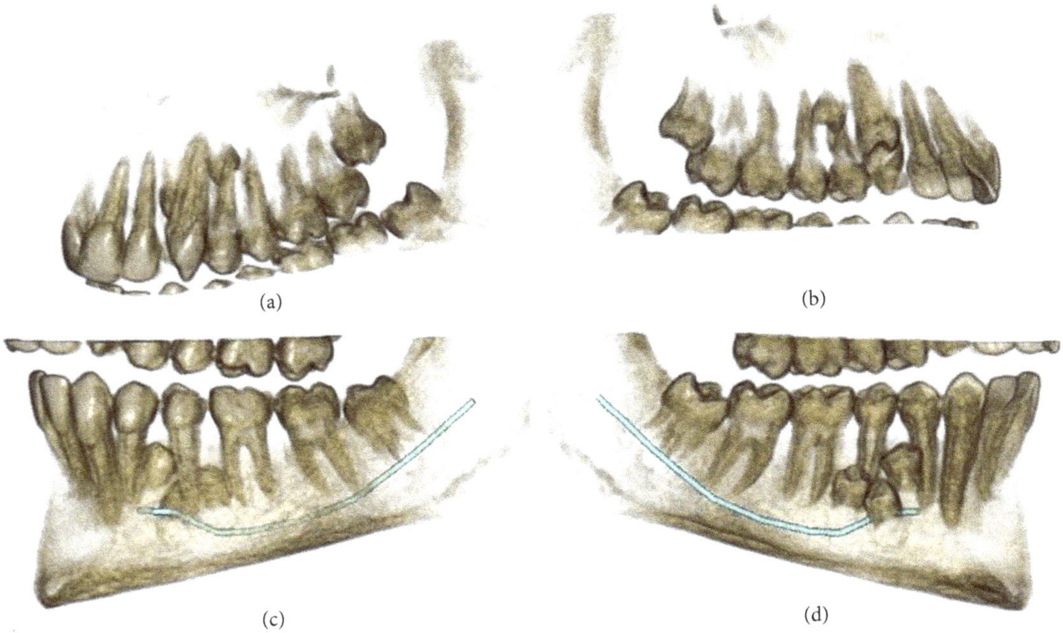

FIGURE 10: 3D reconstructions of the left quadrants in the maxilla and mandible. (a, c) The buccal view. (b, d) The palatal view. The mandibular nerve canal is highlighted.

In this study, all the 10 supernumerary teeth were impacted without any clinical signs or symptoms and without affecting the occlusion; they were found quite accidentally. It was in line with most cases. About 75% of supernumerary premolars usually remain unerupted, with no clinical symptoms or signs, and usually discerned incidentally on radiographs [6, 7, 14–17]. Still, it should be noted that such findings have been mostly reported for cases of sporadic hyperdontia, and having 10 impacted supernumerary teeth is quite rare. All of the supernumerary teeth seen in this study were vertically positioned. In general, hyperdontia can have different directions and positions: they can stand vertically like normal teeth, appear transverse, or even inverted; they also may be ectopic or follow an abnormal eruption path [7].

Moreover, the supernumerary teeth observed in our case had short roots, indicating their late development. This finding was consistent with most supernumerary premolars

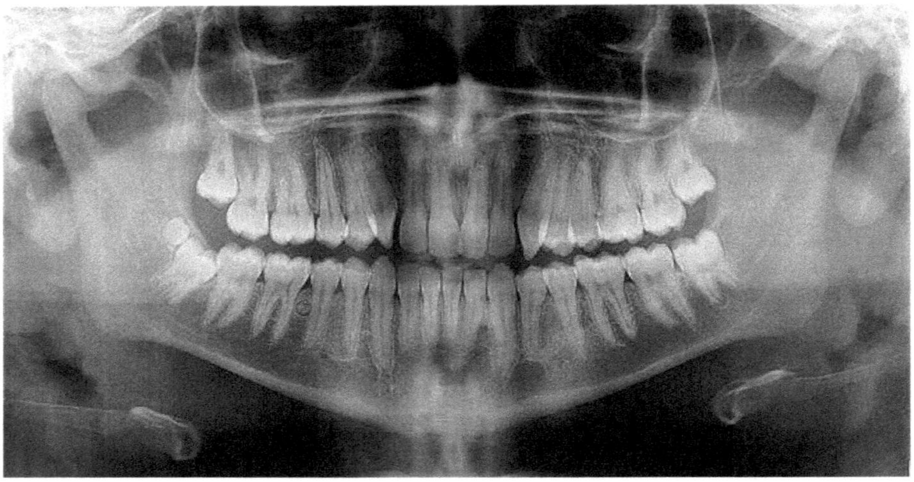

Figure 11: The panoramic radiograph taken after extracting 9 supernumerary teeth (all except the distomolar).

which usually develop late, for instance at the age of 13 years old or later [18]. It should be noted that many supernumerary teeth are prone to recurring after extraction at a later age [6, 8]. Therefore, it is recommended to take follow-up radiographs.

The treatment may vary from author to author. The usual treatment is to conservatively extract such teeth, or if possible, to reposition some of them into the arch [5, 18]. Some suggest that if the supernumerary tooth is erupted in a reasonable alignment and has not affected the occlusion, it might be left unextracted and merely monitor until the supernumerary tooth begins to pose a danger to the neighboring structures. However, if the space is lacking, it should be extracted as early as possible to prevent crowding and occlusal disruptions [5, 19]. For impacted supernumerary teeth, an early extraction before potential orthodontic treatments may be recommended [6, 14]. Nevertheless, some experts suggest that in order to avoid any iatrogenic damage to adjacent teeth or anatomical structures, the practitioner should wait for the supernumerary tooth roots to complete and/or until the normal permanent teeth are fully erupted [5, 6, 20]. In the current case, all the supernumerary teeth except the distomolar were removed before beginning the orthodontic treatment. The distomolar was not extracted because of clinical considerations, i.e., not interfering with orthodontic treatment or occlusion and, at the same time, being traumatic to extract.

4. Conclusions

The possibility of occurrence of multiple unerupted supernumerary teeth without any clinical manifestations and completely hidden to the eye might emphasize the value of preventive radiography.

References

[1] K. Tworkowski, E. Gasowska, D. Baryla, and K. Gabiec, "Supernumerary teeth - literature review," *Journal of Pre-Clinical and Clinical Research*, vol. 14, no. 1, pp. 18–21, 2020.

[2] F. Amini, V. Rakhshan, and S. Jamalzadeh, "Prevalence and pattern of accessory teeth (hyperdontia) in permanent dentition of Iranian orthodontic patients," *Iranian Journal of Public Health*, vol. 42, no. 11, pp. 1259–1265, 2013.

[3] D. Amarlal and M. S. Muthu, "Supernumerary teeth: review of literature and decision support system," *Indian Journal of Dental Research*, vol. 24, no. 1, pp. 117–122, 2013.

[4] S. K. Mallineni, "Supernumerary teeth: Review of the literature with recent updates," *Conference Papers in Science*, vol. 2014, 6 pages, 2014.

[5] F. Ata-Ali, J. Ata-Ali, D. Peñarrocha-Oltra, and M. Peñarrocha-Diago, "Prevalence, etiology, diagnosis, treatment and complications of supernumerary teeth," *Journal of Clinical and Experimental Dentistry*, vol. 6, pp. e414–e418, 2014.

[6] K. Khalaf, S. Al Shehadat, and C. A. Murray, "A review of supernumerary teeth in the premolar region," *International journal of dentistry*, vol. 2018, 6 pages, 2018.

[7] L. D. Rajab and M. A. Hamdan, "Supernumerary teeth: review of the literature and a survey of 152 cases," *International Journal of Paediatric Dentistry*, vol. 12, no. 4, pp. 244–254, 2002.

[8] R. Solares and M. I. Romero, "Supernumerary premolars: a literature review," *Pediatric Dentistry*, vol. 26, no. 5, pp. 450–458, 2004.

[9] M. A. Sawai, M. Faisal, and S. Mansoob, "Multiple supernumerary teeth in a nonsyndromic association: rare presentation in three siblings," *Journal of Oral and Maxillofacial Pathology: JOMFP*, vol. 23, p. 163-, 2019.

[10] M. Scheiner and W. Sampson, "Supernumerary teeth: a review of the literature and four case reports," *Australian Dental Journal*, vol. 42, no. 3, pp. 160–165, 1997.

[11] W. Yusof, "Non-syndrome multiple supernumerary teeth: literature review," *Journal (Canadian Dental Association)*, vol. 56, no. 2, pp. 147–149, 1990.

[12] V. Arikan, B. M. Ozgul, and T. Firdevs, "Prevalence and characteristics of supernumerary teeth in a child population from Central Anatolia-Turkey," *Oral health and dental management*, vol. 12, no. 4, pp. 269–272, 2013.

[13] D. Bowden, "Post-permanent dentition in the premolar region," *British Dental Journal*, vol. 131, no. 3, pp. 113–116, 1971.

[14] L. K. Rubenstein, S. J. Lindauer, R. J. Isaacson, and N. Germane, "Development of supernumerary premolars in an orthodontic population," *Oral Surgery, Oral Medicine, Oral Pathology*, vol. 71, no. 3, pp. 392–395, 1991.

[15] P. Scanlan and S. Hodges, "Supernumerary premolar teeth in siblings," *British Journal of Orthodontics*, vol. 24, no. 4, pp. 297–300, 1997.

[16] C. Turner and C. Hill, "Supernumerary mandibular premolar: the importance of radiographic interpretation," *ASDC Journal of Dentistry for Children*, vol. 53, no. 5, pp. 375–377, 1986.

[17] S. Cochrane, J. Clark, and N. Hunt, "Late developing supernumerary teeth in the mandible," *British Journal of Orthodontics*, vol. 24, no. 4, pp. 293–296, 1997.

[18] A. Parolia, M. Kundabala, M. Dahal, M. Mohan, and M. S. Thomas, "Management of supernumerary teeth," *Journal of Conservative Dentistry*, vol. 14, no. 3, pp. 221–224, 2011.

[19] C. Herath, C. Jayawardena, N. Nagarathne, and K. Perera, "Characteristics and sequelae of erupted supernumerary teeth: a study of 218 cases among Sri Lankan children," *Journal of Investigative and Clinical Dentistry*, vol. 8, no. 4, article e12250, 2017.

[20] T. Saini, J. J. Keene, and J. Whetten, "Radiographic diagnosis of supernumerary premolars: case reviews," *Journal of Dentistry for Children*, vol. 69, no. 2, pp. 184–190, 2002.

10

A Case Report on Endodontic Management of a Rare Vertucci Type III Maxillary Canine

Hrudi Sundar Sahoo, R. Kurinji Amalavathy, and D. Pavani

Department of Conservative Dentistry and Endodontics, Sathyabama Dental College, Chennai, Tamil Nadu, India

Correspondence should be addressed to Hrudi Sundar Sahoo; hrudi21@gmail.com

Academic Editor: Daniel Torrés-Lagares

Success in root canal treatment demands a thorough knowledge of usual root canal anatomy and its variations pertaining to every tooth. Variations in root canal anatomy are often accompanied by complex orientation of pulp tissues making a thorough mechanical and chemical debridement a challenge. Inability to treat such complexities often leads to endodontic failure. Upon a quick review of the literature, it has been noted that very few root canal complexities in maxillary canines have been reported. To be a successful clinician, one must be aware of such rare anatomical instances in maxillary canines. Based on possible branching of the root canal system, root canal configurations of permanent teeth were divided into eight different types by Vertucci. The classification included single to three separate root canals. This case report presents a permanent right maxillary canine which is single rooted having a single canal orifice and a root canal dividing into two canals (buccal and palatal) at the middle third of the root and then joining at the apical third, before exiting with a single apical foramen (Vertucci type III).

1. Introduction

Success in root canal treatment demands a thorough knowledge of usual root canal anatomy and its variations pertaining to every tooth. Variations in root anatomy are often accompanied by complex orientation of pulp tissues making a thorough mechanical and chemical debridement a challenge. Inability to treat such complexities often leads to endodontic failure. One of the major reasons for endodontic failure can be missing extra root canals [1]. With advancements in digital imaging, magnification, instrumentation, and disinfection, treating complicated root canal systems has become more predictable.

The root canal systems include an intricate network of pulp tissues that include blood vessels and nerve tissues. Upon review of the literature, a large number of root canal anatomical variations have been reported in human anterior teeth. The possibility of finding two or three root canals in lower anterior teeth can range between 1% and 43%. Among lower anterior teeth, usually the canines are known to have one root and one root canal. Vertucci and Bellizzi and Hartwell had reported that 15% of mandibular canines had two separate root canals with one or two separate exits [2, 3]. Later on, few case reports cited the occurrence of two roots and three root canals, three root canals and two exits, and two separate roots and two root canals [4–6]. On the contrary, the upper canines are usually single canaled and single rooted. A maxillary canine with a single root canal dividing into two separate canals followed by joining of those two canals to the exit at a single foramen is a rare anatomy. Such aberrant root canal anatomy can result from abnormal development during tooth formation.

Based on possible branching of the root canal system, Vertucci classified root canal configurations of permanent teeth into eight different types. The classification included single to three separate root canals [7].

This case report presents a permanent right maxillary canine which is single rooted having a single canal orifice and root canal dividing into two canals (buccal and palatal) at the middle third of the root and then joining at the apical third, before exiting with a single apical foramen (Vertucci type III).

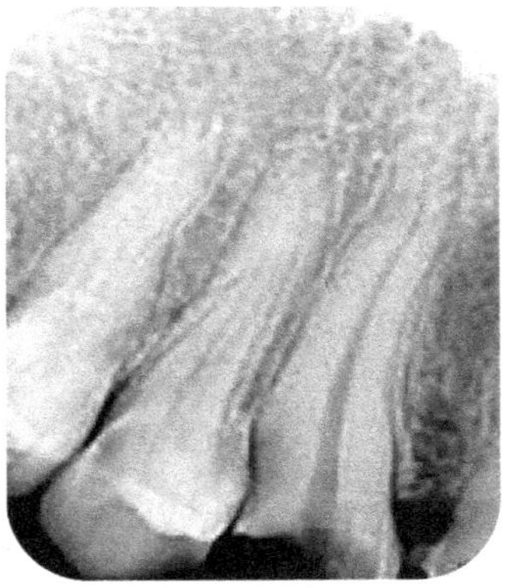

Pre-operative

FIGURE 1

2. Case Report

A 33-year-old male patient was referred from a private practitioner to the Department of Conservative Dentistry and Endodontics of Sathyabama Dental College and Hospital, Chennai, with the chief complaint of sensitivity and occasional pain in the left region of upper front teeth. On clinical examination, the patient had a crown-bridge prosthesis spanning from the left upper canine to the right upper canine. Since the crown-bridge prosthesis had a compromised stability, it was removed and an intraoral radiograph in relation to the #12 and #13 region was taken (Figure 1). The radiograph revealed distoproximal dental caries involving enamel, dentin, and pulp of tooth #13. An electric pulp test suggested symptomatic irreversible pulpitis.

In the first visit, under local anesthesia (Lignox 2%; Indoco Remedies Ltd., Mumbai) and rubber dam (Hygienic, Coltene Whaledent) isolation, root canal treatment was initiated in #13. With the help of an endo-access bur (bur type FG-1; Dentsply, USA), an access cavity was made and a single root canal orifice was located. The tentative working length was found to be 26 mm with an apex locator (Root ZX mini; J Morita, Japan). Hand instrumentation (K-files, Mani Inc., Japan) was done till size #50. A copious saline and sodium hypochlorite (3%) irrigation was done during each instrumentation change. Calcium hydroxide (RC-Cal; Prime Dental Ltd., India) was placed as an intracanal medicament. The access cavity was temporized with Cavit (3M ESPE, Germany), and a second visit was scheduled for further management.

Before the scheduled second visit, the patient reported to the department with severe pain in relation to #13. On reentering into the access cavity, fresh bleeding was noted. Hence, multiple angulated radiographs with two #20-size hand K-files inside the root canal were taken to rule out the presence of any extra root canal. These radiographs were inconclusive of missed canals. According to the AAE and AAOMR Joint Position Statement (2016 update), cone beam computed tomography scanning with a low-field volume, following ALARA principles, was done. On analysing CBCT multiple axial images (Figures 2(a)–2(c)), a second root canal (palatal canal) was seen branching out from the main root canal (buccal canal) at the middle third of the root. The palatal root canal joins the buccal root canal at the apical third, just before the exit suggesting Vertucci type III canal configuration (Figures 3(a) and 3(b)). The palatal canal was negotiated with #10 hand K-files under a dental operating microscope (Seiler Alpha Air 3; St. Louis, USA) at 10x magnification. A working length radiograph was taken to confirm the presence of the palatal canal (Figure 4(a)). After orifice enlargement with a #1 Gates Glidden drill (Mani Inc., Japan), instrumentation was done till #20 hand K-file (Mani Inc., Japan) followed by preparation of the remaining canal using the Self-Adjusting File (SAF; ReDent, Ra'anana, Israel) and the VATEA irrigation pump for chemical debridement with 3.5% sodium hypochlorite during canal preparation.

In the scheduled third visit, the patient was asymptomatic. In view of complicacy of the root canal, the obturation of both root canals (Figure 4(b)) was carried out using thermoplasticized gutta percha (Elements; Sybron Endo, Germany). The follow-up review radiograph (Figure 4(c)) after 6 months revealed no periapical changes, and the patient was found to be asymptomatic.

3. Discussion

A few indications of an aberrant root canal anatomy are a modified coronal access, unusual location and size of the canal orifice, and indistinct X-ray images [8]. In this case, multiple angulated digital X-rays failed to provide definitive information of any variation in the root canal system.

Routine radiographs most often fail to indicate additional root canals or any variation in root canal anatomy whereas CBCT has been highly successful in facilitating a better visualization and three-dimensional imaging of such unusual anatomy. Unlike conventional CT scans, CBCT provides higher resolution with reduced radiation dose [9–11]. The principle of "as low as reasonably achievable" (ALARA) was considered, but the necessity and advantage of using CBCT in this case outweighed the risks of additional exposure. Hence, for better understanding of the root canal system, a judicious use of cone beam computed tomography was required in the current case. CBCT of tooth #13 performed in this case confirmed the existence of two canals (one palatal and one buccal) as well as vividly presented the course of these two canals (Vertucci type III). Hence, CBCT definitively helped in the proper diagnosis and improved the treatment success by enabling the description of such a rare anatomic variation precisely.

Çalişkan et al. [12] studied the root canal number, configuration, and ramifications of permanent teeth in a Turkish population. They reported percentage of Vertucci type III [1 -2 -1] as 4.35% whereas Nikhita et al. [13] studied 250 maxillary canines in an Indian population and reported the occurrence of Vertucci type III as 11.6%.

To probe for an additional canal, a tactile examination of all the walls of the major canal was performed with the tip of a precurved scouting hand K-file (size #10). A catch was felt in the palatal surface of the major canal wall. Hence, the presence of a possible canal bifurcation was suspected. Green [14] reported that on deeper penetration into a canal, if an

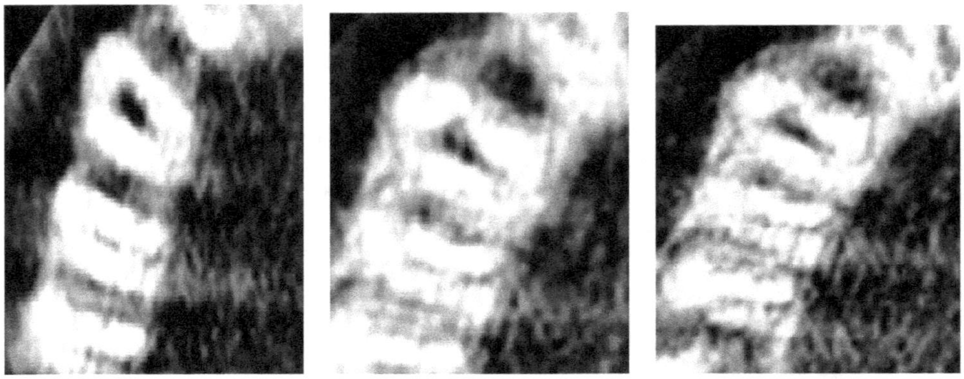

(a) At the orifice (b) At the bifurcation (c) At the root apex

FIGURE 2

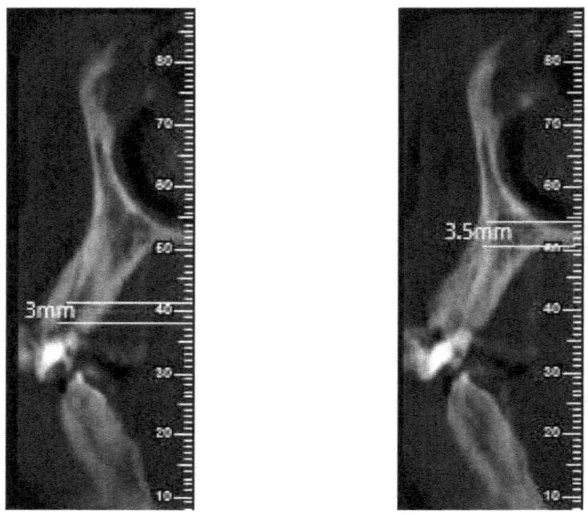

(a) Bifurcation at approx. 3 mm from the canal orifice (b) Both root canals join at approx. 3.5 mm from the root apex

FIGURE 3

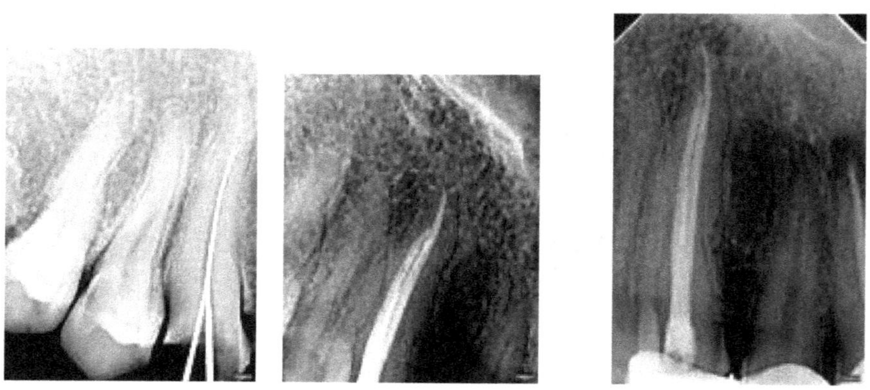

(a) Working length (b) Obturation (c) Follow-up radiograph after 6 months

FIGURE 4

instrument demonstrates eccentric direction, termed directional control, an additional canal should be suspected. With the aid of CBCT axial images, the second root canal orifice was located under a dental operating microscope. The role of a dental microscope in endodontic practice cannot be underestimated as it helped to locate and visualize the second orifice at almost the middle third of the root canal (the point of bifurcation of the main root canal). Such an aberrant anatomy can also be expected to occur in the contralateral maxillary canine. Hence, such findings can also serve as an alert to a clinician while treating the left maxillary canine, if necessary, in the future.

The buccal canal that was in line with the main passage is usually amenable to adequate enlarging and obturation procedures; the preparation and filling of the palatal canal were extremely difficult. Under an endodontic microscope, after scouting and shaping the palatal canal till #20, a self-adjustable file system was used to chemomechanically debride the canal system. The Self-Adjusting File (SAF) (ReDent Nova, Ra'anana, Israel) is a uniquely designed, thin-walled, hollow endodontic file made of a NiTi lattice that is compressible in a canal. The irrigant flow through the hollow file provides chemical debridement with simultaneous enlargement of the canal [15]. Hence, the use of the SAF system in preparing such a complicated root canal system in this case was deemed necessary.

4. Conclusion

The root canal system presents a myriad of complexities. While identifying such variations is a challenge itself, cone beam computed tomography was deemed necessary to understand the complexities present in this case. In addition to such an advanced imaging technique, the use of magnification and the advanced canal preparation system like the Self-Adjusting File system helped us deliver a predictable treatment outcome.

References

[1] M. Hulsmann and E. Schafer, "Problems in gaining access to the root canal system," *Problems in Endodontics: Etiology, Diagnosis and Treatment*, vol. 1, pp. 145–172, 2009.

[2] F. J. Vertucci, "Root canal anatomy of the mandibular anterior teeth," *Journal of the American Dental Association*, vol. 89, no. 2, pp. 369–371, 1974.

[3] R. Bellizzi and G. R. Hartwell, "Clinical investigation of in vivo endodontically treated mandibular anterior teeth," *Journal of Endodontia*, vol. 9, no. 6, pp. 246–248, 1983.

[4] I. Heling, I. Gottlieb-Dadon, and N. P. Chandler, "Mandibular canine with two roots and three root canals," *Endodontics & Dental Traumatology*, vol. 11, no. 6, pp. 301-302, 1995.

[5] A. Orguneser and N. Kartal, "Three canals and two foramina in a mandibular canine," *Journal of Endodontia*, vol. 24, no. 6, pp. 444-445, 1998.

[6] C. D'Arcangelo, G. Varvara, and P. de Fazio, "Root canal treatment in mandibular canines with two roots: a report of two cases," *International Endodontic Journal*, vol. 34, no. 4, pp. 331–334, 2001.

[7] F. J. Vertucci, "Root canal anatomy of the human permanent teeth," *Oral Surgery, Oral Medicine, Oral Pathology*, vol. 58, no. 5, pp. 589–599, 1984.

[8] J. Kottoor, N. Velmurugan, R. Sudha, and S. Hemamalathi, "Maxillary first molar with seven root canals diagnosed with cone-beam computed tomography scanning: a case report," *Journal of Endodontia*, vol. 36, no. 5, pp. 915–921, 2010.

[9] S. Patel, A. Dawood, T. P. Ford, and E. Whaites, "The potential applications of cone beam computed tomography in the management of endodontic problems," *International Endodontic Journal*, vol. 40, no. 10, pp. 818–830, 2007.

[10] M. K. Nair and U. P. Nair, "Digital and advanced imaging in endodontics: a review," *Journal of Endodontia*, vol. 33, no. 1, pp. 1–6, 2007.

[11] T. Cotton, T. Geisler, D. Holden, S. Schwartz, and W. Schindler, "Endodontic applications of cone-beam volumetric tomography," *Journal of Endodontia*, vol. 33, no. 9, pp. 1121–1132, 2007.

[12] M. K. Çalişkan, Y. Pehlivan, F. Sepetçioğlu, M. Türkün, and S. Ş. Tuncer, "Root canal morphology of human permanent teeth in a Turkish population," *Journal of Endodontia*, vol. 21, no. 4, pp. 200–204, 1995.

[13] N. Somalinga Amardeep, S. Raghu, and V. Natanasabapathy, "Root canal morphology of permanent maxillary and mandibular canines in Indian population using cone beam computed tomography," *Anatomy Research International*, vol. 2014, Article ID 731859, 7 pages, 2014.

[14] D. Green, "Double canals in single roots," *Oral Surgery, Oral Medicine, Oral Pathology*, vol. 35, no. 5, pp. 689–696, 1973.

[15] M. A. Dietrich, T. C. Kirkpatrick, and J. M. Yaccino, "*In vitro* canal and isthmus debris removal of the self-adjusting file, K3, and WaveOne files in the mesial root of human mandibular molars," *Journal of Endodontia*, vol. 38, no. 8, pp. 1140–1144, 2012.

11

Ameloblastic Carcinoma with Calcification: A Rare Case Report in the Mandible and Literature Review

Neda Kardouni Khoozestani[1] **Farzaneh Mosavat,**[2] **Mohammad Shirkhoda,**[3] **and Ramtin Azar**[2]

[1]*Departments of Oral and Maxillofacial Pathology, Cancer Institute, Tehran University of Medical Sciences, Tehran, Iran*
[2]*Oral and Maxillofacial Radiology, School of Dentistry, Tehran University of Medical Sciences, Tehran, Iran*
[3]*Department of Onco-Surgery, Cancer Institute, Tehran University of Medical Sciences, Tehran, Iran*

Correspondence should be addressed to Neda Kardouni Khoozestani; nkardouni@tums.ac.ir and Ramtin Azar; dr.ramtinazar@gmail.com

Academic Editor: Leandro Napier de Souza

Ameloblastic carcinoma (AC) is a scarce malignant tumor which is more prevalent in the mandible than the maxilla. It occurs in a wide range of age groups, and there is a sex predilection in males. AC shows specific microscopic features and requires more aggressive surgical treatment plans in comparison with conventional ameloblastoma. Radiographically, AC resembles ameloblastoma except that it rarely represents focal mineralized materials, seemingly reflecting dystrophic calcification. This characteristic is uncommon in typical ameloblastomas, and only few cases reported with such opacities and mineralized materials. Due to this rare radiographic and microscopic presentation, an accurate diagnosis could be challenging, and pathologists should consider a combination of benign and malignant odontogenic tumors occurring in jaws.

1. Introduction

Odontogenic malignancies are rare lesions which comprise one percent of all cysts and tumors happening in the jaws arising from tissues associated with odontogenic epithelium [1–3]. AC is considered a rare entity that shows the histopathological characteristics of ameloblastoma with histological atypia regardless of metastasis occurring or not [2].

Considering the rarity and diverse nomenclature of this lesion, AC has been a topic of diagnostic challenges for a long period of time [3]. The most common sign of AC is swelling; nevertheless, symptoms such as trismus, pain, dysphonia, and rapid growth also may occur [1, 4, 5]. However, in 2017, the World Health Organization announced that there seems to be little justification for dividing such a rare tumor into smaller subsets; therefore, it continues simply as a single entity (ameloblastic carcinoma) [6].

Radiographically, AC looks like ameloblastoma except that it occasionally shows focal radiopaque materials; apparently, it reflects dystrophic calcification itself. This trend does not often appear in typical ameloblastomas [4]. The literature was searched according to the combination of the following terms on PubMed: ((calcifi∗) OR minerali∗) AND (ameloblastoma) [Mesh].

We documented a case of recurrent AC with calcification in a 40-year-old woman who underwent surgery and radiotherapy.

2. Case Report

A 40-year-old woman referred to Imam Khomeini Cancer Institute was complaining of intense lower facial pain and progressive swelling for the period of the last six months. Although she has not had a considerable problem in her past medical history, she has also given us a history of her left second premolar and first molar teeth root canal therapy in which she had not noticed any change in pain and swollen area size. She had also undergone incisional biopsy in another health care center with pathologic results designated as a "malignant Pindborg tumor."

On clinical examination, diffuse swelling causing lower lip tenderness and paresthesia with extension to the left posterior part of the mandible was detected. On examination, a mass that measures approximately 4 cm with a rubbery consistency was found. The overlying skin tissue was intact; however, oral mucosa was ulcerated. No palpable subcutaneous cervical lymph node was found. There was no difficulty in swallowing, dysphagia, trismus, or dysphonia.

On panoramic and cone-beam computed tomography (CBCT), the lesion with a well-defined border and internal focal radiopacities was seen that extended from the periapical area of the mandibular left canine to the mandibular left second molar in an anteroposterior dimension and from the alveolar crest to the inferior border of the mandible in a superoinferior aspect (Figure 1). Buccal and lingual cortical plate perforation was also detected. The inferior alveolar canal (IAC) was involved by the lesion, which confirmed the patient's history of pain and paresthesia (Figure 2). After multidisciplinary evaluations and elucidation of the lesion destructive nature in radiographs, left hemimandibulectomy was performed for the patient (Figure 3).

Microscopic examinations showed odontogenic epithelial neoplasm composed of sheet and island of epithelial cells with malignant features including cellular pleomorphism, hyperchromatism, few atypical mitotic figures, central necrosis, and perineural invasion in a collagenized stroma. At the periphery of the islands, tall columnar cells resembling ameloblast cells with nuclear palisading, reverse polarity, and subnuclear vacuolization are evident. The particular feature of this tumor was the presence of intercellular eosinophilic amorphous materials in extensive areas that had been transformed into mineralized materials in some parts. The lesion was superficially covered by ulcerated stratified squamous epithelium (Figure 4). Besides, Ki-67 immunostaining was performed, and its expression was noticeable (around 45% in HPF), especially at the peripheral cells and occasionally at the central cells of the tumor islands (Figure 4(e)).

3. Discussion

Odontogenic malignancies are rare lesions which are composed of one percent of all cysts and tumors appearing in the jaws emanating from tissue associated with odontogenic epithelium [1, 5, 7, 8]. For the first time in 1984, Shafer described the ameloblastic carcinoma as ameloblastoma that shows some extent of cellular pleomorphism and necrosis [4].

Varying signaling pathways which take part in the progression of ameloblastomas have been recognized highlighting the MAPK signaling pathway with its predominant B-RAF proto-oncogene serine/threonine kinase (BRAF) V600E mutation [9]. Since the presence of B-RAF proto-oncogene serine/threonine kinase (BRAF) V600E mutation in ameloblastoma and some cases of ameloblastic carcinoma has been reported, which may be involved in its behavior, targeted therapies have been used as an alternative in the

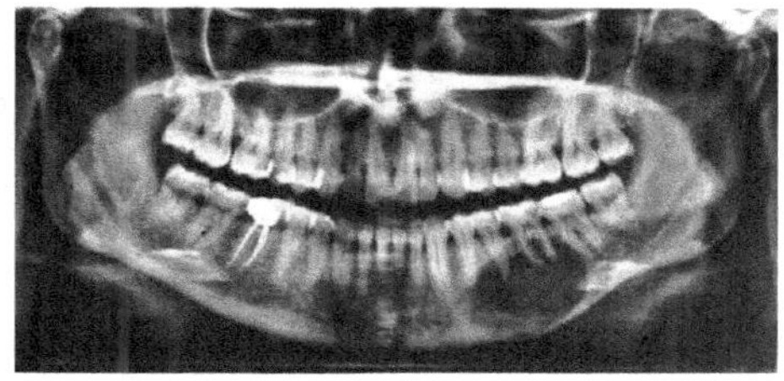

FIGURE 1: Panoramic radiograph showing a radiolucent lesion in the left mandible body containing small radiopaque foci, especially in the lower parts.

case of resistance or recurrent ameloblastoma and ameloblastic carcinoma [9].

Based on a systematic literature review which has been carried out by Deng et al. from January 2000 to July 2018 and our literature review, AC presents a higher male prevalence when compared to females. The most involved site in the jaw is the posterior area of the mandible with a 64% occurrence rate [10]. AC can occur in a wide age range; however, the average age of 45 years is considered in the literature. The most usual symptom of AC is swelling (68%), although AC may be accompanied by pain, fast growth, difficulty in jaw functions, and dysphonia [4, 10]. Our case was conducted more or less in the same age group which revealed no difficulty in swallowing, dysphagia, trismus, and dysphonia.

Based on radiographic view, differential diagnosis of posterior mandibular radiolucency includes odontogenic keratocyst, myxoma, Pindborg tumor, ameloblastoma, and less commonly intraosseous malignancies or metastatic lesions [10, 11]. The radiographic findings do not help the diagnosis, although the destructive nature of the presented case in radiographs is more in favor of malignant neoplasms, including ameloblastic carcinoma as well.

Differentiation between ameloblastic carcinoma and classic ameloblastoma may be impossible based on the radiological aspect solely. Both of the lesions demonstrate a bony hard expansive mass with teeth displacement, loss of lamina dura, root resorption, and occasionally teeth loosening [12, 13]. Like classic ameloblastoma, AC is mostly found in the premolar and molar regions of the mandible. Both of them typically have a well-defined and corticated border, although sometimes a scalloped border can be observed [14]. AC similar to ameloblastoma is unilocular or more commonly multilocular radiolucent. Most of the septa in AC are course and thick, which is seen also in classic ameloblastoma and can lead to a honeycomb- or soap bubble-like pattern in radiographic appearances. However, AC typically shows more features such as dystrophic calcifications and mixed solid and cystic regions [12–15].

As mentioned in the radiographic features of the discussed case, there were severe buccal and lingual cortical plate perforation, root blunting of a mandibular first premolar, and root resorption in a mandibular first molar as well as the appearance of dystrophic calcifications. The notable radiologic feature of this patient was the presence of multiple small internal radiopacities throughout the lesion. Based on our literature review, two cases of AC have been represented

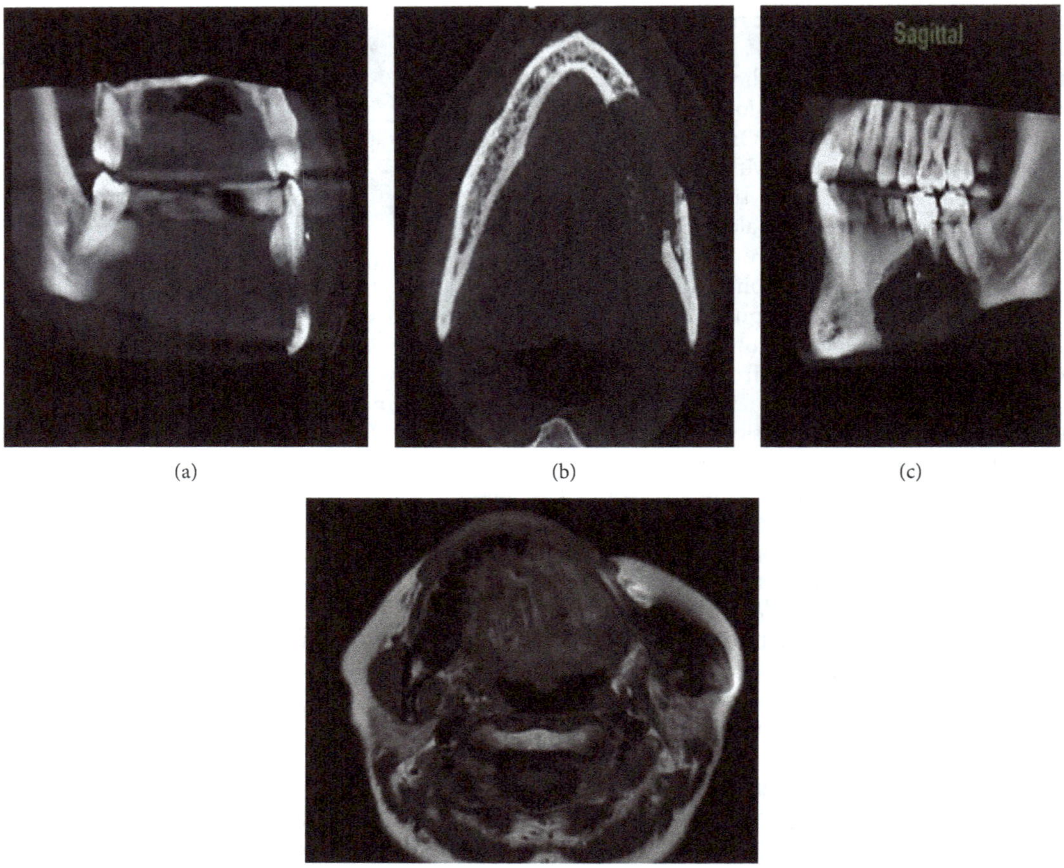

(a) (b) (c)

(d)

Figure 2: (a–c) Coronal, axial, and sagittal CBCT views showing severe buccal and lingual cortical plate perforation and IAC involvement by the tumor. The small radiopaque foci marked with arrows (b, c). (d) T1-weighted MRI showing left hemimandibular excision with its ipsilateral masseter muscle resection from the left lateral incisor area.

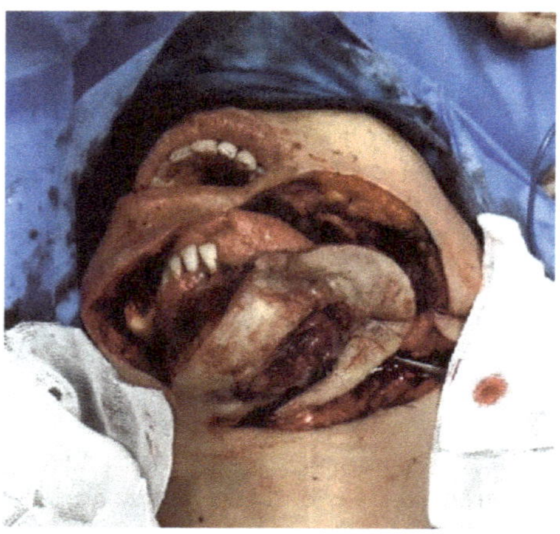

Figure 3: Patient surgical photography showing hemimandibulectomy which provides safe margin removal.

with calcification [10, 16]. Similarly, a systematic literature review published in 2019 which had been done by Deng et al. from 2000 to 2018 strengthens our results [10, 16].

On occasion, calcification may be a result of intensive apoptotic activity, and the final differentiation of keratinocytes is taught out to be a variant of the apoptotic process [7, 10, 17, 18]. Histologically, the main differential diagnosis of AC with cellular atypia, necrosis, and such extensive calcified materials could carry the malignant calcifying epithelial odontogenic tumor, squamous odontogenic tumor with malignant features, and metastatic carcinoma from the unknown primary origin. Due to observation of some calcified foci, our case mistakenly had been reported as a malignant Pindborg tumor. Regarding the existence of palisaded columnar cells at the periphery of neoplastic islands, the malignant Pindborg tumor which was formed from polygonal to squamoid cells with atypical cytologic features can be ruled out [3, 4, 19]. The amyloid stain negativity of eosinophilic amorphous intercellular materials has also verified the diagnosis. The next differential diagnosis which was ruled out was the squamous odontogenic tumor with malignant features. Rare entity neoplasm does not show palisaded tall columnar cells at the periphery of islands; moreover, it lacks stellate reticulum-like cells in the island's center and, the last but not least, lacks intercellular secretions in both the WHO and simple types of this neoplasm [19, 20]. The third pathological differential diagnosis was excluded due to the patient's clinical history and complete metastasis workup that no other origin was detected.

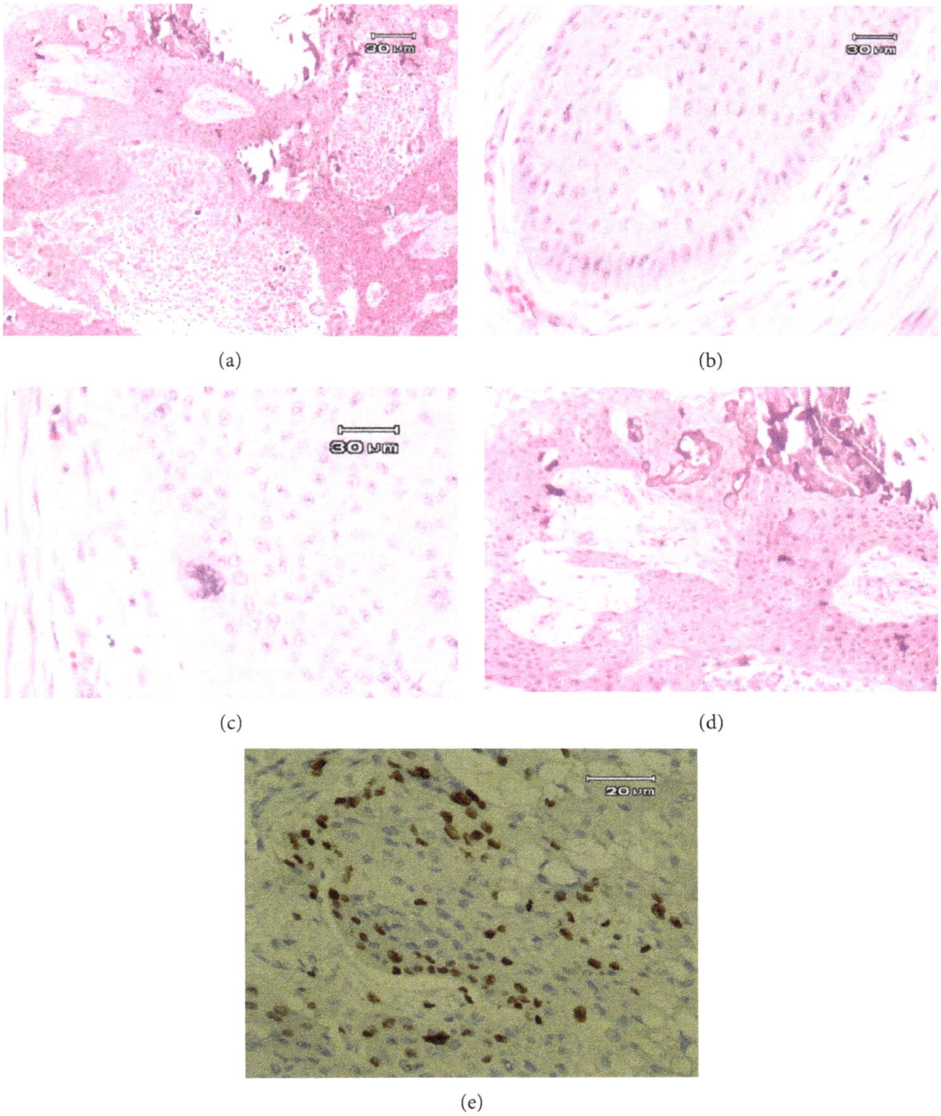

FIGURE 4: Histopathological features of ameloblastic carcinoma. (a) Ameloblastic carcinoma depicting the extensive area of calcified materials at the center of islands as well as in the intracellular areas (hematoxylin and eosin, ×40). (b) Follicles and islands with marked palisaded tall columnar cells at the periphery (hematoxylin and eosin, ×400). (c) Tumoral cells with pleomorphism, cellular atypia, loss of peripheral palisading, nuclear polarity, and presence of tumoral giant cell (hematoxylin and eosin, ×400). (d) Amorphous eosinophilic intercellular secretion which undergoes calcifications in some foci (hematoxylin and eosin, ×100). (e) Ki-67 immunostaining in ameloblastic carcinoma showed a significantly high Ki-67 labeling index especially at the periphery of the islands (×400).

Looking at the microscopic features of this case in a different angle reveals that the tangible absence of stellate reticulum-like cells in the center of islands, trabeculae, and sheets of the neoplastic cells is highly in favor of AC. In this regard, Angiero et al. pointed out that the presence of nests, islands, sheets, or trabeculae of reverse polarized epithelium with scarce or no existence of stellate reticulum-like areas can be considered a diagnostic clue for the pathologist to appraise AC in differential diagnosis [21]. The Ki-67 labeling index shows a statistically significant difference between ameloblastoma and ameloblastic carcinoma, which ranges from 11.87% to 53.29% in the case of the latter [22]. Ameloblastic carcinoma by itself is a rare lesion, and AC with calcification is much more uncommon, and according to the literature review, only a few cases have been reported so far [4, 10]. Loyola et al. noted an infrequent but interesting presence of calcification in the vicinity of malignant odontogenic epithelium in the AC, which in turn can complicate the diagnosis [23]. Fitzpatrick et al. reported a case of ameloblastic carcinoma with features of ghost cell odontogenic carcinoma in the anterior area of the maxilla in a 37-year-old man which revealed multiple calcifications histologically [24]. Casaroto et al. reviewed cases of ameloblastic carcinoma and found that 12.5% of cases exhibited calcification and three (12.5%) had rosette-like structures [25]. Although ghost cells, keratin production, calcifications, and rosette-like structures were rare in AC cases, these features should also be carefully evaluated when present in this tumor [25]. Another study analyzed 14 cases of ameloblastoma, one of which showed calcification. It can be concluded that since calcification in ameloblastoma is rare, the presence of these calcifications must be carefully evaluated [26].

There are different methods to tackle AC, including surgical resection with a safe margin with or without cervical lymph node removal and surgical removal with or without chemotherapy. Having a safe margin can reduce the rate of recurrence to less than 15% [10, 27]. Another treatment modality that had been reported in the literature review for these patients is surgical resection with neck dissection with or without radiotherapy (29.4% recurrence) [10, 27]. The lung is the most prevalent region (9%) for distant metastasis according to the literature review [10, 27].

Our case underwent hemimandibulectomy and radiotherapy. We followed the patient for four years after the initial diagnosis of AC. She is still alive but unfortunately suffering from multiple lung metastases and poor general health quality.

4. Conclusion

Dystrophic calcifications are rare findings in ACs. However, the presence of such materials as an occasional feature can be considered a diagnostic point for pathologists. It seems that more cases are needed to be studied to understand how these calcifications could relate to the patient's outcomes.

References

[1] A. Horváth, E. Horváth, and S. Popşor, "Mandibular ameloblastic carcinoma in a young patient," *Revue Roumaine de Morphologie et Embryologie*, vol. 53, no. 1, pp. 179–183, 2012.

[2] D. Sozzi, V. Morganti, G. M. Valente, F. Moltrasio, A. Bozzetti, and F. Angiero, "Ameloblastic carcinoma in a young patient," *Oral Surgery, Oral Medicine, Oral Pathology, Oral Radiology*, vol. 117, no. 5, pp. e396–e402, 2014.

[3] J. A. Regezi, J. J. Sciubba, and R. C. K. Jordan, *Oral pathology: clinical pathologic correlations*, Elsevier Health Sciences, 2017.

[4] R. L. Corio, L. I. Goldblatt, P. A. Edwards, and K. S. Hartman, "Ameloblastic carcinoma: a clinicopathologic study and assessment of eight cases," *Oral Surgery, Oral Medicine, Oral Pathology*, vol. 64, no. 5, pp. 570–576, 1987.

[5] S. A. M. Mahmoud, H. W. Amer, and S. I. Mohamed, "Primary ameloblastic carcinoma: literature review with case series," *Polish Journal of Pathology*, vol. 69, no. 3, pp. 243–253, 2018.

[6] N. A. Brown and K. S. J. Elenitoba-Johnson, "Update from the 4th edition of the World Health Organization classification of head and neck tumours: hematolymphoid tumours," *Head and Neck Pathology*, vol. 11, no. 1, pp. 96–109, 2017.

[7] T. S. Saluja and R. Hosalkar, "Reconnoitre ameloblastic carcinoma: a prognostic update," *Oral oncology*, vol. 77, pp. 118–124, 2018.

[8] S. Pandey, O. Bhutia, A. Roychoudhury, A. Arora, and K. Bhatt, "Literature review of 86 cases of mandibular ameloblastic carcinoma," *National Journal of Maxillofacial Surgery*, vol. 9, no. 1, pp. 2–7, 2018.

[9] R. González-González, S. López-Verdín, J. Lavalle-Carrasco et al., "Current concepts in ameloblastoma-targeted therapies in B-raf proto-oncogene serine/threonine kinase V600E mutation: systematic review," *World Journal of Clinical Oncology*, vol. 11, no. 1, pp. 31–42, 2020.

[10] L. Deng, R. Wang, M. Yang, W. Li, and L. Zou, "Ameloblastic carcinoma: clinicopathological analysis of 18 cases and a systematic review," *Head & Neck*, vol. 41, no. 12, pp. 4191–4198, 2019.

[11] M. Keerthi, P. R. D. Shyam, R. T. Madhusudan, and P. Ramanand, "An unusual case of capacious ameloblastic carcinoma," *Indian Journal of Dental Advancements*, vol. 5, p. 1134, 2013.

[12] B. Devenney-Cakir, B. Dunfee, R. Subramaniam et al., "Ameloblastic carcinoma of the mandible with metastasis to the skull and lung: advanced imaging appearance including computed tomography, magnetic resonance imaging and positron emission tomography computed tomography," *Dento Maxillo Facial Radiology*, vol. 39, no. 7, pp. 449–453, 2010.

[13] M. Minami, T. Kaneda, K. Ozawa et al., "Cystic lesions of the maxillomandibular region: MR imaging distinction of odontogenic keratocysts and ameloblastomas from other cysts," *AJR American Journal of Roentgenology*, vol. 166, no. 4, pp. 943–949, 1996.

[14] J. Asaumi, M. Hisatomi, Y. Yanagi et al., "Assessment of ameloblastomas using MRI and dynamic contrast-enhanced MRI," *European Journal of Radiology*, vol. 56, no. 1, pp. 25–30, 2005.

[15] S. M. Mallya, E. W. N. Lam, S. C. White, and M. J. Pharoah, "White and Pharoah's oral radiology: principles and interpretation," Elsevier, 2019.

[16] V. Naik and A. D. Kale, *Ameloblastic carcinoma: a case report*, Quintessence international, Berlin, Germany, 2007.

[17] Y. Maruoka, H. Harada, T. Mitsuyasu et al., "Keratinocytes become terminally differentiated in a process involving programmed cell death," *Biochemical and Biophysical Research Communications*, vol. 238, no. 3, pp. 886–890, 1997.

[18] K. M. Kim, "Apoptosis and calcification," *Scanning Microscopy*, vol. 9, no. 4, pp. 1137–1175, 1995.

[19] B. W. Neville, D. D. Damm, C. M. Allen, and A. C. Chi, *Oral and maxillofacial pathology*, Elsevier Health Sciences, 2015.

[20] S. Akrish, A. Buchner, Y. Shoshani, M. Vered, and D. Dayan, "Ameloblastic carcinoma: report of a new case, literature review, and comparison to ameloblastoma," *Journal of Oral and Maxillofacial Surgery*, vol. 65, no. 4, pp. 777–783, 2007.

[21] F. Angiero, R. Borloni, M. Macchi, and M. Stefani, "Ameloblastic carcinoma of the maxillary sinus," *Anticancer Research*, vol. 28, no. 6b, pp. 3847–3854, 2008.

[22] M. Martínez-Martínez, A. Mosqueda-Taylor, R. Carlos-Bregni et al., "Comparative histological and immunohistochemical study of ameloblastomas and ameloblastic carcinomas," *Medicina oral, Patologia Oral y Cirugia Bucal*, vol. 22, no. 3, p. e324, 2017.

[23] A. M. Loyola, S. V. Cardoso, P. R. de Faria et al., "Ameloblastic carcinoma: a Brazilian collaborative study of 17 cases," *Histopathology*, vol. 69, no. 4, pp. 687–701, 2016.

[24] S. G. Fitzpatrick, S. A. Hirsch, C. M. Listinsky, D. J. Lyu, and D. A. Baur, "Ameloblastic carcinoma with features of ghost cell odontogenic carcinoma in a patient with suspected Gardner

syndrome," *Oral Surgery, Oral Medicine, Oral Pathology and Oral Radiology*, vol. 119, no. 4, pp. e241–e245, 2015.

[25] A. R. Casaroto, G. L. Toledo, J. L. Filho, C. T. Soares, M. M. Capelari, and V. S. Lara, "Ameloblastic carcinoma, primary type: case report, immunohistochemical analysis and literature review," *Anticancer Research*, vol. 32, no. 4, pp. 1515–1525, 2012.

[26] J. M. Hall, D. R. Weathers, and K. K. Unni, "Ameloblastic carcinoma: an analysis of 14 cases," *Oral Surgery, Oral Medicine, Oral Pathology, Oral Radiology, and Endodontics*, vol. 103, no. 6, pp. 799–807, 2007.

[27] P. Shah, R. Venkatesh, C. More, and V. Vaishnavee, "Ameloblastic carcinoma: presentation of a rare case," *Journal of Indian Academy of Oral Medicine and Radiology*, vol. 29, no. 3, pp. 213–216, 2017.

12

Multilayer Super-Translucent Zirconia for Chairside Fabrication of a Monolithic Posterior Crown

Sven Rinke,[1,2] Anna Metzger,[1] and Holger Ziebolz[1]

[1]*Dental Clinic Prof. Dr. S. Rinke, Dr. M. Jablonski & Dr. H. Ziebolz, Hanau, Germany*
[2]*University Medical Center Göttingen, Department of Prosthodontics, Göttingen, Germany*

Correspondence should be addressed to Sven Rinke; sven.rinke@med.uni-goettingen.de

Academic Editor: Andrea Scribante

This case report describes the chairside fabrication of a monolithic posterior crown using a multilayer super-translucent zirconia material. According to the manufacturer's information, the newly introduced multilayer zirconia (4-YTZP) offers a unique combination of fracture strength (>850 MPa with speed-sintering) and improved optical properties, thus allowing a reduced minimum material thickness and optional temporary luting. By using up-to-date components of the CEREC system, including superfast dry-milling and a speed-sintering process, the fabrication of a monolithic zirconia crown is possible within an acceptable timeframe for the chairside workflow (60-75 min). The usage of a multilayer super-translucent material allows for the individualization of the restoration, typically in a single combined stain and glaze firing. However, it should be noted that clinical data for this type of restoration are still sparse. Therefore, manufacturer recommendations regarding indication, preparation, and cementation must be followed very strictly.

1. Introduction

Since the introduction of translucent zirconia ceramic materials more than 10 years ago, these materials allow the fabrication of monolithic crowns and fixed partial dentures (FPDs) [1, 2].

Omission of ceramic veneering reduces the risk of fractures in the veneering ceramics to a great extent (Figure 1). Existing clinical data show a significantly reduced technical complication rate in the posterior region in comparison to veneered restorations made of zirconia [3–5]. So far, the use of zirconia ceramic materials for the chairside fabrication of monolithic crowns and FPDs was not considered reasonable due to the comparatively long sintering times [6, 7]. The development of so-called speed-sintering processes in combination with translucent zirconia ceramic materials now offers the option of a chairside processing of zirconia crowns and FPDs [1, 6, 8, 9]. However, the advantage of zirconia materials in the chairside workflow and the choice of materials should be discussed in general [1, 10, 11].

High-strength glass-ceramics are the most frequently used materials in chairside processing (e.g., IPS e.max CAD, Ivoclar Vivadent, Schaan, Liechtenstein; CERECTessera, Dentsply Sirona, Charlotte, USA) [7, 11–14]. Their 3-point flexural strength of more than 450 MPa is sufficient for the fabrication of single crowns and 3-unit FPDs up to the first premolar, provided that the following preconditions are considered: The minimum material thickness required for the restoration is 1.0 mm, the adhesive luting is indispensable, and temporary cementation is not possible [15, 16].

High translucency that allows for a distinct chameleon effect and good conditioning properties for adhesive luting is the main advantage of this group of materials [12, 17]. The present clinical data document high success and survival rates for chairside-fabricated single-tooth restorations over observational periods of up to 10 years [10, 12, 18, 19].

Meanwhile, translucent zirconia ceramic materials are available with different modifications; the translucency is mainly caused by varying percentages of alumina and yttria. Although the first generation of zirconia with a portion of 3 mol% yttrium oxide shows high 3-point flexural strength

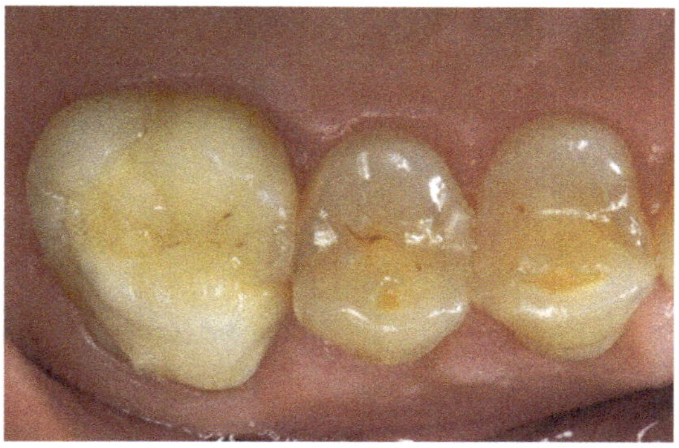

Figure 1: Zirconia materials of the first generation could only be used for veneered restorations, especially the molar region was prone to an increased risk for fractures of the veneering ceramics.

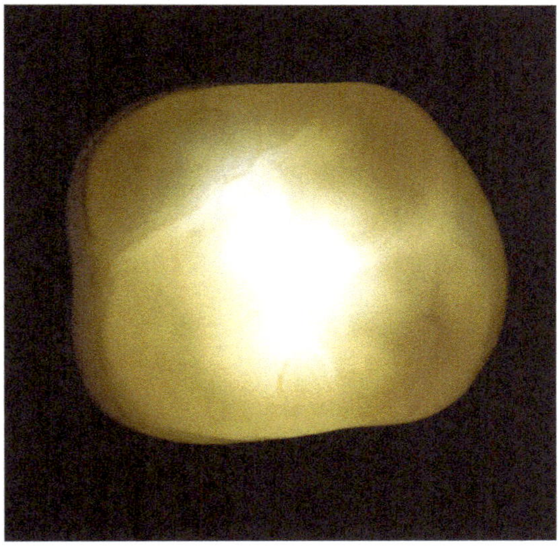

Figure 2: Transillumination of a zirconia crown of the fourth generation (CEREC MTL Zirconia, Dentsply Sirona).

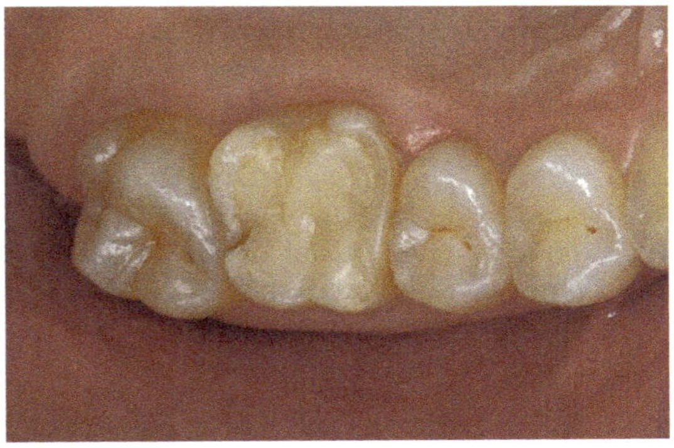

Figure 3: Initial situation: endodontically treated first upper molar with an insufficient composite restoration.

(ISO 6872-2015) in the region of 1,000 to 1,200 MPa, the translucency of this group of materials is relatively low compared to glass-ceramic materials [1]. By reducing the alumina share, an increased translucency could be achieved in zirconia materials of the second generation, leading to nearly unchanged mechanical properties [20]. For monolithic crowns and FPDs of the

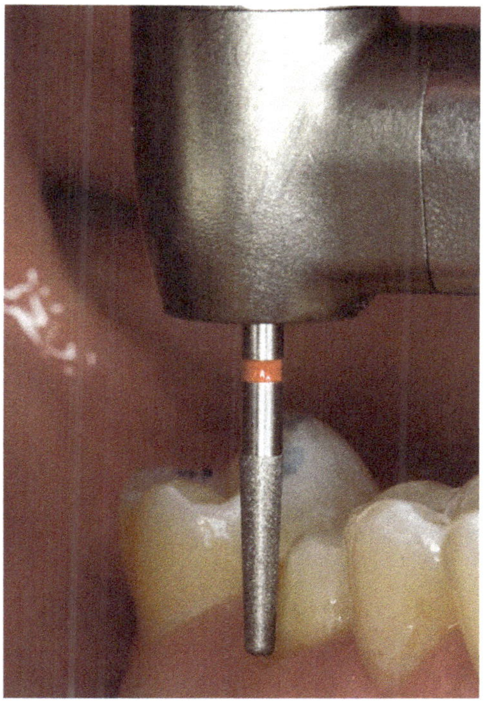

Figure 4: Design of the preparation limit: shoulder with rounded inner angle (8951.314.017, Komet Dental, Lemgo, Germany).

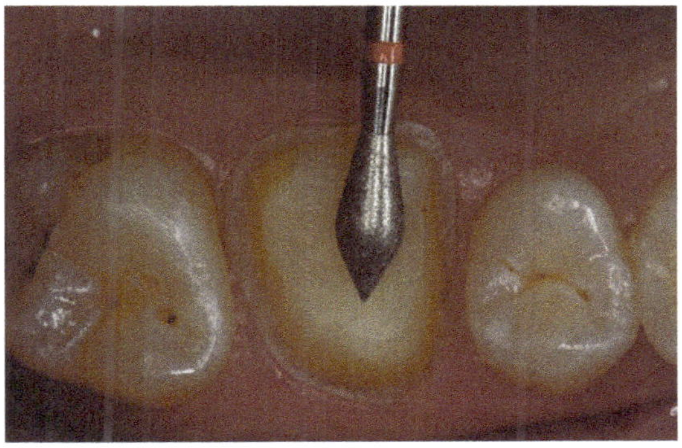

Figure 5: Preparation of the occlusal surface (8899.314.027, Komet Dental, Lemgo, Germany).

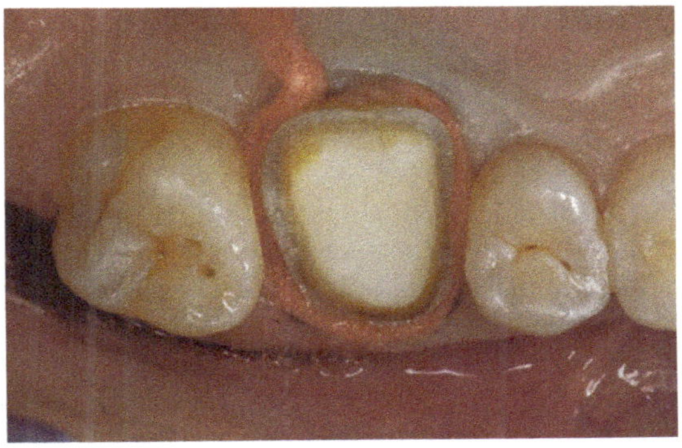

Figure 6: Preparation for the intraoral scan. For increased lateral extrusion of the soft tissues, a layer of cotton is applied after a knitted retraction cord is placed. The cotton is removed immediately prior to oral scanning.

TABLE 1: Clinical and technical procedures (step-by-step) for the chairside fabrication of multilayer zirconia crowns.

Step	Clinical procedures	Technical procedures
1	Adhesive build-up Preparation Soft tissue management Placement of retraction cord	
2	Intraoral scanning Preparation, antagonistic jaw and buccal scan (bite registration)	
3		CAD design Preparation analysis (substance reduction, undercuts, artefacts) Determination of preparation limit Modification of the restoration design
4		CAM process Selection of ceramic block Dry-milling Speed-sintering
5		Staining and glazing of the restoration Conditioning of the intaglio restoration surface (air-abrading process)
6	Try-in Verification of correct shade Occlusal and proximal adjustments if needed	
7	Luting Definitive cementation (e.g., self-adhesive cement) or provisional cementation	

second generation, first clinical studies document a significant reduction in the technical complication rate of tooth- and implant-supported single-tooth restorations in comparison to veneered zirconia restorations [3, 4, 10, 21].

Zirconia materials of the third generation contain 5 mol% yttrium. This allows a translucency comparable with that of high-strength glass-ceramic materials. On the other hand, in comparison with classic zirconia materials with an yttria content of 3 mol%, these materials show a reduced strength [2, 10, 20]. Therefore, these zirconia materials do not offer a wider range of indication in comparison to high-strength glass-ceramics. They are suitable for single crown restorations and 3-unit FPDs up to the first premolar [1, 10].

The fourth generation of zirconia materials contains 4 mol% yttrium. Although this leads to a slight reduction in translucency compared to high-strength glass-ceramics, the mean flexural strength increases to 850–1,000 MPa [1, 2, 20–22] (Figure 2).

This modification results in 3 clinically relevant aspects: First of all, according to the manufacturers' information, these materials are suitable for the fabrication of anterior and molar single crowns and 3-unit FPDs, allowing for a restoration with FPDs to replace the first or second molar. Additionally, due to the increased strength of the material, the minimum material thickness can be reduced to 0.6–0.7 mm. The third clinically relevant advantage is the approval of this material group for temporary cementation [2, 20].

Summarizing these material properties, it is apparent that especially zirconia materials of the fourth generation are a meaningful addition to high-strength glass-ceramics in the chairside workflow, as they allow for a wider range of indications while offering a more minimal-invasive preparation.

In this combination, the main indications for the use of high-strength glass-ceramics are inlays, onlays, partial crowns, crowns, and veneers. Zirconia materials of the fourth generation should preferably be used for the fabrication of single crowns and 3-unit FPDs [1]. For the every-day chairside processing of zirconia materials in a dental practice, the processing time should be shortened to a single appointment. In this context, the following aspects are important:

(a) *Short Processing Times and Dry Processing to Avoid Drying Prior to Sintering*. As zirconia materials are processed in a presintered, chalk-like state, processing times of 5-6 minutes for a single crown can be achieved when using an appropriate milling unit (e.g., Primemill, Dentsply Sirona, Charlotte, USA) [23].

(b) The sintering period should be kept as short as possible. By choosing a speed-sintering program, it can be reduced to less than 20 minutes. In vitro studies show that speed-sintering does not have a negative influence on the material properties (hydrothermal aging behavior, Weibull characteristics, hardness, and translucency) of appropriate zirconia materials [8, 9, 24]

Ideally, individualization of the restoration should be finished in a single stain and glaze process. This can be achieved by using multilayer zirconia blocks. Pigmented

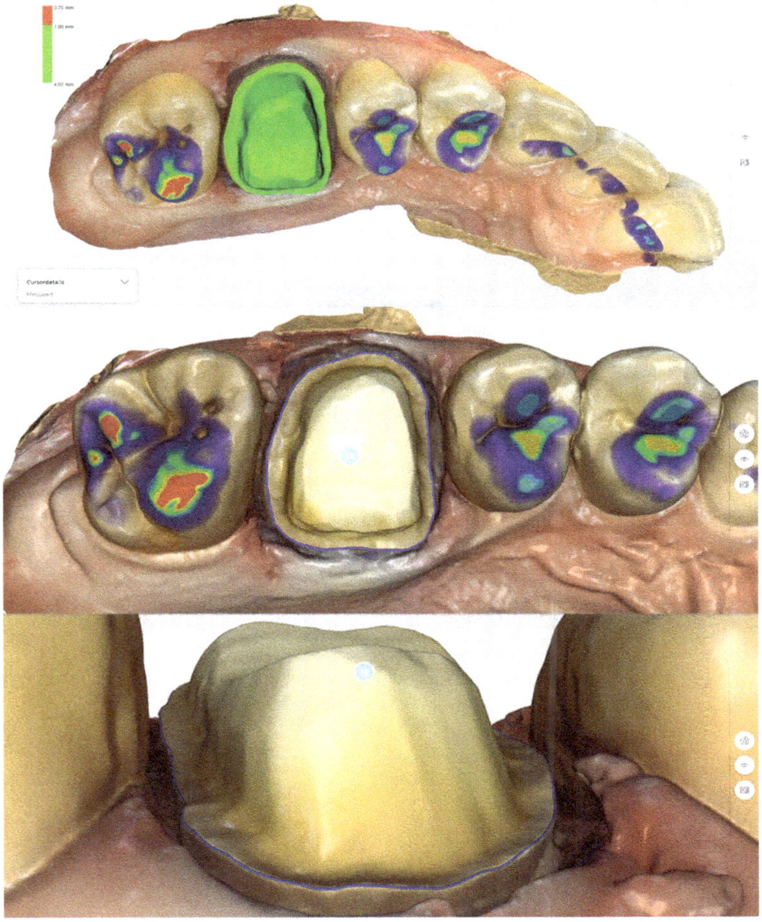

Figure 7: Analysis of preparation and determination of the preparation limit. The entire preparation limit is shown and can be detected automatically.

layers of varying intensities simulate the typical color gradient of a natural tooth. These multilayer zirconia blocks consist of 4–5 color layers in different pigmentations while showing similar translucencies [21]. In comparison with a single-color block, this integrated color gradient simplifies the individual characterization of the restoration significantly. In ideal circumstances, a multilayer material requires only one combined stain and glaze process to achieve an esthetically perfect result [25, 26].

Until now, the mechanical and optical properties, as well as the abrasion and fatigue behavior of multilayer translucent zirconia materials, have been evaluated in several in vitro studies [20, 26–28]. However, reports on clinical experiences are limited to case studies and reports with labside-fabricated restorations with observational periods up to 24 months [29, 30]. Clinical data for chairside-fabricated restorations from multilayer translucent zirconia materials are still sparse [23].

The present case report demonstrates the chairside fabrication of a monolithic single-tooth restoration by using a new multilayer zirconia material of the fourth generation (CEREC MTL Zirconia, Dentsply Sirona, Charlotte, USA) with the current version of the CEREC system (Primescan&-Primemill, Dentsply Sirona, Charlotte, USA).

2. Case Presentation

During a prophylaxis appointment, an insufficient composite restoration of an endodontically treated first upper molar was detected in a 31-year-old female patient (Figure 3). X-ray diagnostics revealed a sufficient endodontic treatment ad-apex without apical findings, thus allowing for a prosthodontic restoration.

After removing the existing restoration, the tooth was prepared and treated with an adhesive build-up (Clearfil DC core plus, Dentin, Kuraray Noritake Dental Inc., Tokyo, Japan).

The equigingival preparation limit was performed as a shoulder with rounded inner angle (Figure 4). The occlusal design was prepared with a rhombic instrument to achieve an aperture angle of 120–140° (Figure 5) [31, 32]. The axioocclusal line angles were rounded with the same instrument. The occlusal reduction was approximately 1 mm, and the cutting depth at the preparation limit was ranging from 0.8 to 1 mm. Thus, a minimum occlusal and axial material thickness of 0.8 mm was ensured.

Before digital impression taking, a retraction cord (Ultrapak Clean Cut, size 1, Ultradent Products, South Jordan, USA) was applied. In order to achieve maximum lateral

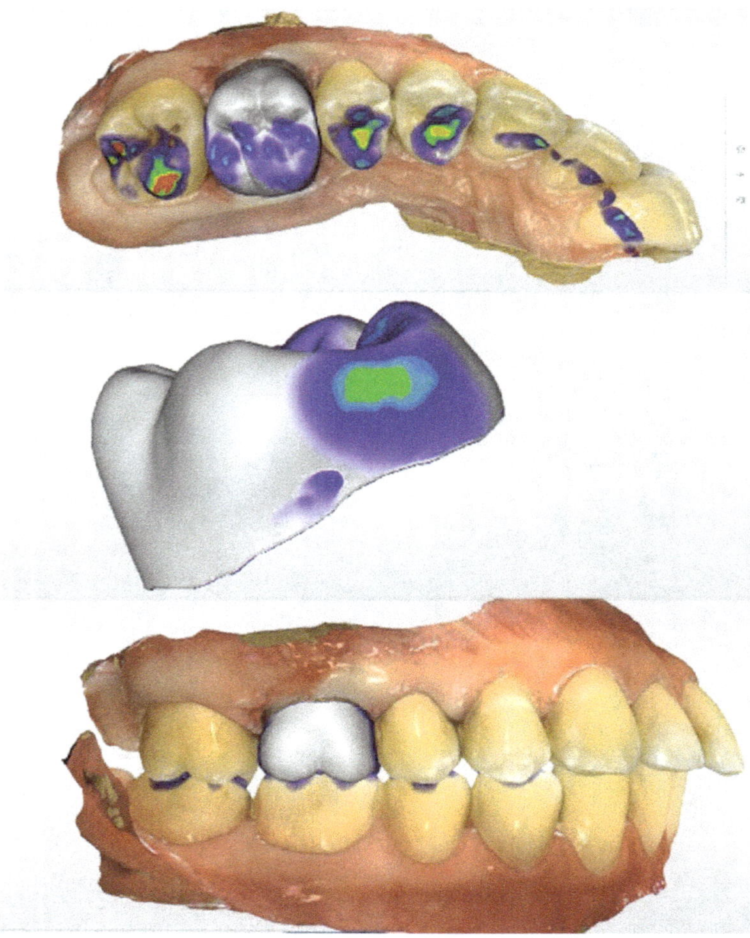

Figure 8: Virtual crown design (CEREC SW 5.2.2., Dentsply Sirona, Charlotte, USA). The occlusal contact points are reduced/built-up until they are depicted in turquoise. The design of the proximal contacts should be optimized to show light green areas.

soft tissue displacement, one layer of hemostatic cotton was placed as top layer (Figure 6). In addition, for a sufficient hemostasis and conditioning of the soft tissues, a compression cap (Roeko Comprecap, size 5, ColteneWhaledent, Cuyahoga Falls, USA) was applied. The patient was instructed to fix the cap by biting down. After a residence time of 10 minutes, the digital impression was taken (Table 1).

Immediately before intraoral scanning (CERECPrimescan AC, Dentsply Sirona, Charlotte, USA) of the preparation quadrant, the compression cap and hemostatic cotton were removed and the scanning area was gently air-dried. Throughout the scanning process, the retraction cord remained in situ. The application of hemostatic cotton caused a pronounced lateral extrusion of the soft tissues, allowing a very good reproduction of the preparation limit. Moreover, the construction software allows the automatic definition of the preparation limit. In the next step, data acquisition of the opposite jaw and a digital bite registration by lateral scanning were performed.

After the final data acquisition, the preparation was analyzed by construction software (CEREC SW 5.2.2, Dentsply Sirona, Charlotte, USA). The occlusal reduction was evaluated as sufficient, and no undercuts were detected (Figure 7). The automatically determined preparation limit could be transferred without modifications (Figure 7). A modification of the restoration design was only necessary by adjusting the occlusal and proximal contacts. As the zirconia restoration requires glazing during the fabrication process, the contacts should be designed as small areas (color of contact point: turquoise, Figure 8). The proximal contacts should be designed more distinct (color of contact point: light green, Figure 8), in order to ensure sufficient contact to the adjacent teeth. If the contacts are too tight, they can be easily adjusted with a diamond-coated polishing lens. A too weak proximal contact point would require comparatively more time for correction, as a new glaze firing is required in this case (Table 1).

In the next step, the vertical position of the restoration within the CEREC MTL Zirconia block was determined. Normally, the restoration is placed in the middle of the block, thus covering the entire color gradient [23, 29, 30]. In the present case, the adjacent teeth showed a pronounced portion of whitish enamel. In order to achieve a distinct visible incisal part, the restoration was placed approximately 1 mm below the surface of the block (Figure 9).

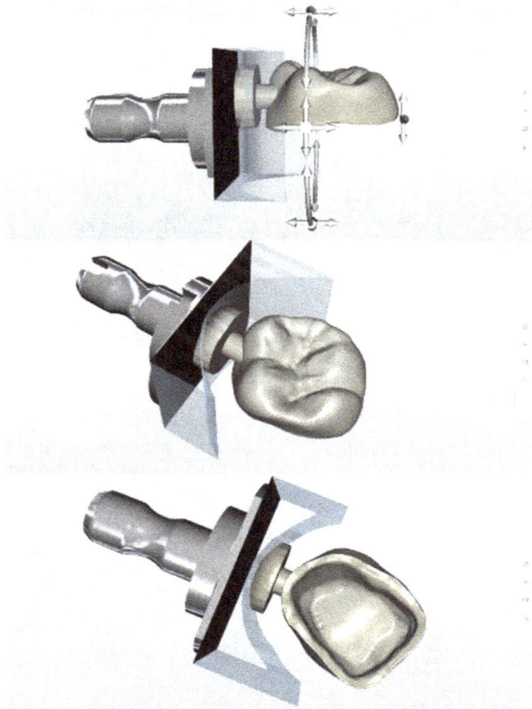

FIGURE 9: Vertical positioning of the restoration to determine the desired color gradient and the fixation area of the restoration.

The crown was fabricated in a dry-milling process (Primemill, Dentsply Sirona, Charlotte, USA) from a multilayer translucent zirconia block (CEREC MTL Zirconia mono, Dentsply Sirona, Charlotte, USA). For fabrication, the milling mode "fine" was selected and the settings for the occlusal and radial spacer were 120 μm (standard settings).

The restoration was milled from a block in color A3. This selection was based on the basic shade of the buccal surfaces of the adjacent teeth.

Apart from the mode "fine," a "superfast" milling mode is available. When using the superfast mode, a zirconia restoration can be dry-milled in 5 to 6 minutes. If this mode is chosen, it is essential to set the minimum material thickness parameter from 0.6 to 0.7 mm before processing. After milling, the retention pin of the crown was removed, and the connecting area was finished with a fine-grid diamond instrument (Figure 10).

Afterwards, the crown was densely sintered in an 18-minute speed-sintering process (CERECSpeedfire, Dentsply Sirona, Charlotte, USA). The CEREC software transferred all the information required for this process directly to the sintering unit (Table 1). If required, a try-in of the restoration is possible at this stage in order to check the occlusal and proximal contacts. The authors' experience shows that only corrections of the proximal contacts are required if the contact points are adjusted during the design process as described. These adjustments can be made after the final glazing of the crown without compromising the esthetic results by using a diamond-impregnated polyurethane polishing instrument for high-

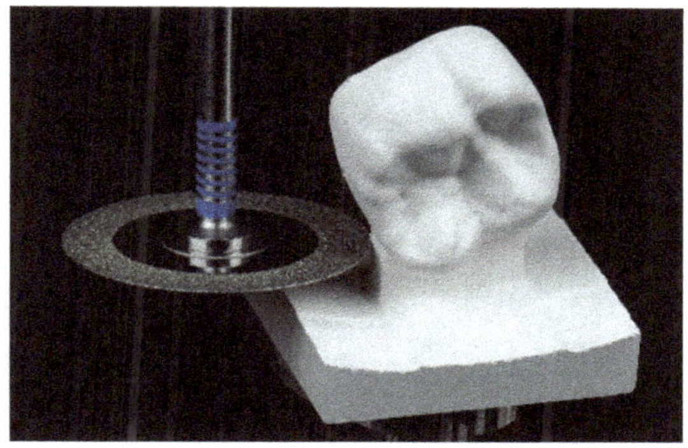

FIGURE 10: Milled restoration made of CEREC MTL Zirconia (Dentsply Sirona, Charlotte, USA). A diamond-coated separating disk is used to remove the retention pin.

strength ceramics (e.g., 94013C, Komet Dental, Lemgo, Germany). Therefore, in the present case, the authors forwent a try-in of the restoration and directly started the color characterization.

For this step, the entire external surface of the crown was covered with a transparent glazing (DS Universal Overglaze, Dentsply Sirona, Charlotte, USA). A layer of effect ceramic was applied to intensify the coloring of the cervical parts of the restoration (DS Universal Body Stain S1, Dentsply Sirona, Charlotte, USA) (Figure 11(a)). Finally, the fissures were color-characterized with a staining liquid (DS Universal Stain Mahogany, Dentsply Sirona, Charlotte, USA). To achieve the best results in coloring, a fine root canal instrument (e.g., reamers, ISO 010) is fit (Figure 11(b)). Finally, the cusp summits and cusp slopes were individualized. In the present case, the whitish parts of the adjacent teeth had to be mocked by a suitable staining liquid (DS Universal Incisal Stain I1, Dentsply Sirona, Charlotte, USA). After color application, the combined glaze-stain firing was performed at 760°C with a holding time of 2 minutes. The total processing time of the glazing was 9 minutes. Finally, the restoration was high-shine polished with a diamond polishing paste (Dura-Polish Dia, Shofu Inc., Kyoto, Japan).

In most cases, an esthetically optimized restoration can be fabricated with a colorless glazing material and 3 staining colors only (DS Body Stain S1, DS Incisal Stain S1, DS Mahogany, Dentsply Sirona, Charlotte, USA) in a single firing process, thus resulting in significantly shorter processing times. Afterwards, the individualized crown was tried in. An occlusal adjustment was not necessary. Only the proximal contacts were a little too tight; they were adjusted with a 2-step polishing system for high-strength ceramics. The contact point was slightly reduced with a prepolishing instrument (94020 C, Komet Dental, Lemgo, Germany) (Figure 12). In a second step, the revised areas were polished with a suitable instrument (94020F, Komet Dental, Lemgo, Germany).

The restoration was conditioned for the final cementation by air-abrading with fine-grained alumina (50 μm) at 0.1-0.2 MPa (Figure 13) and luted with a self-adhesive cement (Calibra Universal translucent, Dentsply Sirona,

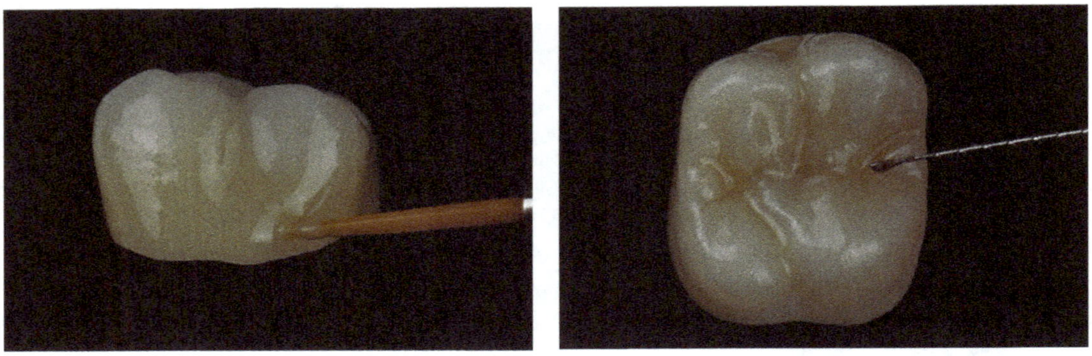

(a) (b)

FIGURE 11: (a) Individualization of the cervical part of the restoration (Dentsply Sirona Universal Stain, color: Body S1, Dentsply Sirona, Charlotte, USA). (b) Fissure characterization with Dentsply Sirona Universal Stain, color Mahogany. A manual endodontic instrument (ISO 015) is ideal for precise application.

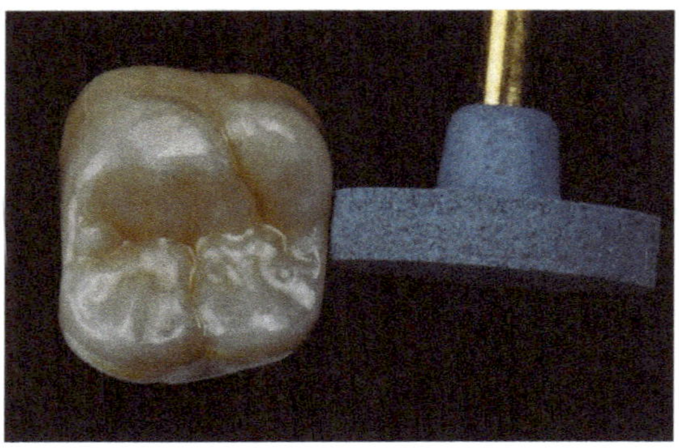

FIGURE 12: Adjustment of proximal contact points with a diamond-coated polyurethane polishing instrument.

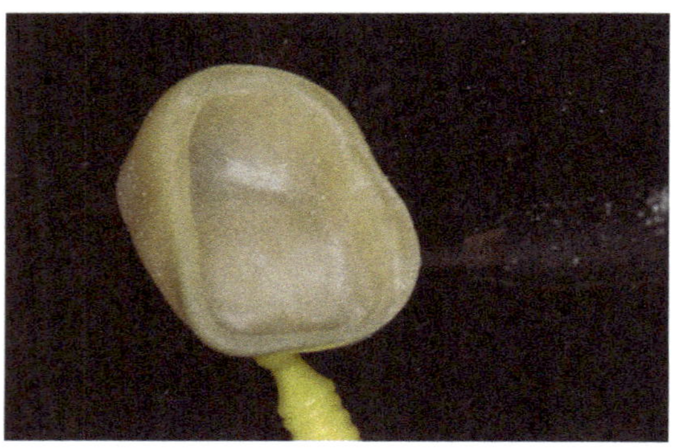

FIGURE 13: Prior to cementation, the internal surface of the crown is air-abraded with fine-particle-size alumina (<50 μm) at a pressure of 0.1–0.2 MPa.

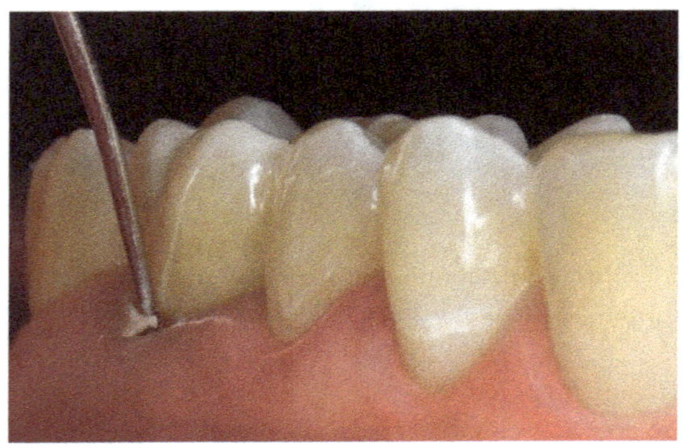

FIGURE 14: The comparatively easy removal of excess cement after a short-time light polymerization (2-3 seconds) is a clinically relevant advantage of self-adhesive cements.

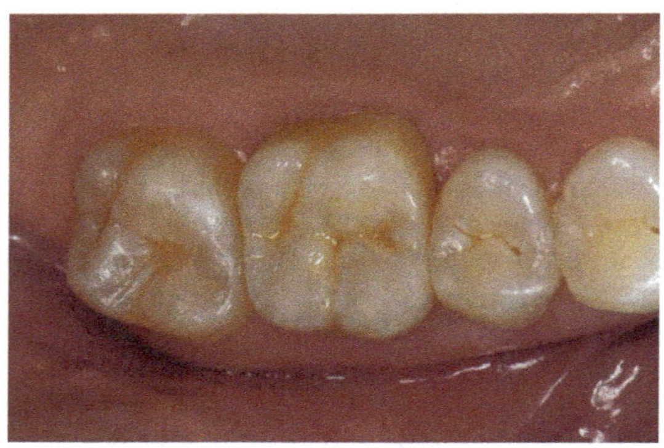

FIGURE 15: Occlusal view of the cemented monolithic zirconia crown.

Charlotte, USA). After a short prehardening of the excess cement (2-3 seconds per surface), the excess material was removed with a probe or a scaler (Figure 14). The final light-curing was performed for 40 seconds each, buccal, occlusal, and lingual. The restoration proved to be a good color match with the adjacent teeth, and the patient was very satisfied with the esthetic results of the treatment (Figures 15 and 16).

3. Discussion

This case report describes the chairside fabrication of a monolithic zirconia crown. This type of restoration can generally be fabricated in a single appointment. However, it should be considered that this process is related to some technical preconditions (superfast milling, speed-sintering process, and multilayer zirconia material) [1, 2, 8, 9].

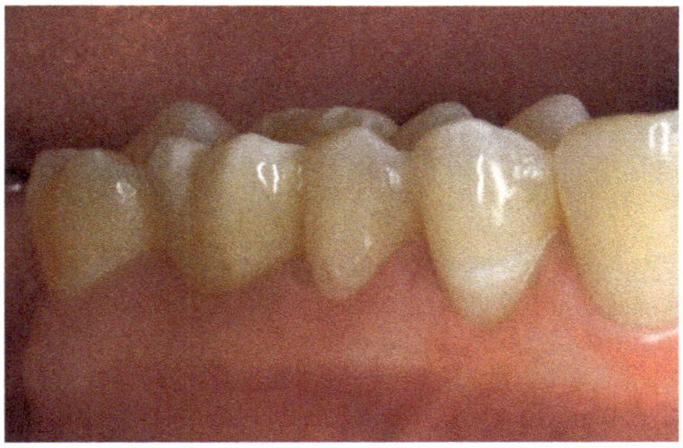

FIGURE 16: Lateral view of the final restoration 2 weeks after final insertion.

The use of a speed-sintering process is an important technical precondition. In the present case report, a special sintering oven for the CEREC system (CERECSpeedfire, Dentsply Sirona, Charlotte, USA) was used [2, 8]. Zirconia materials can only be speed-sintered while they are dry. This requires new equipment that allows for dry processing, e.g., the newer CEREC milling and grinding units (e.g., CEREC-Primemill, Dentsply Sirona, Charlotte, USA). If zirconia is grinded in a wet state, a 20-minute drying process is required before sintering [8, 9]. This prolongation is considered counterproductive in the chairside fabrication of dental restorations. The "superfast" mode of the CERECPrimemill leads to a significant reduction in grinding time. In this mode, a full crown restoration can be fabricated in 5-6 minutes [16, 23].

It has to be considered that speed-sintering is a relatively new processing technique. Several in vitro studies have demonstrated that for suitable zirconia materials, this cost- and time-effective processing technique has no negative influence on the mechanical and optical properties such a hardness, fracture toughness, Weibull characteristics, hydrothermal aging behavior, and translucencies [8, 9, 24, 27, 28]. Nevertheless, up to date some possible aspects on clinical relevant factors (e.g., biocompatibility) remain unclear [26, 30]. Using a multilayer zirconia material offers the advantage that the typical color gradient in teeth, from the cervix to the incisal area, is already integrated with the finally sintered restoration. This specific precoloring allows for an esthetically satisfying individualization in a combined stain and glaze firing—this is an essential feature in the chairside fabrication of dental restorations because it leads to a reduced processing time compared to single-color zirconia materials [13, 14, 26].

Due to the constant development of the design software, the current version (CEREC SW 5.2.2, Dentsply Sirona, Charlotte, USA) offers practical design proposals that mainly only need minor adjustments at the occlusal and proximal contact points [14]. This adds to the significant reduction in design process times [16].

With the procedures and materials presented in this case report, a monolithic zirconia crown can technically be fabricated in approximately 75-90 minutes. Compared to previous fabrication processes, this is a significant shortening of chairside processing times for zirconia restorations [16]. However, independent from the fabrication procedure, the individual aspects of material choice have to be considered. Above all, this applies to the color choice of the zirconia block. When using zirconia of the fourth generation, the color of the restoration might be influenced by the color of the prepared stump. As the translucency of the material increases with decreasing layer thickness, the risk of a shining-through of the stump must be addressed, especially in the cervical area. High-translucent ceramic materials have limited applicability for the restoration of discolored stumps [2, 17, 21, 26].

For optimal performance in molar restorations, it is helpful to choose the block color (CEREC MTL Zirconia) one shade darker than the tooth color if the restoration has a wall thickness of approximately 1 mm. This is based on the clinical experience that the sintered restorations were too light when the determined target shade was used. Although color adaptation was possible, it required a second stain firing. In contrast, when choosing a block in a darker shade, the correct color match could be obtained in one combined stain and glaze [2, 21, 23]. However, this standard of choosing a color should not be applied in restorations with thick walls, as the crowns appear darker with an increased wall thickness [2, 21]. In these cases, the restoration should be milled from the color that was determined to be the target shade.

According to the manufacturer, the minimum material thickness of multilayer zirconia of the fourth generation can be reduced to 0.6-0.7 mm due to the comparably high flexural strength (>850 MPa) compared to glass-ceramic materials. This would present a major advantage of this new material, as the minimum required wall thickness allows for a minimum-invasive preparation. Moreover, the strength of the material offers the option of temporary cementation, which is not possible for high-strength glass-ceramics and zirconia of the third generation [6, 12, 16].

Nevertheless, as it happens with other restorative esthetic materials, also the flexural resistance of zirconia frameworks could be altered by several factors over time (e.g., acidic environment or cyclic load) [33, 34]. These variables should be evaluated in future tests before a general recommendation of these reduced material thicknesses can be given.

Moreover, it is necessary to mention that the fabrication process presented in this report is based on comprehensive in vitro data [1, 16, 20, 21], whereas results from clinical studies are still not available. This represents a limitation of the present case report. Therefore, the manufacturer's instructions, especially regarding the indication range, the recommended preparation design, cementation, and technical processing parameters, must be carefully observed [2]. An alternative treatment option for the case presented would have been the chairside fabrication of a crown made from a high-strength glass-ceramics (e.g., IPS e.max CAD, Ivoclar Vivadent, Schaan, and Liechtenstein). This treatment alternative has the advantage of less prerequisites regarding the milling process and the postprocessing as no dry-milling or speed-sintering is necessary. On the other hand, the minimum material thickness for glass-ceramic restorations is slightly higher than for the multilayer zirconia, and a temporary luting of these restorations is not possible.

4. Conclusions

Overall, if the technical prerequisites (superfast dry-milling and speed-sintering processes) are given, the fabrication of a zirconia restoration can easily be performed in a dental practice. The use of a multilayer zirconia block of the fourth generation facilitates the process and allows for a time-saving esthetic individualization of the restoration.

References

[1] T. A. Sulaiman, "Materials in digital dentistry-a review," *Journal of Esthetic and Restorative Dentistry*, vol. 32, no. 2, pp. 171–181, 2020.

[2] E. Kontonasaki, A. E. Rigos, C. Ilia, and T. Istantsos, "Monolithic zirconia: an update to current knowledge. Optical properties, wear, and clinical performance," *Dental Journal*, vol. 7, no. 3, p. 90, 2019.

[3] B. E. Pjetursson, I. Sailer, A. Latyshev, K. Rabel, R. J. Kohal, and D. Karasan, "A systematic review and meta-analysis evaluating the survival, the failure, and the complication rates of veneered and monolithic all-ceramic implant-supported single crowns," *Clinical Oral Implants Research*, vol. 32, Suppl 21, pp. 254–288, 2021.

[4] C. I. M. B. Leitão, G. V. O. Fernandes, L. P. P. Azevedo, F. M. Araújo, H. Donato, and A. R. M. Correia, "Clinical performance of monolithic CAD/CAM tooth-supported zirconia restorations: systematic review and meta-analysis," *Journal of Prosthodontic Research*, 2021.

[5] M. F. Solá-Ruiz, M. Baixauli-López, A. Roig-Vanaclocha, J. Amengual-Lorenzo, and R. Agustín-Panadero, "Prospective study of monolithic zirconia crowns: clinical behavior and survival rate at a 5-year follow-up," *Journal of Prosthodontic Research*, vol. 65, no. 3, pp. 284–290, 2021.

[6] M. B. Blatz and J. Conejo, "The current state of chairside digital dentistry and materials," *Dental Clinics of North America*, vol. 63, no. 2, pp. 175–197, 2019.

[7] K. Baroudi and S. N. Ibraheem, "Assessment of chair-side computer-aided design and computer-aided manufacturing restorations: a review of the literature," *Journal of International Oral Health*, vol. 7, no. 4, pp. 96–104, 2015.

[8] J. U. Jansen, N. Lümkemann, I. Letz, R. Pfefferle, B. Sener, and B. Stawarczyk, "Impact of high-speed sintering on translucency, phase content, grain sizes, and flexural strength of 3Y-TZP and 4Y-TZP zirconia materials," *The Journal of Prosthetic Dentistry*, vol. 122, no. 4, pp. 396–403, 2019.

[9] F. Mayinger, R. Pfefferle, A. Reichert, and B. Stawarczyk, "Impact of high-speed sintering of three-unit 3Y-TZP and 4Y-TZP fixed dental prostheses on fracture load with and without artificial aging," *The International Journal of Prosthodontics*, vol. 34, no. 1, pp. 47–53, 2021.

[10] F. Zarone, M. I. Di Mauro, P. Ausiello, G. Ruggiero, and R. Sorrentino, "Current status on lithium disilicate and zirconia: a narrative review," *BMC Oral Health*, vol. 19, no. 1, p. 134, 2019.

[11] N. Bustamante-Hernández, J. M. Montiel-Company, C. Bellot-Arcís et al., "Clinical behavior of ceramic, hybrid and composite onlays. A systematic review and meta-analysis," *International Journal of Environmental Research and Public Health*, vol. 17, no. 20, 2020.

[12] A. Aziz, O. El-Mowafy, and S. Paredes, "Clinical outcomes of lithium disilicate glass-ceramic crowns fabricated with CAD/CAM technology: a systematic review," *Dental and Medical Problems*, vol. 57, no. 2, pp. 197–206, 2020.

[13] R. Kallala, M. H. Chaouch, K. Nasr, and T. Courset, "Step-by-step esthetic rehabilitation with chairside system," *Case Reports in Dentistry*, vol. 2021, Article ID 5558158, 6 pages, 2021.

[14] S. Rinke, A.-K. Pabel, M. Rödiger, and D. Ziebolz, "Chairside fabrication of an all-ceramic partial crown using a zirconia-reinforced lithium silicate ceramic," *Case Reports in Dentistry*, vol. 2016, Article ID 1354186, 7 pages, 2016.

[15] M. B. Blatz, M. Vonderheide, and J. Conejo, "The effect of resin bonding on long-term success of high-strength ceramics," *Journal of Dental Research*, vol. 97, no. 2, pp. 132–139, 2018.

[16] G. Marchesi, A. Camurri Piloni, V. Nicolin, G. Turco, and R. di Lenarda, "Chairside CAD/CAM materials: current trends of clinical uses," *Biology*, vol. 10, no. 11, 2021.

[17] P. Baldissara, V. F. Wandscher, A. M. E. Marchionatti, C. Parisi, C. Monaco, and L. Ciocca, "Translucency of IPS e.max and cubic zirconia monolithic crowns," *The Journal of Prosthetic Dentistry*, vol. 120, no. 2, pp. 269–275, 2018.

[18] A. Rauch, S. Reich, L. Dalchau, and O. Schierz, "Clinical survival of chair-side generated monolithic lithium disilicate crowns: 10-year results," *Clinical Oral Investigations*, vol. 22, no. 4, pp. 1763–1769, 2018.

[19] F. Le, H. Engqvist, and W. Xia, "Glass-ceramics in dentistry: a review," *Materials*, vol. 13, no. 5, 2020.

[20] E. Kontonasaki, P. Giasimakopoulos, and A. E. Rigos, "Strength and aging resistance of monolithic zirconia: an update to current knowledge," *Japanese Dental Science Review*, vol. 56, no. 1, pp. 1–23, 2020.

[21] S. M. Fathy, W. Al-Zordk, M. E. Grawish, and M. V. Swain, "Flexural strength and translucency characterization of aesthetic monolithic zirconia and relevance to clinical indications: a systematic review," *Dental Materials*, vol. 37, no. 4, pp. 711–730, 2021.

[22] G. K. R. Pereira, L. F. Guilardi, K. S. Dapieve, C. J. Kleverlaan, M. P. Rippe, and L. F. Valandro, "Mechanical reliability, fatigue strength and survival analysis of new polycrystalline translucent zirconia ceramics for monolithic restorations," *Journal of the Mechanical Behavior of Biomedical Materials*, vol. 85, pp. 57–65, 2018.

[23] M. J. Skramstad, "A new milling unit for an efficient workflow," *International Journal of Computerized Dentistry*, vol. 23, no. 1, pp. 83–91, 2020.

[24] E. Jerman, F. Wiedenmann, M. Eichberger, A. Reichert, and B. Stawarczyk, "Effect of high-speed sintering on the flexural strength of hydrothermal and thermo-mechanically aged zirconia materials," *Dental Materials*, vol. 36, no. 9, pp. 1144–1150, 2020.

[25] F. Tabatabaian, "Color aspect of monolithic zirconia restorations: a review of the literature," *Journal of Prosthodontics*, vol. 28, no. 3, pp. 276–287, 2019.

[26] N. Kolakarnprasert, M. R. Kaizer, D. K. Kim, and Y. Zhang, " New multi-layered zirconias: composition, microstructure and translucency," *Dental Materials*, vol. 35, no. 5, pp. 797–806, 2019.

[27] S. M. Cokic, J. Vleugels, B. van Meerbeek et al., "Mechanical properties, aging stability and translucency of speed-sintered zirconia for chairside restorations," *Dental Materials*, vol. 36, no. 7, pp. 959–972, 2020.

[28] H. Liu, M. Inokoshi, K. Nozaki et al., "Influence of high-speed sintering protocols on translucency, mechanical properties, microstructure, crystallography, and low-temperature degradation of highly translucent zirconia," *Dental Materials*, vol. 38, no. 2, pp. 451–468, 2022.

[29] S.-N. Yoon, J.-S. Han, I.-S. Yeo, and H. I. Yoon, "Full mouth rehabilitation of a severely worn dentition using intraoral scanner and the CAD/CAM double scanning technique," *Journal of Korean Academy of Prosthodontics*, vol. 58, no. 1, p. 67, 2020.

[30] M. Gseibat, P. Sevilla, C. Lopez-Suarez, V. Rodríguez, J. Peláez, and M. J. Suárez, "Prospective Clinical Evaluation of Posterior Third-Generation Monolithic Zirconia Crowns Fabricated with Complete Digital Workflow: Two-Year Follow-Up," *Materials*, vol. 15, no. 2, p. 672, 2022.

[31] M. O. Ahlers, G. Mörig, U. Blunck, J. Hajtó, L. Pröbster, and R. Frankenberger, "Guidelines for the preparation of CAD/CAM ceramic inlays and partial crowns," *International Journal of Computerized Dentistry*, vol. 12, no. 4, pp. 309–325, 2009.

[32] D. Edelhoff and M. O. Ahlers, "Occlusal onlays as a modern treatment concept for the reconstruction of severely worn occlusal surfaces," *Quintessence International*, vol. 49, no. 7, pp. 521–533, 2018.

[33] A. Scribante, M. Bollardi, M. Chiesa, C. Poggio, and M. Colombo, "Flexural properties and elastic modulus of different esthetic restorative materials: evaluation after exposure to acidic drink," *BioMed Research International*, vol. 2019, 2019.

[34] S. Kuroda, A. Shinya, P. K. Vallittu, Y. Nakasone, and A. Shinya, "Effect of water temperature on cyclic fatigue properties of glass-fiber-reinforced hybrid composite resin and its fracture pattern after flexural testing," *The Journal of Adhesive Dentistry*, vol. 15, no. 1, pp. 19–26, 2013.

13

B.P.F.C.® Bio-Plasma® with Pure Growth Factors (BioPlasma®) Used for the Treatment of a Persistent Great Periapical Lesion of an Endodontically Treated Tooth: A New Therapeutic Option

Raffaello Viganò,[1,2] Mirko Disconzi,[2] Edoardo Bertini,[2] Luca Viganò,[3] and Cinzia Casu[4]

[1]*DDS, Freelancer in Varese, Italy*
[2]*University of Milano, Milano, Italy*
[3]*Department of Oral Radiology, San Paolo Dental Building, University of Milano, Milano, Italy*
[4]*Private Dental Practice, Cagliari, Italy*

Correspondence should be addressed to Cinzia Casu; ginzia.85@hotmail.it

Academic Editor: Giuseppe Alessandro Scardina

The aim of this case report was to evaluate the efficacy of a new platelet-rich plasma preparation and its regenerative capacity of bone periapical tissue for the treatment of a very compromised endodontic treated tooth, with a periapical lesion of 1.5 cm in diameter, using a pure platelet concentrate. This is made without the use of anticoagulant or any type of activator, e.g., bovine thrombin, calcium chloride. For this reason, it has been called "Pure"; it is the B.P.F.C.® Bio-Plasma® with Pure Growth Factors (BioPlasma®) designed and developed by Dr. Raffaello Viganò. The patient has read and signed a written consent form. The study protocol was approved by the Ethics Committee for Human Studies, University of Varese. X-ray at 2 and 6 months and 4 years after endodontic surgery demonstrated the success of the treatment.

1. Introduction

Recent literature reviews have shown that the survival of endodontically treated teeth is very high. Some studies reported that the success rate for endodontic surgery is between 82 and 94%, and it is considered an effective treatment before the replacement by a single-tooth implant [1, 2]. The majority of teeth with adequate root fillings, adequate restorations, and included in a recall program remained functional and healthy for more than 20 years [3]. However, around 10% of the patients who had an endodontic surgery 10 years before develop periapical lesions, due to several factors like missed canals, age, treatment sessions, and density of root filling [1]. Periapical lesions consistently undermine the tooth retention, suggesting subsequent extraction of the element.

Platelet concentrates (PCs) are biological autologous products obtained after various processing of a whole blood sample, mostly through centrifugation, and consist mainly of great concentration of platelets and growth factors (GFs) [4, 5]. The objective of the processing is to separate the blood components in order to discard elements considered as not usable (mostly the red blood cells, heavy and easily separated) and to gather and concentrate the elements that may be used for therapeutic applications such as fibrinogen/fibrin, platelets, growth factors, leukocytes, and other forms of circulating cells, in solution in liquid plasma [5]. In short, these products are extracts of the blood circulating tissue. They are tissues themselves and not pharmaceutical preparations. PCs are used on a surgical or wounded site in order to stimulate, improve, and accelerate healing [5]. In all wounds, the coagulation of blood to form a fibrin/platelet clot and matrix is the initial step of the natural healing process. The use of platelet concentrates was designed to reinforce this natural process. With time, this concept of optimization of healing evolved to a more sophisticated concept of tissue regeneration promoted by the growth factors and the cells contained in these preparations [5].

In modern surgery, PCs seem to enhance bone and soft tissue healing in alveolar ridge augmentation, periodontal surgery, socket preservation, implant surgery, endodontic regeneration, sinus augmentation, bisphosphonate-related osteonecrosis of the jaw (BRONJ), osteoradionecrosis, closure of oro-antral communication (OAC), and oral ulcers [4].

There are two main types of PCs, platelet-rich plasma (PRP) and platelet-rich fibrin (PRF), that contain anticoagulant citrate and the activation takes place with calcium chloride [5, 6]. There are several subclassifications of them.

Leukocyte-poor platelet-rich plasma products are preparations without leukocytes and with a low-density fibrin network after activation.

Leukocyte- and platelet-rich plasma (L-PRP) products are preparations with leukocytes and with a low-density fibrin network after activation.

Leukocyte-poor platelet-rich fibrin products are preparations without leukocytes and with a high-density fibrin network.

Leukocyte- and platelet-rich fibrin (L-PRF) products are preparations with leukocytes and with a high-density fibrin network [5].

The PRF families had several applications in oral and maxillofacial surgery and, in general, are usable in other disciplines with interesting results, particularly for the treatment of skin wound ulcers [5].

This article proposes a case of very compromised tooth with a big periapical lesion treated with a pure platelet-rich plasma concentrate, used to regenerate the bone. The aim of the study is to report the regenerative ability of this platelet concentrate, called Bio-Plasma®, described for the first time by Dr. Raffaello Viganò [6], and to show its possible use as a bone healing promoter in those cases where the bone and soft tissues have undergone a resorption process.

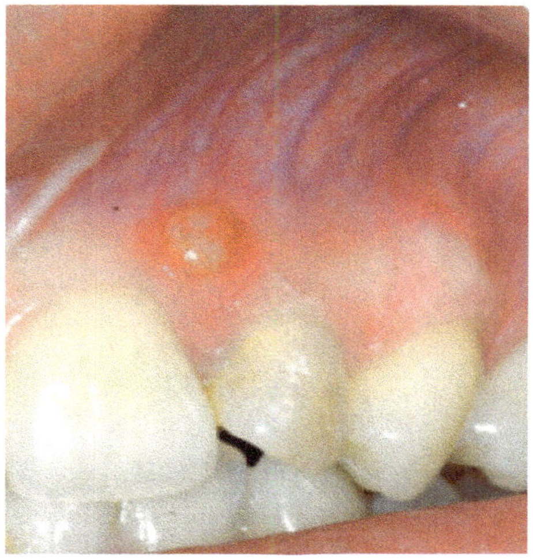

Figure 1: Starting clinical situation.

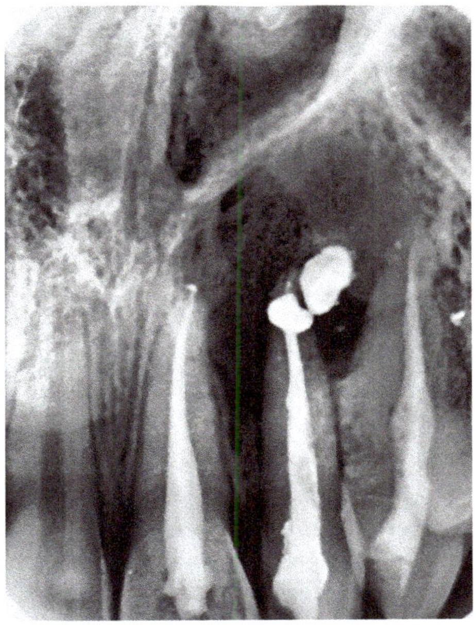

Figure 2: Starting X-ray.

2. Case Presentation

A 20-year-old female patient had come to our attention for the evaluation of the previously treated element 2.2. She reported good health without systemic disease. The patient was submitted 12 months earlier to an endodontic treatment because element 2.2 was necrotic. A local big trauma could be the reason of the necrosis, but the patient was asymptomatic at the time when the necrotic tooth was discovered. She presented a fistula in correspondence of tooth 2.2 (Figure 1), and with an X-ray, it was possible to see the previous endodontic treatment and a radiolucent lesion greater than 1.5 cm in diameter (Figure 2). A computed tomography was performed (Figure 3). A diagnosis of periapical lesion was made. It was decided to maintain the dental element through an endodontic retreatment of the element by endodontic surgery with the positioning of the B.P.F.C. product. The patient has read and signed a written consent form. The study protocol was approved by the Ethics Committee of the Circolo Macchi Foundation Hospital of Varese with deliberative act no. 53 dated 08/02/2013.

Endodontic retreatment was made with a retrograde endodontics. Local anesthesia was performed with mepivacaine with adrenaline 1 : 100,000, 1.8 ml with a 32 mm needle. A flap with 45 degree relief incision was performed. The incision was made with a number 15 blade. The flap produced had been carried out at partial thickness in order to ensure the greatest possible mobility (Figure 4). After removal of the inflammatory-infected material, a horizontal cut of the last 3 mm of the root apex had been performed with a diamond bur. K-files with sequence 15-20-25 taper 0.2 were used at first, then Pro file (Procad, Karlsruhe, Germany) from file 15 to file 40 (Figure 5). At the change of each instrument, irrigation with a solution of 5% sodium hypochlorite was performed. The root canal was closed with MTA (Dentsply Maillefer, Pennsylvania, USA) (Figure 6). After endodontic retreatment and curettage of the periapical site, the B.P.F.C. was prepared and inserted in the bone cavity.

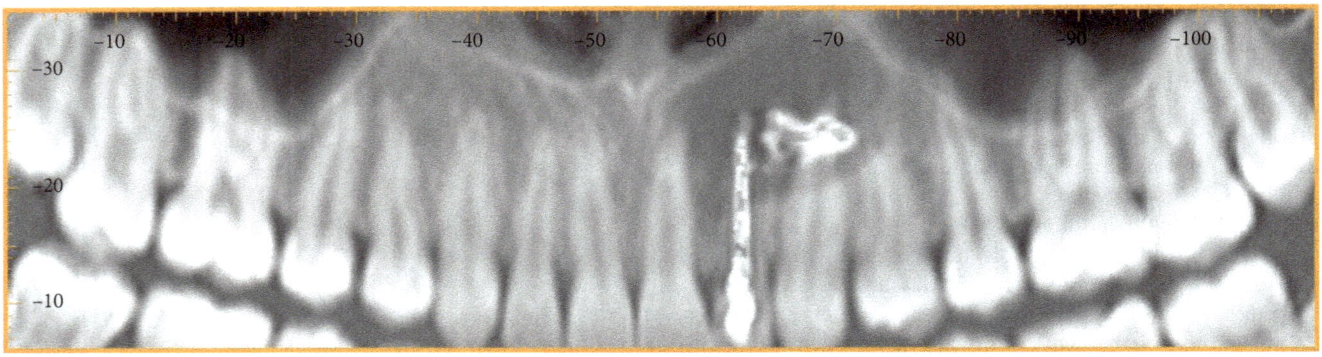

FIGURE 3: Starting CT.

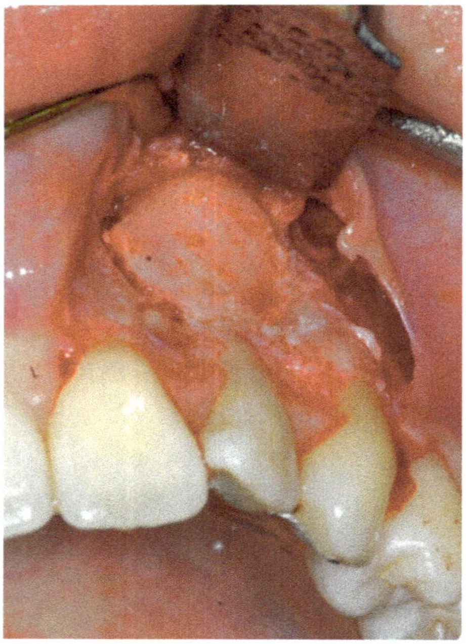

FIGURE 4: Preparation of the flap.

The phases of the protocol with B.P.F.C. were as follows:

(1) 54 ml blood was taken from the patient by venepuncture of the antecubital vein

(2) The blood was collected in 6 sterile Vacuette tubes (Greiner) with white cap; this indicates that they do not contain anticoagulant and/or subjected to any type of processing

(3) Fractionation of the blood material: take 3 cc with 4/5 aspirations with a 500 μl pipette and place the fraction obtained in the empty and numbered Vacuette. The protocol was provided for the elimination of leukocytes and red blood cells. This product was prepared with a special device designed and developed by Dr. Viganò

(4) Creation of a membrane with a mixture of fibrin and poor plasma (the protocol does not include the use of any activator such as calcium chloride and bovine thrombin to obtain gelation) (Figure 7)

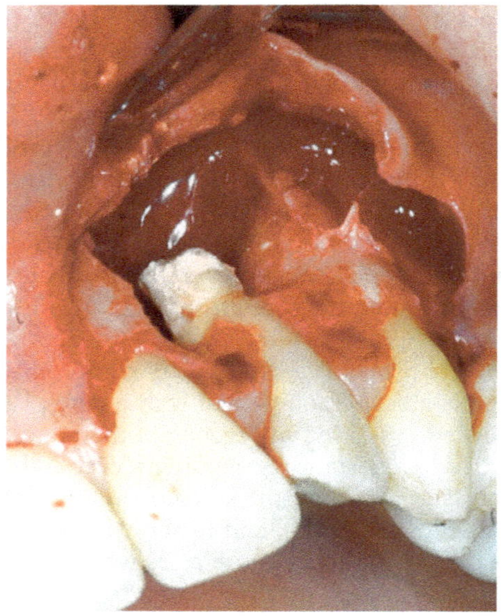

FIGURE 5: Endodontic surgery.

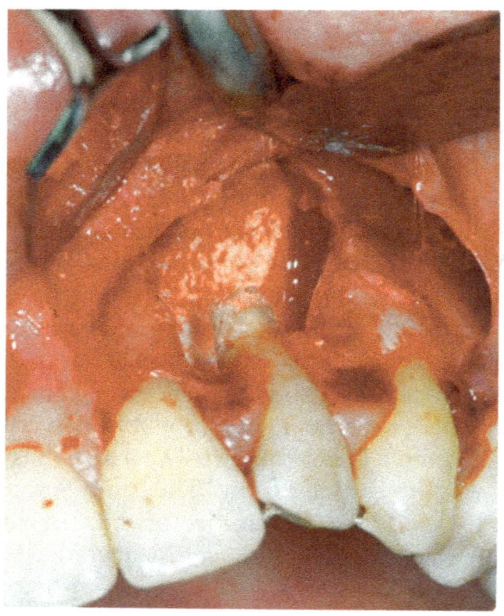

FIGURE 6: Bone curettage.

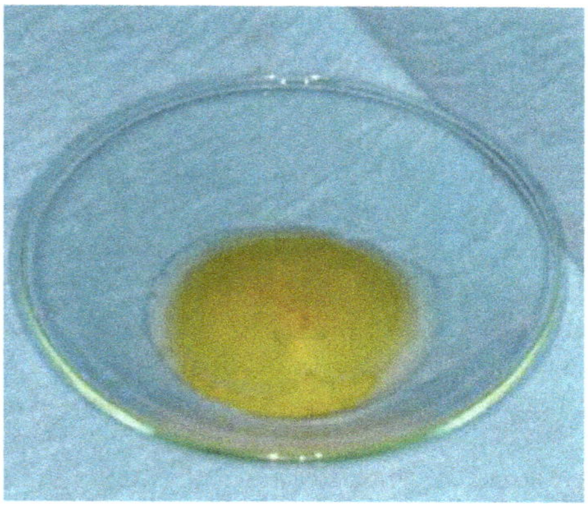

FIGURE 7: Membrane of a mixture of fibrin and poor plasma created.

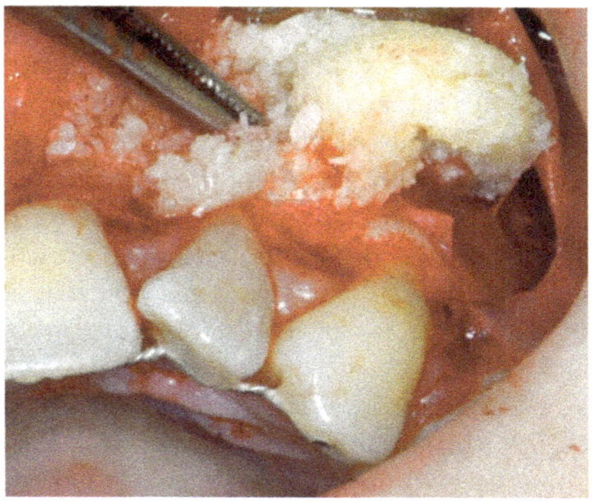

FIGURE 8: Positioning of the membrane.

(5) Preparation of rich gelled plasma and placement at the bone site (Figure 8)

(6) Positioning of the membrane above the rich plasma (Figure 9)

(7) Final suture (Vicryl wire 0000) (Figure 10)

It is important to underline that to prepare the membrane we need a minimum of 2 cc of fibrin. We had transferred the contents into a glass sterile container according to the quantity and size of the membrane to be obtained. This has to stand for 10-15 minutes on the thermostat at room temperature or 20-30 minutes without thermostat, before to place it. An X-ray was performed (Figure 11).

After 2 months, the apical lesion completely healed (Figure 12). Follow-up at 2 and 6 months and 4 years demonstrated the success of the treatment (Figures 13 and 14).

3. Discussion

Our case report showed that the Bio-Plasma® with Pure Growth Factors, inserted in the bone cavity after removal of periapical lesion, could be an interesting therapeutic proposal for very compromised retreated elements instead of implantology.

The therapeutic objective of utilizing growth factors in oral surgery is to improve upon the body's regenerative

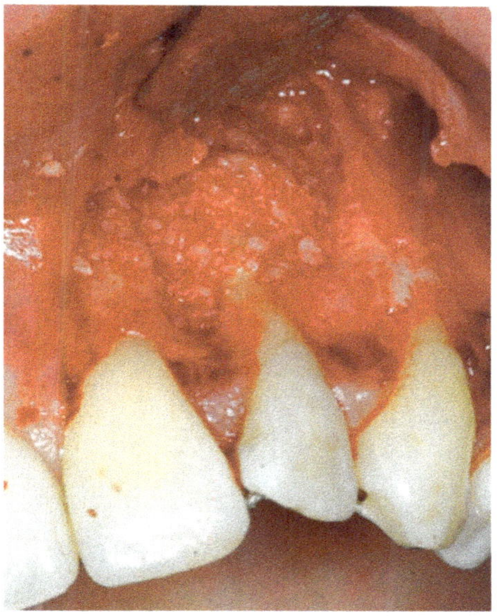

FIGURE 9: Membrane positioned.

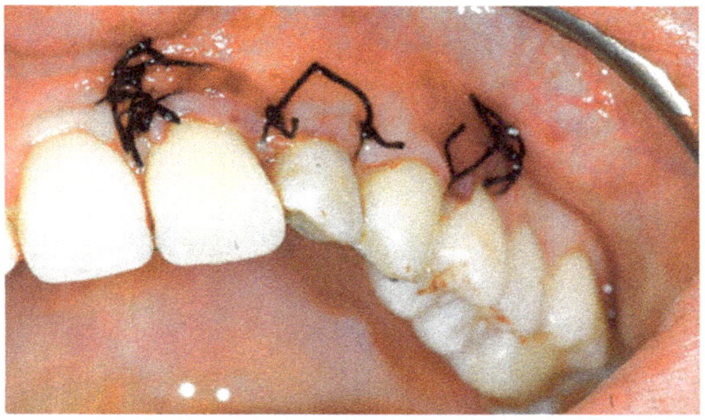

FIGURE 10: Final suture.

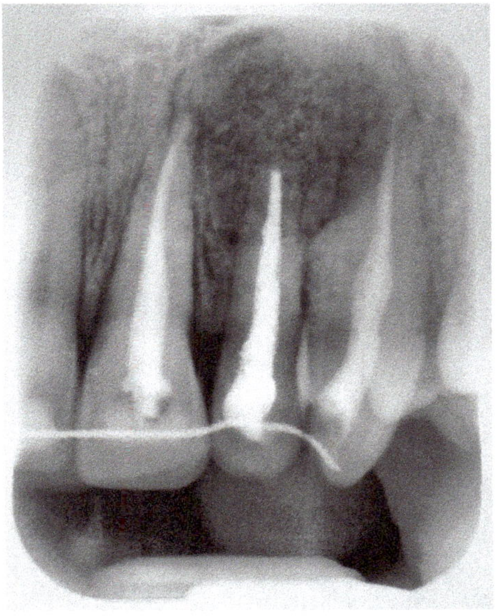

FIGURE 11: Postoperative X-ray.

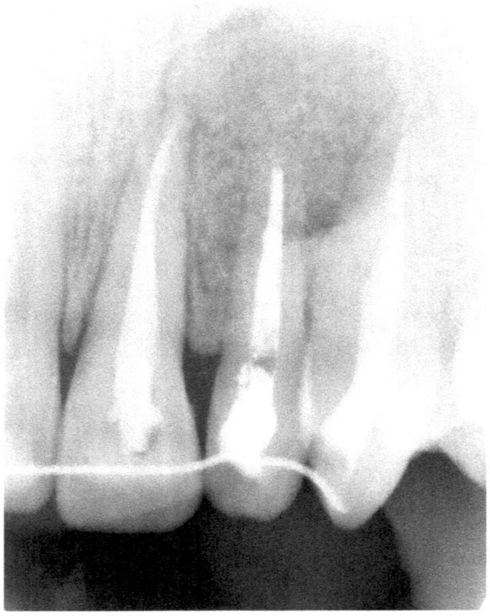

FIGURE 12: Healing after 3 months, clinical situation.

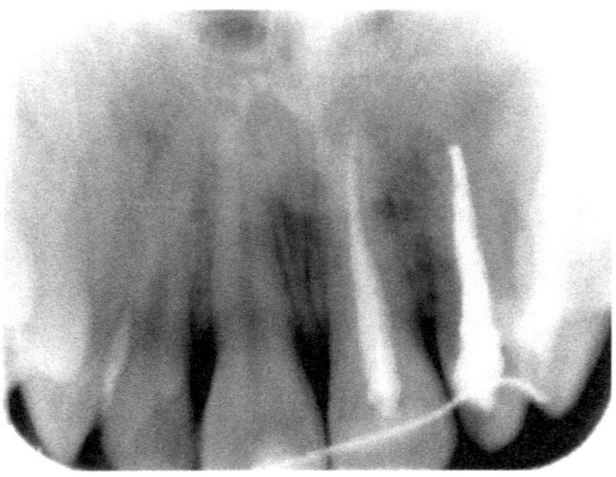

FIGURE 13: Healing at 6-month follow-up, X-ray.

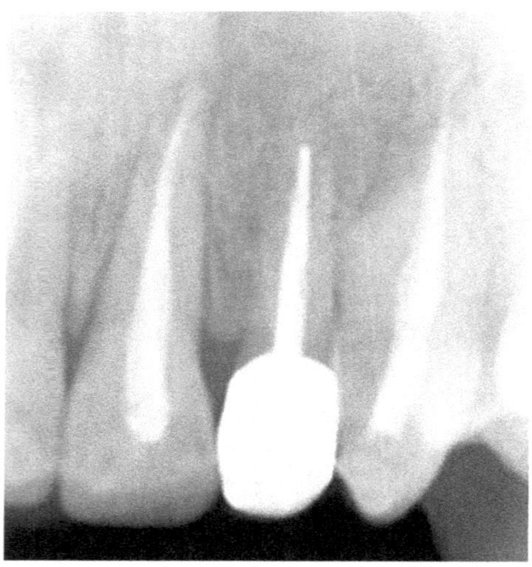

FIGURE 14: X-ray at 4-year follow-up.

capacity. In many situations, the unaided regeneration process is insufficient to allow complete repair of both bone and soft tissues [7].

With the advent of implantology, there is an increasing tendency to avoid dental retreatment of very complex elements and to prefer replacing it with a dental implant, but it is important to evaluate what are the prognoses of the two treatments (endodontics or implant surgery). The survival rate of dental implants varies from 91.8% to 100% after 1 to 10 years. No apparent differences on survival rates were noted depending on the time of placement. The quantitative synthesis of the success rate of zirconia implants was reported as 91.6% similar to that of titanium implants [8]. Sutter et al. in a very recent study (March 2020) reported that at the 1-year follow-up, 91.4% of the 81 teeth included in this retrospective study exhibited successful clinical and radiographic healing. They concluded that the type of tooth was significantly associated with the success of the surgery, but not other variables such as radiological severity of periapical inflammation, lesion histopathology, administration of antibiotics, smoker status, the quality of the root canal treatment, and preoperative pain and clinical signs of inflammation [9]. Alghamdi et al. in their review found that in previous works authors stressed that the healing of periapical lesions after endodontic surgery is faster than other surgery treatment, although it is very difficult to make a comparison with different works in the literature which report different follow-up times [10]. For this reason, the endodontic surgery seems better for our case. To improve the speed of healing of endodontic lesions, reduce postoperative symptoms, and improve bone quality, several researchers have tried to combine devices such as laser and photodynamic therapy with endodontic surgery, obtaining good results. However, there are still too few studies on these fascinating principals [11, 12].

The use of PRF to improve the healing of endodontic lesion was successfully documented in recent literature by Popowicz et al., with 2 case reports at 1-year follow up [13], and also by Goyal et al. with 3 case reports in a study in March 2020 [14]. However, in larger studies where the use of PRP was added to endodontic surgery, the difference in terms of bone quality compared to that of the control group was not statistically significant [15]. Betancourt et al. used other platelet derivatives for this purpose such as L-PRF on a case of severe endoperiodontal injury, in which there was an important improvement only from the periodontal point of view [16]. The long-term success of endodontic surgery is high, and it is currently preferable to tooth extraction and implant positioning. However, healing for damage greater than 1 cm takes several months [1, 2], while in our case it was already visible at 2 months. A good curettage of the residual bone cavity, the instrumentation, and the seal with MTA have certainly helped to determine an improvement in bone quality and speed of healing. The properties of the MTA are widely supported by several articles in the most recent review [17]. The limits of this protocol are related to the formation of a prepared team (assistant, nurse, etc.) and the patient's fear of needle. Several studies demonstrate how a well-trained staff is a strong predictable factor for the outcome of medical treatments [18].

Further clinical trials are needed to validate this starting result.

References

[1] R. Fernández, J. A. Cardona, D. Cadavid, L. G. Álvarez, and F. A. Restrepo, "Survival of endodontically treated roots/teeth based on periapical health and retention: a 10-year retrospective cohort study," *Journal of Endodontia*, vol. 43, no. 12, pp. 2001–2008, 2017.

[2] M. Torabinejad and S. N. White, "Endodontic treatment options after unsuccessful initial root canal treatment," *The Journal of the American Dental Association*, vol. 147, no. 3, pp. 214–220, 2016.

[3] C. Prati, C. Pirani, F. Zamparini, M. R. Gatto, and M. G. Gandolfi, "A 20-year historical prospective cohort study of root canal treatments. A multilevel analysis," *International Endodontic Journal*, vol. 51, no. 9, pp. 955–968, 2018.

[4] F. S. Al-Hamed, M. Mahri, H. Al-Waeli, J. Torres, Z. Badran, and F. Tamimi, "Regenerative effect of platelet concentrates in oral and craniofacial regeneration," *Frontiers in Cardiovascular Medicine*, vol. 6, p. 126, 2019.

[5] D. M. Dohan Ehrenfest, I. Andia, M. A. Zumstein, C. Q. Zhang, N. R. Pinto, and T. Bielecki, "Classification of platelet concentrates (platelet-rich plasma-PRP, platelet-rich fibrin-PRF) for topical and infiltrative use in orthopedic and sports medicine: current consensus, clinical implications and perspectives," *Muscles, Ligaments and Tendons Journal*, vol. 4, no. 1, pp. 3–9, 2014.

[6] R. Viganò, L. Viganò, and C. Casu, "B.P.F.C.® Bio-plasma® with pure growth factors (bioPlasma®) for the surgical treatment of patients at risk of maxillary osteonecrosis, related to bisphosphonates (BRONJ)," *Minerva Stomatologica*, vol. 67, Supplement 3, p. 25, 2018.

[7] T. Bielecki and D. M. Dohan Ehrenfest, "Platelet-rich plasma (PRP) and platelet-rich fibrin (PRF): surgical adjuvants, preparations for in situ regenerative medicine and tools for tissue engineering," *Current Pharmaceutical Biotechnology*, vol. 13, no. 7, pp. 1121–1130, 2012.

[8] K. I. Afrashtehfar and M. Del Fabbro, "Clinical performance of zirconia implants: a meta-review," *The Journal of Prosthetic Dentistry*, vol. 123, no. 3, pp. 419–426, 2020.

[9] E. Sutter, S. Valdec, D. Bichsel, D. Wiedemeier, M. Rücker, and B. Stadlinger, "Success rate 1 year after apical surgery: a retrospective analysis," *Oral and Maxillofacial Surgery*, vol. 24, no. 1, pp. 45–49, 2020.

[10] F. Alghamdi, A. J. Alhaddad, and S. Abuzinadah, "Healing of periapical lesions after surgical endodontic retreatment: a systematic review," *Cureus*, vol. 12, no. 2, article e6916, 2020.

[11] B. P. de Oliveira, A. C. Câmara, G. S. Ferreira, S. P. S. Neto, P. F. C. Silva, and C. M. Aguiar, "Photodynamic therapy: a novel ally for surgical endodontic treatment? Case report," *Journal of Lasers in Medical Sciences*, vol. 9, no. 4, pp. 288–290, 2018.

[12] R. Metin, U. Tatli, and B. Evlice, "Effects of low-level laser therapy on soft and hard tissue healing after endodontic surgery," *Lasers in Medical Science*, vol. 33, no. 8, pp. 1699–1706, 2018.

[13] W. Popowicz, A. Palatyńska-Ulatowska, and M. R. Kohli, "Targeted endodontic microsurgery: computed tomography-based guided stent approach with platelet-rich fibrin graft: a report of 2 cases," *Journal of Endodontia*, vol. 45, no. 12, pp. 1535–1542, 2019.

[14] L. Goyal, N. Gupta, and N. D. Gupta, "Autologous platelet-rich derivatives along with alloplastic bone substitute in the management of complex perio-endo cases," *Journal of Indian Society of Periodontology*, vol. 24, no. 2, pp. 182–185, 2020.

[15] N. B. Karan and B. Aricioğlu, "Assessment of bone healing after mineral trioxide aggregate and platelet-rich fibrin application in periapical lesions using cone-beam computed tomographic imaging," *Clinical Oral Investigations*, vol. 24, no. 2, pp. 1065–1072, 2020.

[16] P. Betancourt, R. Elgueta, and R. Fuentes, "Treatment of endo-periodontal lesion using leukocyte-platelet-rich fibrin. A case report," *Colombia Médica*, vol. 48, no. 4, pp. 204–207, 2017.

[17] K. Zafar, S. Jamal, and R. Ghafoor, "Bio-active cements-mineral trioxide aggregate based calcium silicate materials: a narrative review," *The Journal of the Pakistan Medical Association*, vol. 70, no. 3, pp. 497–504, 2020.

[18] A. Chércoles-Ruiz, A. Sánchez-Torres, and C. Gay-Escoda, "Endodontics, endodontic retreatment, and apical surgery versus tooth extraction and implant placement: a systematic review," *Journal of Endodontia*, vol. 43, no. 5, pp. 679–686, 2017.

14

Facial Line Angles: A Key to Tooth-like Rehabilitation

Rim Kallala,[1,2,3] **Yosra Gassara,**[2,3] **Ines Azouzi,**[2,4] **Amani Adli,**[2,3] **Dalenda Hadyaoui,**[2,3] **Zohra Nouira,**[2,3] **Chiraz Baccouche,**[1] **Soumaya Touzi,**[1,2] **Belhassen Harzallah,**[2,3] **and Mounir Cherif**[2,3]

[1]*University of Monastir, Faculty of dental Medicine, Department of dental anatomy, Monastir, Tunisia*
[2]*University of Monastir, Research Laboratory of Occlusodontics and Ceramic Prostheses LR16ES15, 5000 Monastir, Tunisia*
[3]*Department of Fixed Prosthodontics of the Dental Clinic of Monastir, Monastir, Tunisia*
[4]*Department of Fixed Prosthodontics of the Military Hospital of Instruction of Tunis, Tunis, Tunisia*

Correspondence should be addressed to Rim Kallala; dr.kallalarim@gmail.com

Academic Editor: Estella Musacchio

Recently, improvement of appearance and a quest for beauty have become a primary concern for patients. It is a challenging task for a clinician to achieve esthetic integration of prosthetic pieces for anterior teeth, particularly for highly demanding patients who give attention to particular details. The challenge is harder when only one tooth has to be restored. The objective is to achieve a fully and perfectly integrated rehabilitation with natural dentition. Poorly described, facial line angles are key to the success of achieving the desired tooth shape, especially for the maxillary central incisor. They influence both the shape and color of the tooth through optical illusion. Their misplacement could certainly spoil the esthetic outcome. Thus, it is mandatory to respect and recreate them. The objective of the present study was to define and then to highlight their importance. It also aimed to give some tips on how to perfect the shape of prosthetic teeth through a clinical case of central incisor esthetic rehabilitation.

1. Introduction

Recently, improvement of appearance and a quest for beauty have become a primary concern of patients. Esthetic dentistry is one of the most concerned fields by this vogue. The smile is a means of expression and communication. Having a perfect one is a purpose, nowadays [1]. For anterior teeth, it is a challenging task for a clinician to succeed esthetic integration of prosthetic pieces, particularly for highly demanding patients who give attention to particular details [1]. This challenge is harder when only one tooth has to be restored. Here, the purpose is to achieve unnoticed and unremarkable rehabilitation. Poorly described, facial line angles are key to the success of achieving the desired tooth shape [2], especially for the maxillary central incisor. Their misplacement could certainly spoil the esthetic outcome. Thus, it is mandatory to respect and recreate these lines during wax-up and prosthesis design [2]. The objective of the present paper was to define and then to highlight their importance. It also aimed to give some tips to perfect the shape of prosthetic teeth through a clinical case of central incisor esthetic rehabilitation.

2. Definition and Features

Line angles are defined as the lines that mark the transition from the buccal and lingual surface to the proximal one [2]. Each tooth exhibits four lines angles: mesiofacial, distofacial, mesiopalatal, and distopalatal.

From a morphological point of view, these lines are formed by the conjunction of the cervical line to the contact area [3]. They obey the symmetry rule in regard to a straight line on the contact zone [3]. Consequently, the mesial transition line is symmetrical in regard to the distal one of the proximal teeth [3] (Figure 1). Interacting with each other, line angles create both cervical and facial embrasures [3, 4].

According to Sesemann, a line angle is defined as the line at which two planes intersect [4]. Geographical size and

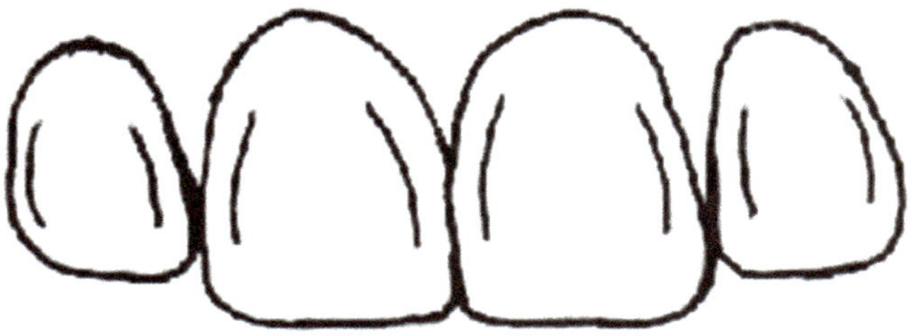

FIGURE 1: Facial Line angles symmetry with contralateral tooth.

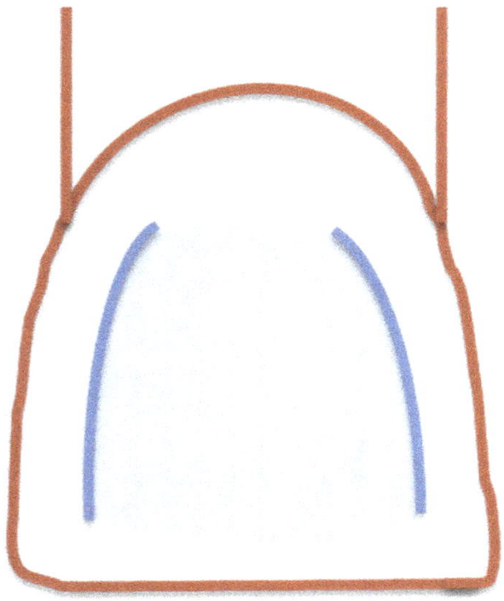

FIGURE 2: Tooth facial reflexive surface bounded by mesial and distal line angles.

magnitude of both reflexive and deflective surfaces are defined by the tooth line angle. Thus, the visual perception the tooth labial surface is significantly dependent on the teeth (Figure 2). When viewed from the frontal plane, both mesial and distal line angles are slightly curved, whereas, when viewed from the sagittal plane, they are straight [4].

3. Clinical Presentation

A 31-years-old healthy woman consulted the Fixed Prosthetic Department of the Clinical Dentistry of Monastir, Tunisia. The patient asked to replace her prosthetic upper-right central incisor. She was unsatisfied, especially with the shape of the tooth.

The intraoral examination showed that the crowned tooth exhibited triangular shape, while the contralateral one was oval (Figure 3). An evident over-contour, spoiling the smile, was responsible of the plaque retention at that area. Both edges were not aligned: the one of the left central incisor was irregular (Figure 3). The patient reported that her two incisors were fractured when she was young.

The first step was the crown removal. The loss of dental tissue was very important, and the abutment did not have enough walls to provide an adequate ferrule effect [5] (Figure 4). For this reason, the orthodontic extrusion was proposed to the patient [5]. Because of a lack of time, she refused this alternative. So, she was clearly informed that lack of a ferrule tooth structure may affect the abutment's strength resistance to fracture [5]. Thus, the metallic post and core was the most suitable solution due to its better fracture resistance than prefabricated glass fiber posts [6]. Once the informed consent to the treatment was obtained, it was carefully placed (Figure 5).

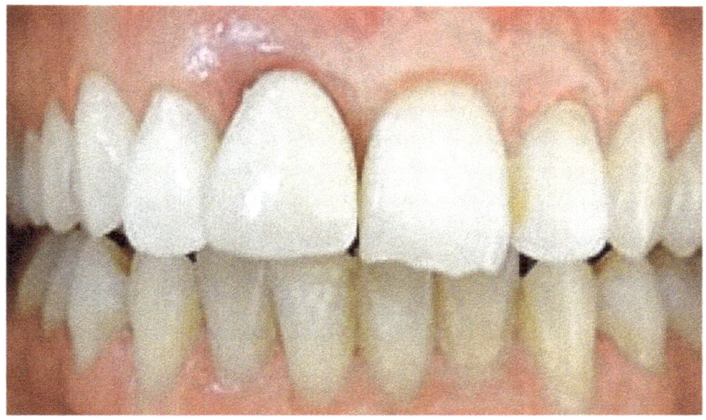

FIGURE 3: Initial situation: The upper right central incisor is crowned and displays triangular shape.

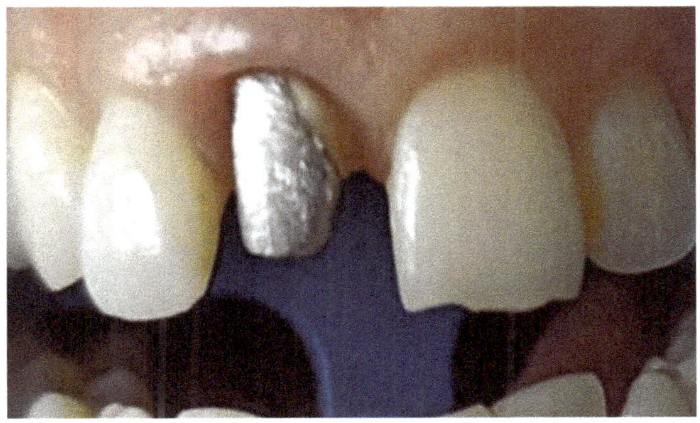

FIGURE 4: After the cementation of the metallic post and core.

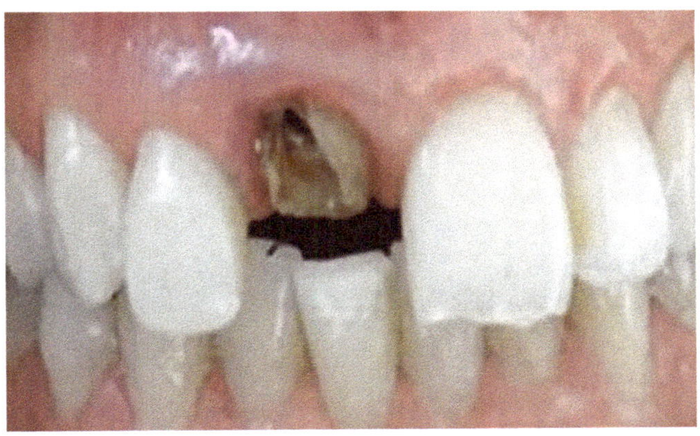

FIGURE 5: After the crown removal: dental tissue loss was subtotal and margins were deep.

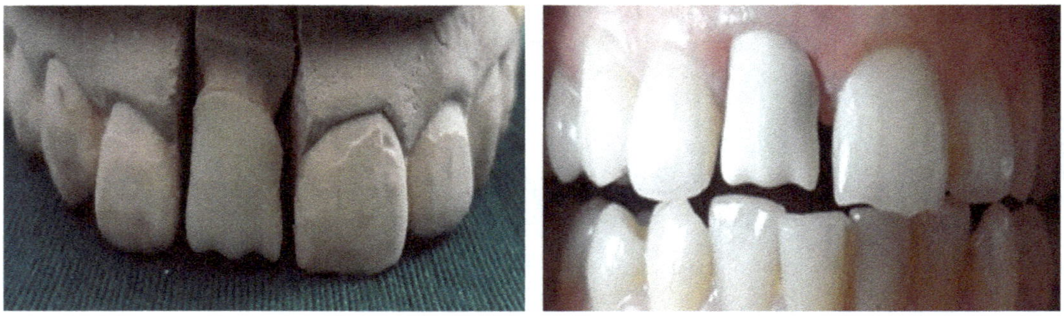

Figure 6: The checking of zirconia framework.

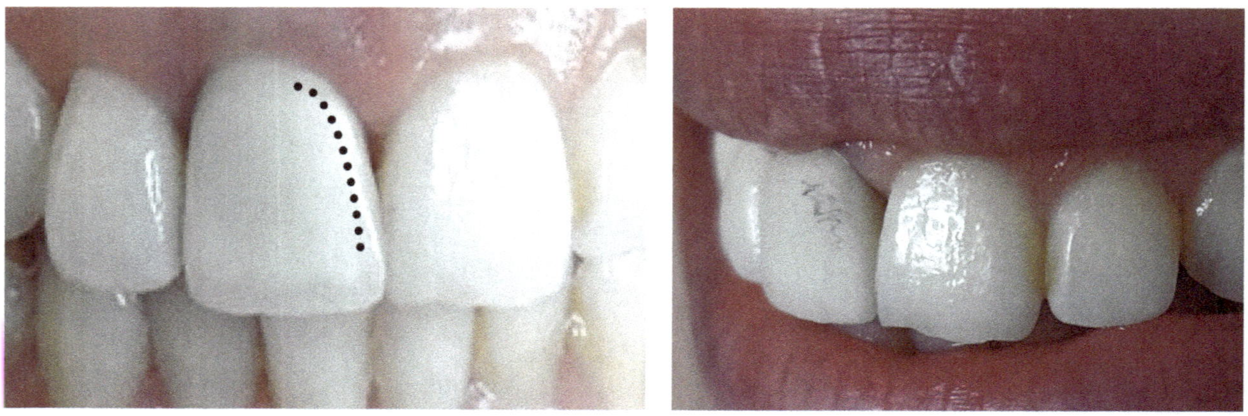

(a) (b)

Figure 7: The intra oral checking of the crown after ceramic stratification showing inappropriate mesial line angle (a) from the frontal view and (b) from the lateral view.

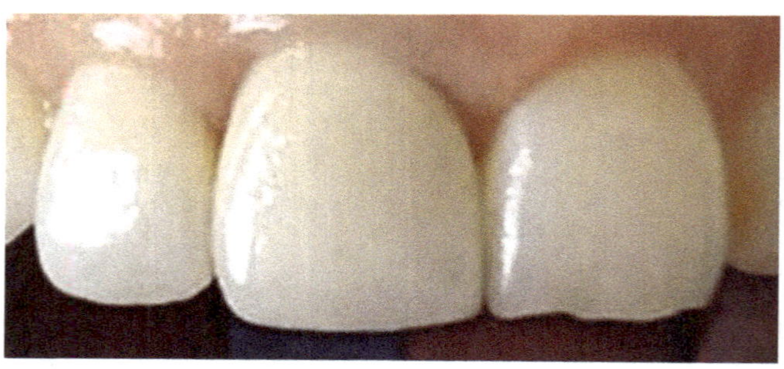

Figure 8: The shape improvement after line angle displacement.

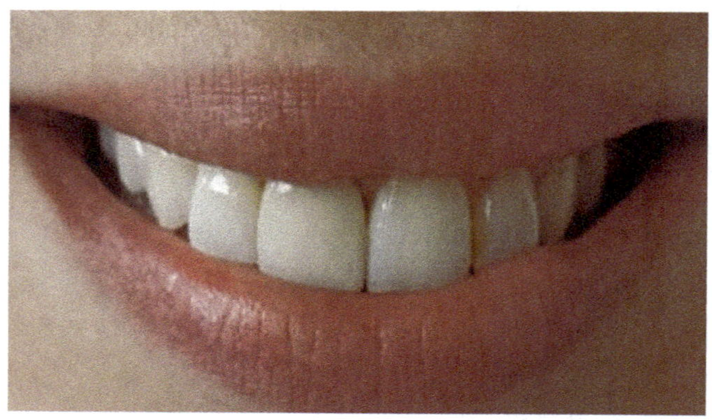

Figure 9: Final outcome showing unnoticed rehabilitation.

The zirconia material was chosen in order to hide the metallic post and core color.

The framework was checked, intraorally (Figure 6), and the space left for ceramic was validated (Figure 6). Then, it was sent to the laboratory to perform the ceramic stratification. Once received, the insertion and cervical adaptation of the prosthetic crown were checked. The tooth shape was also carefully evaluated. The crown shape was triangular compared with the oval homologue one. The mesial line angle was regulated, and the shape was optimized. As the patient was anxious about her teeth, the incisal edge of left central incisor was just regularized (Figures 7 and 8). After glazing, the esthetic outcome was pleasant and the patient was satisfied (Figure 9).

4. Discussion

The American Academy of Cosmetic Dentistry has included line angles among the 44th criterion used by accreditation examiners to assess clinical cases submission [4]. They emphasized the fact that facial morphology of prosthetic rehabilitation have to mimic, at most, the natural one.

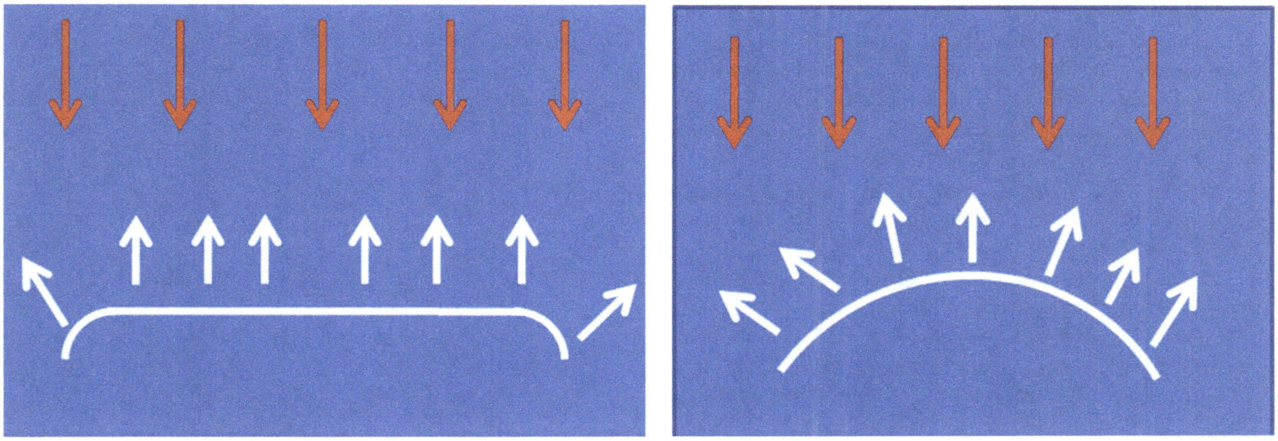

(a) (b)

Figure 10: The light incidence on tooth surface leading to optical illusion [10]. (a) Plate surface. (b) Rounded surface.

Authors consider that the tooth's perceived [7] dimensions are those measured between mesial and distal line angles, which is called the virtual width [7]. Others attributed them to the apparent tooth width, apparent face width, and perceived tooth width [7, 8]. Some others recommended the use of the distance between facial line angles as a tool to check the tooth size and symmetry [8].

Understanding the tooth morphology is considered the first key step to achieving esthetic integration. It is important to recognize that line angles are anatomical structures that provide the tooth shape, which is called the primary anatomy [9]. Their ignorance could lead to bulky shape and under-contoured proximal areas. That is why drawing them directly on the restoration seems to be useful (Figure 7).

Mainly, three shapes of maxillary central incisors are described: triangular, oval, and square. According to Paulo Monteiro [9], four guidelines are essential to define the tooth shape: the outline silhouette, lines angles or primary anatomy, macro texture or secondary anatomy and micro texture or tertiary anatomy.

Due to facial line angles, clinician could display on tooth dimension, and it is called illusion phenomenon [2, 4]. Thus, the area between them, when light strikes directly, is reflected back [2]. However, the outside area deflects less the light and consequently, it is less noticeable (Figure 10). This feature is used, generally, to increase or decrease the tooth width [10] (Figure 10).

The improper placement of facial line angles would make the restoration or the prostheses appear different, although it exhibited the same size of the contralateral tooth [2]. The closer the lines to the tooth's center are, the narrower the tooth appears, while the further the lines to the tooth's center are, the wider the tooth would appear [4, 7].

Also, rounded surface produces optical width reduction. However, plate surface increases it (Figure 10) [10].

Also, when tooth anatomy is not respected, the light deflection is different from the that of the contralateral tooth. Consequently, both the shade and shape would be inappropriate [4, 7].

Sesemann [4] has reported that the 20 square millimeters in smile design occurs between mesiofacial line angles of the central incisors at proximal contact area. He added that when they are bilaterally asymmetrical, the midline would appear canted even when it was perfectly parallel to the face midsagittal midface [4]. The reported case showed the midline discrepancy at the stage of ceramic trying (Figure 7a). The simple removal of the mesial line angle was sufficient to optimize the shape and to recreate a respected midline between central incisors (Figure 8).

The clinician has to carefully evaluate the tooth shape and line placement at the stage of ceramic trying. Embrasures and incisal edge, have to be checked as well. All these characteristics have to be checked from different views (Figure 7).

On the other hand, for fixed monolithic milled prostheses, the innovation of biogeneric model could solve such a problem. This innovative tool, based on mathematic algorithms, would give the ideal tooth morphology [11]. Various studies were conducted comparing the biogeneric tooth morphology with natural ones [11]. Others have compared them with wax done by a laboratory technician [12]. They affirmed the contribution of the biogeneric model in both morphology and occlusion improvement.

5. Conclusions

The tooth morphology understanding is the first step to the success of esthetic dentistry for both composite restoration and fixed prostheses. The placement of line angles is crucial to achieving a natural outcome. Respecting the symmetry is very useful. For milled restorations, the biogeneric model could facilitate their creation and respect. The clinician has to be wise and attentive to achieve the esthetic outcome [10].

References

[1] R. Kallala, S. Nasri, A. Adli et al., "Peg-shaped lateral incisors treated with ceramic three-quarter crown," *Case Reports in Dentistry*, vol. 2021, 5 pages, 2021.

[2] C. Wen, H. Ye, H. Chen, Y. Zhou, M. Huang, and Y. Sun, "Biometry of width between labial transitional line angles in anterior teeth: an observational study," *Journal of Advanced Prosthodontics*, vol. 14, no. 1, pp. 1–11, 2022.

[3] J. Romerowski and G. Bresson, *Anatomie dentaire fonctionnelle. Relations statiques*, CdP édit, Paris, 1988.

[4] M. R. Sesemann, "Understanding and providing appropriate line angles to optimize smile design restorations," *Journal of Cosmetic Dentistry*, vol. 33, no. 3, pp. 66–75, 2017.

[5] J. S. Mamoun, "On the ferrule effect and the biomechanical stability of teeth restored with cores, posts, and crowns," *European Journal of Dentistry*, vol. 8, no. 2, pp. 281–286, 2014.

[6] M. A. Gutiérrez, C. A. Guerrero, and P. A. Baldion, "Efficacy of CAD/CAM glass fiber posts for the restoration of endodontically treated teeth," *International Journal of Biomaterials*, vol. 2022, Article ID 8621835, 2022.

[7] G. O. Gallucci, P. Guex, D. Vinci, and U. C. Belser, "Achieving natural-looking morphology and surface textures in anterior ceramic fixed rehabilitations," *The International Journal of Periodontics & Restorative Dentistry*, vol. 27, no. 2, pp. 117–125, 2007.

[8] C. K. B. N. Scotti, M. M. Velo, G. S. Zabeu, L. S. Bueno, J. F. Bombonatti, and R. F. Mondelli, "Understanding the interaction of resin composite with light for predictable aesthetic results in anterior teeth: a case report," *Brazilian Dental Science*, vol. 21, no. 2, pp. 257–265, 2018.

[9] P. Monteiro, *Essential Shape: The Key to a Tooth-Like Restoration*, Styleitaliano, 2020.

[10] R. C. Rufenacht, *Principles of Esthetic Integration*, I. Co, Ed., Guintessence Publishing, Germany, 2000.

[11] M. Kollmuss, F. M. Jakob, H. G. Kirchner, N. Ilie, R. Hickel, and K. C. Huth, "Comparison of biogenerically reconstructed and waxed-up complete occlusal surfaces with respect to the original tooth morphology," *Clinical Oral Investigations*, vol. 17, no. 3, pp. 851–857, 2013.

[12] C. Ellerbrock and B. Kordass, "Comparison of computer generated occlusal surfaces with functionally waxed-on surfaces," *International Journal of Computerized Dentistry*, vol. 14, no. 1, pp. 23–31, 2011.

15

Postextractive Alveolar Ridge Preservation using L-PRF: Clinical and Histological Evaluation

Giorgio Serafini,[1] **Marco Lollobrigida**,[1] **Lorenzo Fortunato**,[1] **Giulia Mazzucchi**,[1] **Luca Lamazza**,[1] **Dario Di Nardo**,[1] **Iole Vozza**,[1] **Mara Riminucci**,[2] **and Alberto De Biase**[1]

[1]*Department of Oral and Maxillo Facial Sciences, "Sapienza" University of Rome, Italy*
[2]*Department of Molecular Medicine, "Sapienza" University of Rome, Italy*

Correspondence should be addressed to Giorgio Serafini; giorgio.serafini@uniroma1.it

Academic Editor: Kevin Seymour

Leukocyte- and platelet-rich fibrin (L-PRF) is an autologous platelet concentrate rich in growth factors and plasma proteins, obtained by centrifugation of patient whole blood, and widely used in oral surgery. This report describes a case of alveolar ridge preservation with L-PRF membranes. Postextractive alveolar healing was then assessed through a histologic and histomorphometric analysis. A patient requiring tooth extraction and subsequent implant rehabilitation was treated with simple extraction and socket filling with L-PRF membranes. Implant placement was performed at 3 months, and a bone biopsy was obtained for histomorphometric analysis. Histological examination of the grafted sites showed that the use of L-PRF could achieve good results in terms of bone dimension and quality and soft tissue healing. The results of this study support the use of L-PRF membranes to preserve hard and soft tissues after tooth extraction.

1. Introduction

Several techniques have been described in the literature to maintain alveolar bone volume after tooth extraction and facilitate subsequent restorative procedures with endosseous implants.

Tooth extractions are common dental procedures used to remove decayed, damaged, or periodontally compromised teeth. Though associated with few adverse effects, most tooth extractions result in alveolar atrophy due to bone resorption and soft tissue remodeling. The most relevant alterations occur during the first three months after tooth loss, in particular in the buccal plate where bone is generally thinner. In a systematic review, Tan et al. [1] reported a 29-63% of horizontal and 11-22% of vertical bone loss during the first 6 months after tooth extraction without a ridge preservation technique. As a result, these volumetric changes often require bone augmentation techniques for correct implant placement.

Several techniques have been proposed to reduce bone resorption after tooth extraction. In particular, several bone substitutes (autografts, allografts, xenografts, or alloplastic materials) have been tested combined with resorbable or nonresorbable membranes [2, 3]. A recent systematic review [4] reported xenografts as the most beneficial for ridge preservation due to their resorption rate, followed by allografts and alloplastic materials when compared to natural healing. Though graft materials can reduce alveolar bone resorption, grafted sites often have poor vascularization and nonvital residual particles can negatively affect the bone to implant contact [5]. Furthermore, the exposure of resorbable or nonresorbable membranes, often used in combination with bone substitutes, could compromise bone regeneration and wound healing [6]. Finally, the high costs often limit the use of biomaterials in the clinical practice. In this context, autografts may represent an alternative but involve donor site morbidity and a rapid resorption [7].

New biologically active materials have been developed to overcome the disadvantages of conventional bone substitutes. These include first- and second-generation platelet concentrates, respectively, platelet-rich plasma (PRP) gel and leukocyte- and platelet-rich fibrin (L-PRF). L-PRF was

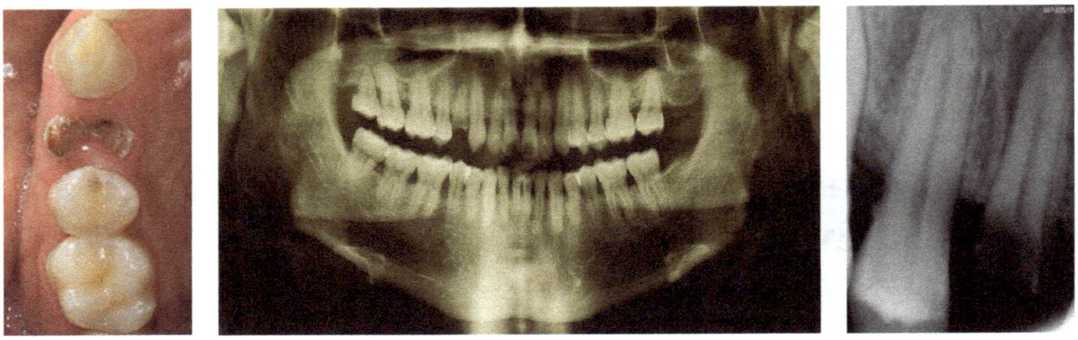

(a) (b) (c)

FIGURE 1: (a) Preoperative occlusal view; (b) orthopantomography; (c) preoperative periapical radiograph.

described for the first time in France by Dohan et al. in 2006 [8] and includes both fibrin clots and liquid components [9]. L-PRF is obtained by centrifugation of patient whole blood without the addition of any additive or anticoagulants, like thrombin, calcium chloride, or EDTA. Once the clot is separated from the supernatant (Platelet Poor Plasma, PPP) and the red blood cells (Red Corpuscle Base, RCBs), it can be compressed into membranes. L-PRF membranes are composed of a dense, high cross-linked, fibrin mesh in which are embedded platelets and leucocytes. This biological scaffold releases growth factors (particularly, PDGF-AB, TGF-β, and VEGF), adhesion molecules (fibronectin, vitronectin, and thrombospondin-1), and pro- and anti-inflammatory cytokines, for up to 7 days [10, 11], which modulate reparative inflammatory process; increase tissue regeneration, angiogenesis, and neovascularization; and reduce postoperative pain and edema [12]. These characteristics make L-PRF suitable as grafting material for postextraction sockets, especially considering the modest costs, simple preparation, and no risk for cross infections. The aim of this study was then to report a case of postextraction socket grafted with L-PRF membranes through a clinical and radiographic evaluation after a 3-month healing period.

2. Case Report

A 35-year-old nonsmoker systemically healthy patient was referred to the Unit of Oral Surgery of the Department of Oral and Maxillo Facial Sciences, Sapienza University of Rome (Italy).

The intraoral exam revealed a nonrestorable carious lesion in the upper right first premolar (Figure 1(a)), confirmed with orthopantomography (Figure 1(b)) and periapical radiograph performed with Rinn holder (Figure 1(c)), in which a periapical periodontitis was highlighted. Before proceeding with tooth extraction, alternative therapeutic solutions, such as orthodontic extrusion or crown lengthening followed by endodontic therapy and prosthetic rehabilitation, were explained to the patient. Considering the advantages and disadvantages of these therapies, in agreement with the patient, the treatment plan included tooth extraction and socket grafting with L-PRF membranes from blood centrifugation, followed by a single unit implant rehabilitation.

The patient was treated in accordance with the Declaration of Helsinki of 1975, as revised in 2013, according to a specific protocol approved by the Ethics Committee for Human Research of Sapienza University of Rome (approval number: 981/17). A written informed consent was obtained from the patient before the treatment.

Seven days before tooth extraction, the patient was undergone scaling and root planing and trained to correct hygiene procedures.

On the day of the surgery, blood samples were collected from the patient in four tubes of 9 mL for a few minutes and immediately centrifuged. Centrifugation (Intra-Spin L-PRF kit, Intra-Lock® International Inc., Boca-Raton, Florida, USA) was performed for 12 minutes at 2700 rpm. Tubes did not contain any additive or anticoagulants. After centrifugation, L-PRF clots were collected from each tube and separated from the red thrombus (composed of red cells), obtaining a fibrin clot with a small red portion in order to include the intermediate portion rich in leucocytes and platelets [13]. L-PRF clots were then placed in a sterile box and slightly compressed for about 5 minutes under a stainless steel plate to form 4 membranes (Figures 2(a) and 2(b)).

Before surgery, the patient rinsed with 0.20% chlorhexidine for 1 minute and local anesthesia (2% mepivacaine with 1 : 100000 adrenaline) was administered. Atraumatic extraction was performed using a piezoelectric device (Piezosurgery®, Mectron, Genova, Italy) to preserve the buccal bone and avoid soft tissue laceration, followed by alveolar debridement and irrigation with sterile saline solution (Figure 2(c)). After tooth extraction, the buccal and palatal bone walls were both preserved. The patient had a thick biotype with a keratinized tissue width of 3 mm and buccal bone thickness of 1 mm. All the measures were recorded with a PCP-15-UNC probe (Hu-Friedy, Chicago, IL, USA). The socket was then filled with three L-PRF membranes previously folded and condensed with a sterile gauze (Figure 2(d)). Finally, one membrane folded in triple layer was placed to cover the socket. Soft tissues were sutured (4/0 nylon suture, 20 mm needle) at the mesial, median, and distal aspects of the socket, without primary closure (Figure 2(e)).

The patient was prescribed an analgesic/anti-inflammatory therapy (ketoprofen 100 mg or acetaminophen 1000 mg as needed), antiseptic mouth rinses (0.20% chlorhexidine

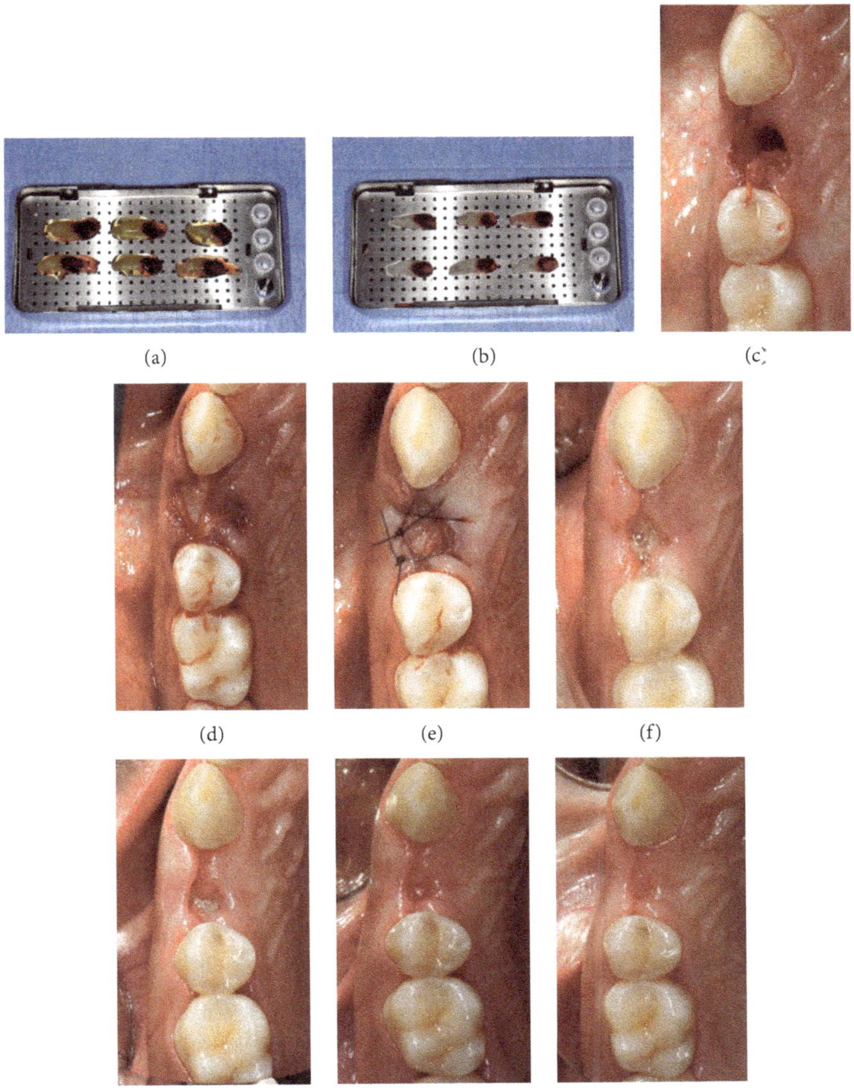

(a) (b) (c) (d) (e) (f) (g) (h) (i)

FIGURE 2: (a) L-PRF clots placed on a plate; (b) L-PRF membranes; (c) postextractive socket; (d) socket grafted with L-PRF membranes; (e) suture; (f) suture removal; (g) 14 days after tooth extraction; (h) 28 days after tooth extraction; (i) 60 days after tooth extraction.

twice daily for 7 days), and postoperative recommendations. The patient was advised to follow a soft and liquid diet, avoiding smoking and hot food for the following hours.

Sutures were removed at 7 days (Figure 2(f)), and the patient underwent a follow-up (14 days, 28 days, and 60 days) monitoring the wound healing (Figures 2(g)–2(i)).

Three periodontal indices (Plaque Index, PI; Gingival Index, GI; and Bleeding on Probing, BoP) were recorded on both the tooth to be extracted and the adjacent teeth the day of the surgery, at 14 days, 28 days, and 3 months in order to monitor the periodontal health conditions at the grafted site and adjacent teeth. According to Silness and Löe, PI was measured at 4 points (buccal, mesial, distal, and palatal) for each tooth [14]. According to Löe and Silness, GI was recorded to assess gingival inflammation through a visual evaluation with a value from 0 (healthy gum) to 3 (obvious inflammation and spontaneous bleeding) [15]. BoP (present or absent) was measured at 4 points (buccal, mesial, distal, and palatal) for each tooth [16]. After tooth extraction and before implant placement, the ridge width was measured at the median points of the alveolar crest in the buccal-palatal direction. A PCP-15-UNC probe was used for recording both alveolar and periodontal parameters. Alveolar ridge width in the buccal-palatal direction was 8 mm immediately after extraction and 7 mm at 3 months showing a minimal reduction. The numerical reduction in periodontal indices during the follow-up indicates a reduction of gingival inflammation (Table 1), which can be explained with an increased compliance of the patient with postoperative hygiene instructions and, as for the 14-dayfollow-up, possibly also due to the antimicrobial action of leukocytes.

After 3 months, before implant placement, a bone biopsy was performed with a surgical trephine bur (2.0 mm internal diameter) at the center of the ridge for histomorphometric

Table 1: Periodontal index measures.

Periodontal indices		Baseline 1.3	Baseline 1.4	Baseline 1.5	14 days 1.3	14 days 1.5	28 days 1.3	28 days 1.5	3 months 1.3	3 months 1.5
GI		1	1	1	1	0	0	0	0	0
PI	B	2	2	2	1	1	0	0	0	0
	M	1	1	1	1	1	0	0	0	0
	D	1	1	1	1	1	1	0	1	0
	P	2	2	2	1	1	1	1	0	0
BoP	B	-	+	-	-	-	-	-	-	-
	M	-	+	+	-	+	-	-	-	-
	D	+	+	+	+	+	-	+	-	-
	P	-	+	+	-	-	-	-	-	-

GI: Gingival Index; PI: Plaque Index; BoP: Bleeding on Probing; B: buccal; M: mesial; D: distal: P: palatal.

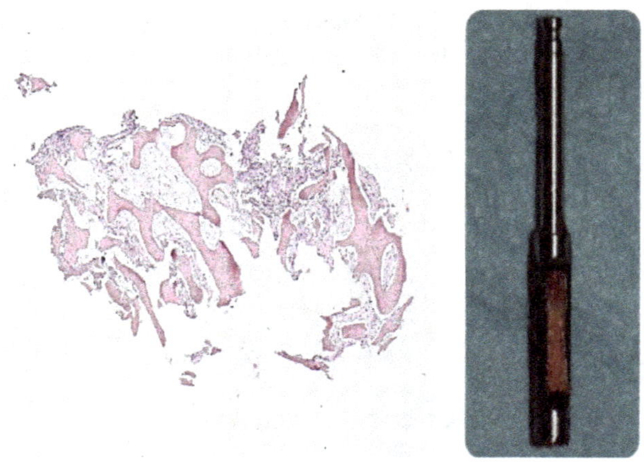

(a) (b)

Figure 3: Histological specimen of the bone tissue taken at the center of the grafted site showing bone tissue surrounded by connective tissue matrix. Hematoxylin-eosin staining; (a) original magnification ×5; (b) surgical trephine bur with bone tissue sample.

analysis of the grafted site (Figures 3(a) and 3(b)) according to Corsi et al. [17]. The tissue specimen was fixed in 4% neutral buffered formaldehyde for 24 hours at 4°C. After fixation, the sample was repeatedly washed in phosphate buffer (pH 7.0), decalcified with 4% EDTA in phosphate buffer (pH 7.0) at 4°C for 48 hours, and routinely embedded in paraffin. Sections of 3 μm thickness were cut from paraffin blocks and used for hematoxylin-eosin stain. The analysis of the bone sample showed newly formed trabecular bone in the grafted site. The trabecular architecture of the bone sample indicates a physiological healing of the postextraction site. At histomorphometric analysis, the bone tissue with osteocytes was 41.8% while the remaining part was composed by connective tissue.

After bone biopsy (Figure 4(a)), a 3.7 × 10 mm implant (Intra-Lock®, Boca Raton, Florida, USA) was placed (Figure 4(b)) and soft tissues sutured (4/0 nylon suture, 20 mm needle) with primary closure (Figure 4(c)). A periapical radiograph was also performed at this time to check correct implant placement (Figure 4(d)). Sutures were then removed 7 days after implant surgery, and a healing abutment was positioned during the second surgery two months later to obtain soft tissue conditioning (Figure 4(e)). A silicone impression with individual tray was taken one month later to fabricate a screw-retained zirconia crown (Figure 4(f)). After 6 months from final restoration, the patient came back for a follow-up, which revealed a stability of the peri-implant soft tissues.

3. Discussion

In the present study, a patient requiring tooth extraction and implant rehabilitation was treated with simple extraction and socket filling with L-PRF membranes. Implant placement was performed three months after ridge preservation, and a bone biopsy was obtained for histomorphometric analysis.

Maintaining an adequate alveolar ridge volume is essential for successful implant placement. However, several internal and external changes of the extraction socket occur after tooth extraction, in particular in the buccal plate, causing a loss of hard and soft tissues [18].

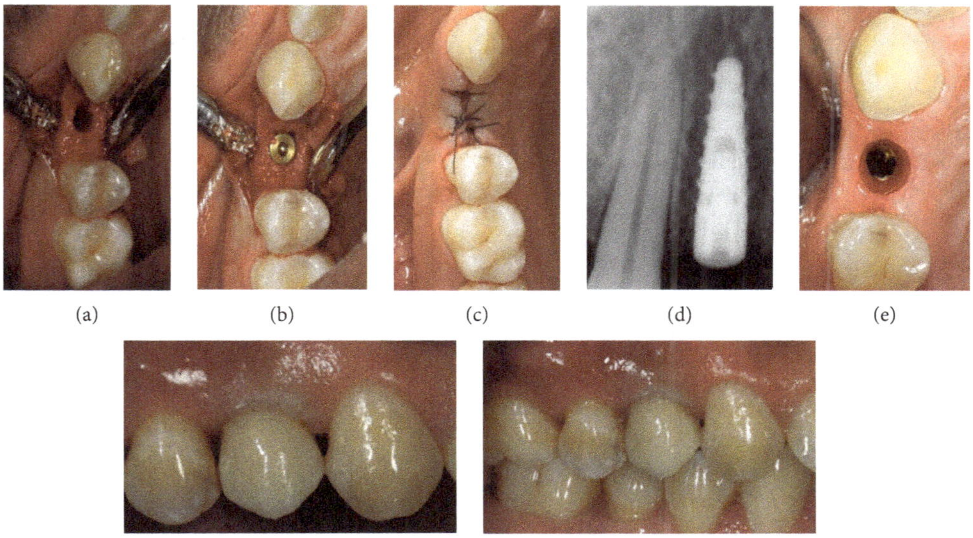

(a) (b) (c) (d) (e) (f) (g)

FIGURE 4: (a) Implant site preparation; (b) implant placement; (c) suture; (d) periapical radiograph after implant placement; (e) soft tissue conditioning; (f) screw-retained zirconia crown; (g) follow-up 6 months after final restoration.

Alveolar ridge preservation includes several techniques to reduce the dimensional changes of hard and soft tissues following tooth extraction. During the last years, several techniques have been proposed [18]. Though graft materials were proven to reduce alveolar bone resorption, they often have poor vascularization and less vital bone formation compared to spontaneous healing [6]. Furthermore, the exposure of resorbable or nonresorbable membranes, often used in combination with bone substitutes, could compromise bone regeneration and wound healing [6]. Finally, the high costs often limit the use of biomaterials in the clinical practice.

Leukocyte- and platelet-rich fibrin (L-PRF) was first described by Dohan et al. in 2006 [8]. It is considered a second-generation platelet concentrate obtained by centrifugation of patient whole blood without the addition of any additive or anticoagulants. With this kind of preparation technique, at least 95% of platelets are embedded into the fibrin network of L-PRF [19]. High concentrations of platelets allow the slow release of growth factors from their alpha granules [20]. These growth factors include Platelet-Derived Growth Factor (PDGF), Vascular Endothelium Growth Factor (VEGF), Transforming Growth Factor-beta (TGF-beta), Fibroblast Growth Factor (FGF), Epidermal Growth Factor (EGF), Insulin-like Growth Factor (IGF), and Hepatocyte Growth Factor (HGF). All of these play an important role in wound healing, in particular improving hemostasis, angiogenesis, and epithelialization. L-PRF has been then used in several surgical procedures, such as oral and maxillofacial surgery and periodontal surgery [21], in order to enhance wound healing process.

The results of this report are consistent with those found in other studies [22, 23], where L-PRF showed to be effective in preserving hard and soft tissues without interfering with physiological bone healing process. Ridge preservation techniques are always desirable when functional and aesthetic results are demanded. Such procedures also facilitate implant placement according to the prosthetic project and with a proper macrogeometry. The beneficial effects of L-PRF in reducing dimensional changes may derive from its capacity to promote tissue regeneration. The dimensional remodeling observed in this study is comparable to those reported with other techniques [24] where bone substitutes were used. However, a recent randomized controlled trial [25] has suggested that PRF may not significantly enhance bone formation after tooth extraction, as compared to spontaneous healing. Even though studies with larger population will be required to reach valid conclusions, current results may provide the base to investigate the combined use of PRF and bone substitutes. Notwithstanding, differently from other techniques, the use of L-PRF is relatively simple and requires minimal costs, no need for primary closure and no risk for membrane exposure. In addition, as an autologous product, there is no risk of disease transmission or graft infection.

Within the limitations of this report, our results support the use of L-PRF in alveolar ridge preservation when implant placement is scheduled after tooth extraction. Additional studies with a larger sample size, randomization, and a split-mouth design are needed to confirm our findings and investigate possible specific indications of L-PRF compared to other biomaterials.

References

[1] W. L. Tan, T. L. T. Wong, M. C. M. Wong, and N. P. Lang, "A systematic review of post-extractional alveolar hard and soft tissue dimensional changes in humans," *Clinical Oral Implants Research*, vol. 23, Supplement 5, pp. 1–21, 2012.

[2] D. Laurito, M. Lollobrigida, F. Gianno, S. Bosco, L. Lamazza, and A. De Biase, "Alveolar ridge preservation with nc-HA and d-PTFE membrane: a clinical, histologic, and histomorphometric study," *International Journal of Periodontics and Restorative Dentistry*, vol. 37, no. 2, pp. 283–290, 2017.

[3] D. Laurito, R. Cugnetto, M. Lollobrigida et al., "Socket preservation with d-PTFE membrane: histologic analysis of the newly formed matrix at membrane removal," *International Journal of Periodontics and Restorative Dentistry*, vol. 36, no. 6, pp. 877–883, 2016.

[4] S. Jambhekar, F. Kernen, and A. S. Bidra, "Clinical and histologic outcomes of socket grafting after flapless tooth extraction: a systematic review of randomized controlled clinical trials," *Journal of Prosthetic Dentistry*, vol. 113, no. 5, pp. 371–382, 2015.

[5] N. U. Zitzmann, P. Schärer, and C. P. Marinello, "Long-term results of implants treated with guided bone regeneration: a 5-year prospective study," *International Journal of Oral and Maxillofacial Implants*, vol. 16, no. 3, pp. 355–366, 2001.

[6] J. M. Iasella, H. Greenwell, R. L. Miller et al., "Ridge preservation with freeze-dried bone allograft and a collagen membrane compared to extraction alone for implant site development: a clinical and histologic study in humans," *Journal of Periodontology*, vol. 74, no. 7, pp. 990–999, 2003.

[7] G. F. Rogers and A. K. Greene, "Autogenous bone graft: basic science and clinical implications," *Journal of Craniofacial Surgery*, vol. 23, no. 1, pp. 323–327, 2012.

[8] D. M. Dohan, J. Choukroun, A. Diss et al., "Platelet-rich fibrin (PRF): a second-generation platelet concentrate. Part II: platelet-related biologic features," *Oral Surgery, Oral Medicine, Oral Pathology, Oral Radiology and Endodontology*, vol. 101, no. 3, pp. e45–e50, 2006.

[9] M. Lollobrigida, M. Maritato, G. Bozzuto, G. Formisano, A. Molinari, and A. De Biase, "Biomimetic implant surface functionalization with liquid L-PRF products: in vitro study," *Biomed Research International*, vol. 2018, Article ID 9031435, 7 pages, 2018.

[10] D. M. Dohan, J. Choukroun, A. Diss et al., "Platelet-rich fibrin (PRF): A second-generation platelet concentrate. Part III: Leucocyte activation: A new feature for platelet concentrates?," *Oral Surgery Oral Medicine Oral Pathology Oral Radiology and Endodontology*, vol. 101, no. 3, pp. e51–e55, 2006.

[11] S. Roy, J. Driggs, H. Elgharably et al., "Platelet-rich fibrin matrix improves wound angiogenesis via inducing endothelial cell proliferation," *Wound Repair and Regeneration*, vol. 19, no. 6, pp. 753–766, 2011.

[12] J. Choukroun, A. Diss, A. Simonpieri et al., "Platelet-rich fibrin (PRF): a second-generation platelet concentrate. Part IV: clinical effects on tissue healing," *Oral Surgery Oral Medicine Oral Pathology Oral Radiology and Endodontology*, vol. 101, no. 3, pp. e56–e60, 2006.

[13] D. M. Dohan Ehrenfest, G. M. de Peppo, P. Doglioli, and G. Sammartino, "Slow release of growth factors and thrombospondin-1 in Choukroun's platelet-rich fibrin (PRF): a gold standard to achieve for all surgical platelet concentrates technologies," *Growth Factors*, vol. 27, no. 1, pp. 63–69, 2009.

[14] J. Silness and H. Löe, "Periodontal disease in Pregnancy II. correlation between oral hygiene and periodontal condition," *Acta Odontologica Scandinavica*, vol. 22, no. 1, pp. 121–135, 2009.

[15] H. Löe and J. Silness, "Periodontal disease in pregnancy I. Prevalence and severity," *Acta Odontologica Scandinavica*, vol. 21, pp. 533–551, 2009.

[16] N. P. Lang, A. Joss, T. Orsanic, F. A. Gusberti, and B. E. Siegrist, "Bleeding on probing. A predictor for the progression of periodontal disease?," *Journal of Clinical Periodontology*, vol. 13, no. 6, pp. 590–596, 1986.

[17] A. Corsi, M. T. Collins, M. Riminucci et al., "Osteomalacic and hyperparathyroid changes in fibrous dysplasia of bone: core biopsy studies and clinical correlations," *Journal of Bone and Mineral Research*, vol. 18, no. 7, pp. 1235–1246, 2003.

[18] I. Darby, S. T. Chen, and D. Buser, "Ridge preservation techniques for implant therapy," *The International Journal of Oral & Maxillofacial Implants*, vol. 24, pp. 260–271, 2009.

[19] D. M. Dohan Ehrenfest, M. Del Corso, A. Diss, J. Mouhyi, and J. B. Charrier, "Three-dimensional architecture and cell composition of a Choukroun's platelet-rich fibrin clot and membrane," *Journal of Periodontology*, vol. 81, no. 4, pp. 546–555, 2010.

[20] C. Y. Su, Y. P. Kuo, Y. H. Tseng, C. H. Su, and T. Burnouf, "In vitro release of growth factors from platelet-rich fibrin (PRF): a proposal to optimize the clinical applications of PRF," *Oral Surgery Oral Medicine Oral Pathology Oral Radiology and Endodontology*, vol. 108, no. 1, pp. 56–61, 2009.

[21] M. Del Corso, A. Vervelle, A. Simonpieri et al., "Current knowledge and perspectives for the use of platelet-rich plasma (PRP) and platelet-rich fibrin (PRF) in oral and maxillofacial surgery part 1: periodontal and dentoalveolar surgery," *Current Pharmaceutical Biotechnology*, vol. 13, no. 7, pp. 1207–1230, 2012.

[22] A. B. Castro, N. Meschi, A. Temmerman et al., "Regenerative potential of leucocyte- and platelet-rich fibrin. Part B: sinus floor elevation, alveolar ridge preservation and implant therapy. A systematic review," *Journal of Clinical Periodontology*, vol. 44, no. 2, pp. 225–234, 2017.

[23] A. Temmerman, J. Vandessel, A. Castro et al., "The use of leucocyte and platelet-rich fibrin in socket management and ridge preservation: a split-mouth, randomized, controlled clinical trial," *Journal of Clinical Periodontology*, vol. 43, no. 11, pp. 990–999, 2016.

[24] S. Das, R. Jhingran, V. K. Bains, R. Madan, R. Srivastava, and I. Rizvi, "Socket preservation by beta-tri-calcium phosphate with collagen compared to platelet-rich fibrin: a clinico-radiographic study," *European Journal of Dentistry*, vol. 10, no. 2, pp. 264–276, 2016.

[25] K. Areewong, M. Chantaramungkorn, and P. Khongkhunthian, "Platelet-rich fibrin to preserve alveolar bone sockets following tooth extraction: a randomized controlled trial," *Clinical Implant Dentistry and Related Research*, vol. 21, no. 6, pp. 1156–1163, 2019.

16

Endodontic Retreatment of Maxillary Second Molar with Four Roots

Gabriel Magnucki

Zahnzentrum Schomaker & Magnucki, Bahnhofstrasse 16-18, 27211 Bassum, Germany

Correspondence should be addressed to Gabriel Magnucki; gabriel_magnucki@gmx.de

Academic Editor: Antonio Miranda Cruz-Filho

The present communication describes the endodontic retreatment of a rare four-rooted maxillary second molar. A 25-year-old patient was referred to our dental practice requesting an apicoectomy because of continuous and permanent pain reaction six months after the first endodontic treatment. The sent radiograph demonstrated three filled root canals (one mesial, two distal) and four radiographically superimposing roots (two mesial, two distal). Due to the diagnosed chronic apical periodontitis and based on the visible untreated root canal, we decided to endodontically re-treat the quadrangular tooth against the referred apicoectomy. In the first session, only the previously untreated mesiopalatal root canal was mechanically prepared and filled with a corticosteroid- and tetracycline-containing paste. After two symptom-free weeks, the gutta-percha was removed from the other canals and calcium hydroxide was applied. Another two weeks later, the four root canals, whose orifices were "irregular quadrilateral" shaped on the pulp chamber floor representing Versiani Type A, were obturated. After the verification of this rare anatomy by cone beam computed tomography, the tooth was classified as Christie's radicular type II. One characteristic of this type is parallel running buccal and palatal roots, which caused a radiographic superimposition and probably led to the endodontic mistreatment in the first case.

1. Introduction

Clear understanding of dental anatomy including root number and canal morphology is an essential prerequisite in endodontic therapies. In particular, anticipation of rare anatomical variations should be crucial for endodontic specialists. Such a dental anomaly is the presence of two palatal roots in human maxillary second molars. Libfeld and Rotstein described in 1200 investigated teeth the frequency of a four-rooted maxillary second molar at 0.4% [1]. Peikoff et al. identified in a retrospective study, containing 520 maxillary second molars with completed endodontic treatments, that 1.4% of the canadian patients had two palatal roots [2]. These results were recently confirmed by Martins et al. in 2018, who reported a similar occurrence rate in the Portuguese population using cone beam computed tomography [3]. Despite this rare incidence, publications concerning tooth anatomy describe several classifications for four-rooted maxillary molars [4–7]. The first characterization was indicated by Christie et al., who characterized maxillary molars with four roots (commonly two buccal and palatal) according to their shape and degree of separation of the palatal roots in three subtypes [4]. Baratto-Filho et al. suggested an additional class IV by demonstrating an endodontic case of fused mesiobuccal and mesiopalatal roots [8]. Furthermore, Versiani et al. indicated that Christie's classification is not feasible while studying four-rooted second maxillary molars [5]. They introduced a new type III, which is based on less divergent and short palatal roots along with widely divergent buccal roots by combining Christie's types II and III [4, 5]. Nevertheless, another classification exists for this rare anatomical anomaly conceived by Carlsen and Alexandersen (2000). They defined the additional palatal root as radix mesio- or distolingualis according to its direct affinity to the pronounced part of the crown [6]. Furthermore, they identified one case exhibiting three buccal roots in a maxillary first molar and classified it as radix paramolaris [7]. However,

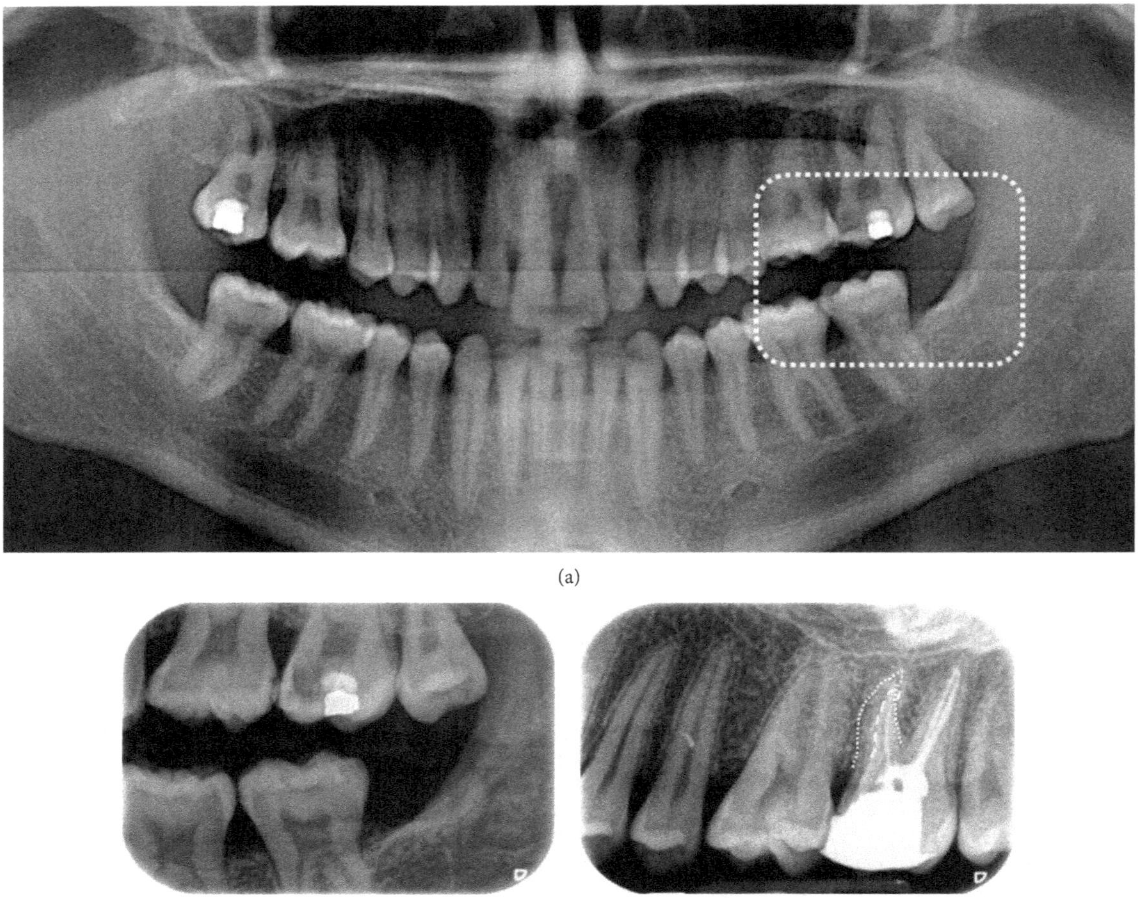

(a) (b) (c)

Figure 1: (a) Panoramic radiograph of the referred patient. (b) Bitewing view of the interesting tooth, which showed a deep carious lesion. (c) X-ray after the first endodontic treatment. In the distal roots, two root fillings are visible, whereas only one filled root canal can be identified in the mesial roots. Note two mesial roots. Buccal: dotted line; palatal: scored line.

not all dental professionals are aware of this anomaly resulting in failed endodontic treatments. Therefore, the following case report describes an endodontic retreatment of a maxillary second molar with two palatal roots.

2. Case Report

A 25-year-old male patient was referred to our Department in Bassum, Lower Saxony, Germany, to receive apicoectomy on the maxillary left second molar. Together with the referral, the radiographic history of the relevant tooth was provided (Figures 1(a)–1(c)). The patient, whose medical history was noncontributory, complained of persistent pain reactions and tenderness of this tooth after a first endodontic treatment six months ago. Clinical examination showed a sufficient composite restoration, a painful tenderness to percussion, and no reaction to cold test. Tooth mobility and periodontal pockets were inconspicuous. No submucosal swelling was observed. The pretreatment radiograph showed an apical radiolucency on the mesial root and three radiopaque root fillings (two distal and one mesial), which led to the diagnosis of a chronic apical periodontitis. This straight radiographic evaluation of the examined tooth revealed no unusual anatomy (Figure 2(a)). But the X-ray image after the first endodontic treatment was taken mesial angulated, and here, a second previously untreated mesial root is visible (Figure 1(c)). Therefore, instead of the proposed apicoectomy, the decision was made to re-treat the root canals.

After the injection of 1 ml local anesthesia containing 40 mg articaine hydrochloride and 0.005 mg epinephrine (Septanest, Septodont, Saint-Maur-des-Fossés, France) and isolation with a rubber dam, the occlusal filling was removed. During the access preparation, the second (mesial), untreated palatal root canal orifices were found. Due to issues in the time management in the first treatment session, only the previously untreated root canal was explored with a manual instrument ISO 15, irrigated with 2.5% NaOCl, and corticosteroid- and tetracycline-containing paste (Ledermix®, RIEMSER Pharma, Greifswald, Germany) was applied with a lentulo spiral filler (ISO 25, Dentsply DeTrey, Konstanz, Germany). The access cavity was filled with Cavit (ESPE, Seefeld, Germany). Two weeks later, the patient described a symptom-free and painless period since the last treatment. During the second session, the gutta-percha in the coronal third of the root canals was removed with a diamond-

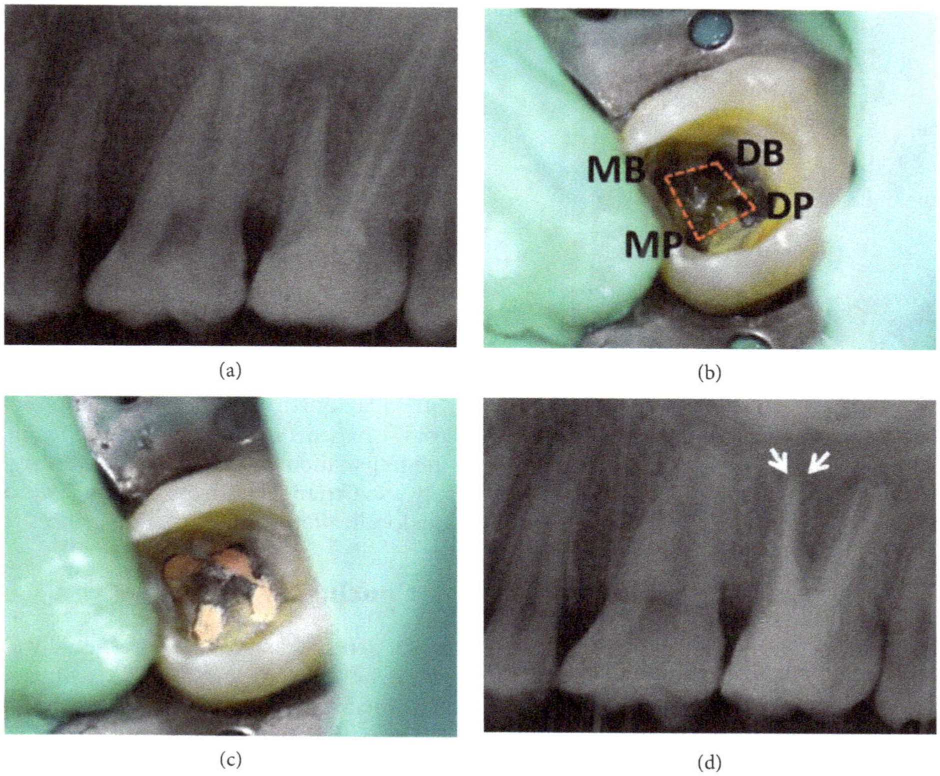

FIGURE 2: (a) The pretreatment radiograph showed an apical radiolucency on the mesial root. Due to the buccal-palatal superimposition, the second mesial root is not visible. (b) Photograph of the pulp chamber floor after removal of the gutta-percha. Root canal orifices were "irregular quadrilateral" shaped on the pulp chamber floor representing Versiani Type A. (c) Photograph after the canal obturation. (d) The posttreatment radiograph showed two mesial filled root canals (arrows).

coated ultrasonic tip (Komet Dental, Lemgo, Germany) and eucalyptus oil (Apotheke Gesundheitszentrum, Bassum, Germany) was applied for ten minutes. Afterwards, the gutta-percha was removed from the three filled canals (mesiobuccal, distobuccal, and distopalatal), and the canals were cleaned as well as shaped with a reciprocating instrument (R25, Reciproc®, VDW, Munich, Germany). The files were cleaned from the gutta-percha debris every three reciprocating units ("pecks") according to the manufacturer's protocol. After the working length was reached (19 mm each canal (apex to the corresponding tooth cusps)), which was determined using an electronic apex locator (VDW.GOLD® RECIPROC®, VDW, Munich, Germany), the residual obturation material was removed ultrasonically (REDO setting, VDW.ULTRA®, VDW, Munich, Germany). The previously untreated canal (mesiopalatal) was also cleaned and shaped with a reciprocating instrument (R25, Reciproc®, VDW, Munich, Germany). Then, the root canals and especially the apical region were enlarged (R40, Reciproc®, VDW, Munich, Germany). During the instrumentation process, the canals were irrigated with 2.5% NaOCl, 2% CHX, and 18% EDTA and the liquids were activated ultrasonically (IRRI setting, VDW.ULTRA®, VDW, Munich, Germany). Afterwards, the disinfection was carried out with $Ca(OH)_2$ (Calcicur®, VOCO, Cuxhaven, Germany), and the coronal seal was performed with Cavit (3M ESPE, Seefeld, Germany). Two weeks later, the canals were reentered and $Ca(OH)_2$ was removed by using 2.5% NaOCl, 2% CHX, and 18% EDTA and obturated with appropriate gutta-percha mastercones (ISO 40, VDW, Munich, Germany) along with an AH plus sealer (Dentsply DeTrey, Konstanz, Germany) using the lateral condensation technique (Figure 2(c)). The permanent restoration was carried out using Tetric EvoCeram (Ivoclar Vivadent, Schaan, Liechtenstein). The postendodontic radiograph demonstrated two mesial-located apices (Figure 2(d)). To verify this rare anatomy, a 3D cone beam computed tomography (CBCT) (KaVo OP 3D DVT, KaVo Dental, Biberach an der Riβ, Germany) was performed and analyzed (Figure 3). The patient gave his informed consent for the publication of this communication.

3. Discussion

The incidence in the literature of four-rooted maxillary second molars varies between 0.22% in Thailand (n (number of investigated teeth) = 457) [9] and 2.4% in France ($n = 167$) [10]. Interestingly, also in other European populations, higher occurrence rates for two palatal roots in maxillary second molars were found in CBCT studies. In Italy, the frequency of upper second molars with four roots was described with 1.27% ($n = 157$) [11]. Comparable results were demonstrated in Greece (1.24%, $n = 402$) [12], in Cyprus (1.37%, $n = 438$) [13], and in the Portuguese study mentioned above (1.44%, $n = 277$) [3]. On the other

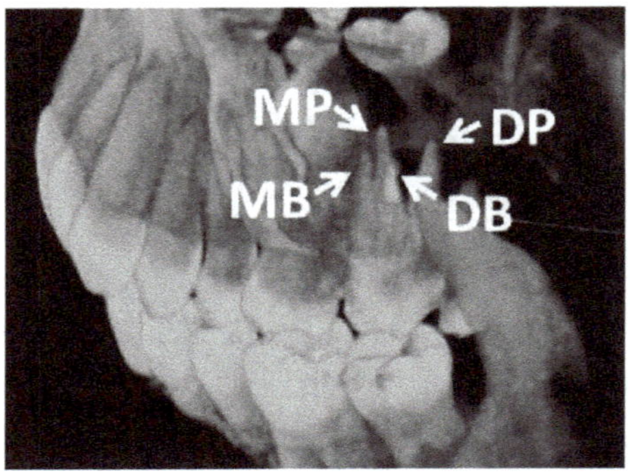

FIGURE 3: Cone beam computed tomographic 3D reconstruction of the treated tooth from a disto-buccal-apico angulation verifies the rare anatomy of four roots. MB: mesiobuccal; DB: distobuccal; MP: mesiopalatal; DP: distopalatal.

hand, in East Asia, lower occurrence rates of this rare morphological anomaly were identified in population-based CBCT studies in Thailand (0.22%, $n = 457$) [9], South Korea (0.49%, $n = 820$) [14], and China (0.28%, $n = 1066$ [15]; 0.77%, $n = 519$ [16]; 0.98%, $n = 1226$ [17]; and 1.12%, $n = 979$ [18]). To clarify the root and canal anatomy of maxillary second molars and especially the global distribution of quadrangular teeth, a meta-analytical literature review would be supportive for the dental community. However, every dental professional and especially endodontists should be aware of the anatomical anomaly of a second palatal root to avoid treatment failures like the one reported in the present case. The rarity of this morphological aberration leads to the expectation of one case every three years in full-time endodontic practice [4]. For example, last year, we extracted a four-rooted maxillary first molar and analyzed its external and internal anatomy in our dental office [19]. After studying this anomaly intensively, we were able to interpret the sent radiographic images correctly. Hence, we decided for an endodontic retreatment against the proposed apicoectomy. Importantly, prior to an endodontic retreatment, all available information and especially radiographic examinations of the first root canal treatment should be obtained. In the present communication, four roots are only visible on the sent X-ray image of the referring colleague.

In clinical case documentations, Christie's classification is commonly used for the description of quadrangular teeth [4]. Christie et al. classified four-rooted maxillary molars according to shape, degree, fusion, and separation of the palatal roots [4]. Due to four separated roots and the parallel running morphology of the buccal and palatal roots, the presented tooth was identified as type II. A further characteristic for type II teeth is shorter roots, which explains the reduced working length in this case report. Remarkably, radiographic superimposition of the buccal and lingual roots in this type can lead to clinical misinterpretation such as in the present case [4]. In contrast, Christie's type I shows widely divergent, long, and tortuous palatal roots and the "cow horn"-shaped buccal roots demonstrate mainly four separate apices on radiographs [4]. Therefore, the diagnosis of this type is more feasible for experienced endodontists. Type III maxillary molars are "constricted in root morphology with the MB, MP and DP canals encaged in a web of root dentin." In radiographs of this type, the DB root appears to stand alone [4]. In summary, the radiographic identification of quadrangular type II molars could be challenging and could complicate a correct diagnosis. However, in diagnostically difficult posterior regions, additional angulated radiographs could help the dentist to determine four-rooted molars. Nowadays, the endodontic usage of cone beam computed tomography can support the diagnosis of root and canal aberrations (Figure 3) [20].

After the correct diagnosis, the preparation of the trepanation cavity is the next endodontic challenge. Versiani pointed out that the root canal orifices were located mainly "irregular quadrilateral" (as in the present case) or "trapezoid" shaped on the pulpal chamber floor [5]. Therefore, the trepanation cavities have to be enlarged from the generally used triangular shape to trapezoid or quadrilateral for the localization of all root canal orifices [5].

4. Conclusion

Every dental practitioner and especially endodontists should possess deep knowledge of all existing anatomical variants and their radiographic characteristics to avoid treatment failures. Before the beginning of an endodontic retreatment, all available information of the first root canal treatment and the radiographic history of the tooth of interest should be obtained for the identification of possible radicular abnormalities.

Acknowledgments

The author would like to thank Mrs. Salome Magnucki for the proofreading of the manuscript. Furthermore, I thank Dr. Kai Witte, Bassum, for performing and analyzing the cone beam computed tomography.

References

[1] H. Libfeld and I. Rotstein, "Incidence of four-rooted maxillary second molars: literature review and radiographic survey of 1,200 teeth," *Journal of Endodontics*, vol. 15, no. 3, pp. 129–131, 1989.

[2] M. D. Peikoff, W. H. Christie, and H. M. Fogel, "The maxillary second molar: variations in the number of roots and canals," *International Endodontic Journal*, vol. 29, no. 6, pp. 365–369, 1996.

[3] J. N. R. Martins, D. Marques, H. Francisco, and J. Caramês, "Gender influence on the number of roots and root canal system configuration in human permanent teeth of a Portuguese subpopulation," *Quintessence International*, vol. 49, no. 2, pp. 103–111, 2018.

[4] W. H. Christie, M. D. Peikoff, and H. M. Fogel, "Maxillary molars with two palatal roots: a retrospective clinical study," *Journal of Endodontics*, vol. 17, no. 2, pp. 80–84, 1991.

[5] M. A. Versiani, J. D. Pécora, and M. D. de Sousa-Neto, "Root and root canal morphology of four-rooted maxillary second molars: a micro-computed tomography study," *Journal of Endodontics*, vol. 38, no. 7, pp. 977–982, 2012.

[6] O. Carlsen and V. Alexandersen, "Radix mesiolingualis and radix distolingualis in a collection of permanent maxillary molars," *Acta Odontologica Scandinavica*, vol. 58, no. 5, pp. 229–236, 2000.

[7] O. Carlsen and V. Alexandersen, "Radix paramolaris and radix distomolaris in Danish permanent maxillary molars," *Acta Odontologica Scandinavica*, vol. 57, no. 5, pp. 283–289, 1999.

[8] F. Baratto-Filho, L. F. Fariniuk, E. L. Ferreira, J. D. Pecora, A. M. Cruz-Filho, and M. D. Sousa-Neto, "Clinical and macroscopic study of maxillary molars with two palatal roots," *International Endodontic Journal*, vol. 35, no. 9, pp. 796–801, 2002.

[9] R. Ratanajirasut, A. Panichuttra, and S. Panmekiate, "A cone-beam computed tomographic study of root and canal morphology of maxillary first and second permanent molars in a Thai population," *Journal of Endodontics*, vol. 44, no. 1, pp. 56–61, 2018.

[10] P. Monsarrat, B. Arcaute, O. A. Peters et al., "Interrelationships in the variability of root canal anatomy among the permanent teeth: a full-mouth approach by cone-beam CT," *PLoS One*, vol. 11, no. 10, article e0165329, 2016.

[11] G. Plotino, L. Tocci, N. M. Grande et al., "Symmetry of root and root canal morphology of maxillary and mandibular molars in a white population: a cone-beam computed tomography study *in vivo*," *Journal of Endodontics*, vol. 39, no. 12, pp. 1545–1548, 2013.

[12] G. E. Nikoloudaki, T. G. Kontogiannis, and N. P. Kerezoudis, "Evaluation of the root and canal morphology of maxillary permanent molars and the incidence of the second mesiobuccal root canal in Greek population using cone-beam computed tomography," *The Open Dentistry Journal*, vol. 9, no. 1, pp. 267–272, 2015.

[13] A. Kalender, B. Celikten, P. Tufenkci et al., "Cone beam computed tomography evaluation of maxillary molar root canal morphology in a Turkish Cypriot population," *Biotechnology & Biotechnological Equipment*, vol. 30, no. 1, pp. 145–150, 2016.

[14] Y. Kim, S. J. Lee, and J. Woo, "Morphology of maxillary first and second molars analyzed by cone-beam computed tomography in a Korean population: variations in the number of roots and canals and the incidence of fusion," *Journal of Endodontics*, vol. 38, no. 8, pp. 1063–1068, 2012.

[15] H. Wang, B. W. Ci, H. Y. Yu et al., "Evaluation of root and canal morphology of maxillary molars in a Southern Chinese subpopulation: a cone-beam computed tomographic study," *International Journal of Clinical and Experimental Medicine*, vol. 10, no. 4, pp. 7030–7039, 2017.

[16] Y. N. Jing, X. Ye, D. G. Liu, Z. Y. Zhang, and X. C. Ma, "Cone-beam computed tomography was used for study of root and canal morphology of maxillary first and second molars," *Beijing Da Xue Xue Bao Yi Xue Ban*, vol. 46, no. 6, pp. 958–962, 2014.

[17] Y. Gu, W. Wang, and L. Ni, "Four-rooted permanent maxillary first and second molars in a northwestern Chinese population," *Archives of Oral Biology*, vol. 60, no. 6, pp. 811–817, 2015.

[18] B. Yang, Q. Lu, Q. X. Bai, Y. Zhang, X. J. Liu, and Z. J. Liu, "Evaluation of the prevalence of the maxillary molars with two palatal roots by cone-beam CT," *Zhonghua kou Qiang yi xue za zhi*, vol. 48, no. 6, pp. 359–362, 2013.

[19] G. Magnucki and W. A. Kahl, "Four rooted maxillary first molar with five root canals and two enamel pearls," *International Journal of Dental and Health Sciences*, vol. 5, no. 4, pp. 600–605, 2018.

[20] T. Venskutonis, G. Plotino, G. Juodzbalys, and L. Mickevičienė, "The importance of cone-beam computed tomography in the management of endodontic problems: a review of the literature," *Journal of Endodontics*, vol. 40, no. 12, pp. 1895–1901, 2014.

17

Osteomyelitis of the Mandible Caused by Late Fracture following Third Molar Extraction

Shinsuke Yamamoto,[1] Naoki Taniike,[1] Daisuke Yamashita,[2] and Toshihiko Takenobu[1]

[1]*Department of Oral and Maxillofacial Surgery, Kobe City Medical Center General Hospital, Kobe, Hyogo 650-0047, Japan*
[2]*Department of Pathology, Kobe City Medical Center General Hospital, Kobe, Hyogo 650-0047, Japan*

Correspondence should be addressed to Shinsuke Yamamoto; s.yamamoto@kcho.jp

Academic Editor: Jose López-López

The common postoperative complications of the extraction of third molars are frequently reported; however, reports about osteomyelitis of the mandible caused by late fracture following third molar extraction are rare. Here, we report a case of osteomyelitis of the mandible caused by late fracture following third molar extraction. A 38-year-old Japanese man was referred to the surgery department with chief complaints of dull pain and swelling in the right masseteric region and paresthesia of his lower lip and mental region in March 2018. A family dentist removed his lower third molar in the right side in January 2018. When the patient was chewing an innards stew 23 days after the procedure, he heard a cracking sound from the right mandible. Thus, we diagnosed the patient as having osteomyelitis of the mandible caused by late fracture following third molar extraction and performed sequestrectomy and curettage under general anesthesia in April 2018. In conclusion, it is necessary to recognize the possibility that late fracture following third molar extraction can cause osteomyelitis. Furthermore, once osteomyelitis of the mandible caused by late fracture occurred, early and appropriate treatment is necessary because the osteomyelitis may progress rapidly and in some cases may result in pathological fracture.

1. Introduction

The common postoperative complications of third molar extraction are alveolar osteitis, secondary infection, bleeding, and paresthesia [1–10]. On the other hand, major complications, such as mandibular fracture, severe hemorrhage, or iatrogenic displacement of the third molar teeth, are rarely reported [6]. Among them, the incidence of mandibular fracture during or after a third molar extraction has been reported to be 0.0046% to 0.0049% [11, 12].

We report herein a case of osteomyelitis of the mandibular caused by late fracture in a Japanese man.

2. Case Report

A 38-year-old Japanese man was referred to the Department of Oral and Maxillofacial Surgery at Kobe City Medical Center General Hospital with chief complaints of dull pain and swelling in the right masseteric region and paresthesia of his lower lip and mental region in March 2018. He had no medical history and was not taking any medication. His lower third molar in the right side was removed due to pericoronitis under local anesthesia by a family dentist in January 2018. The tooth was partially and horizontally impacted (Pell and Gregory Class I, position A) (Figure 1). The method of the extraction involved local anesthesia administration, surgical incision, elevation of a mucoperiosteal flap, ostectomy, tooth sectioning, dislocation, curettage of granulation tissue, irrigation with saline, and suturing. The surgical procedure was uneventful, and he was administered amoxicillin for 3 days. At 7 days after the procedure, he only had mild postoperative pain and had no paresthesia of the lower lip and mental region, as confirmed by his family dentist. At 23 days after the procedure, when the patient was chewing an innards stew, he heard a cracking sound from his right mandible and felt mild pain, and his right masseteric region began to swell. The dentist found no abnormalities on his occlusion and panoramic radiograph. However, he was

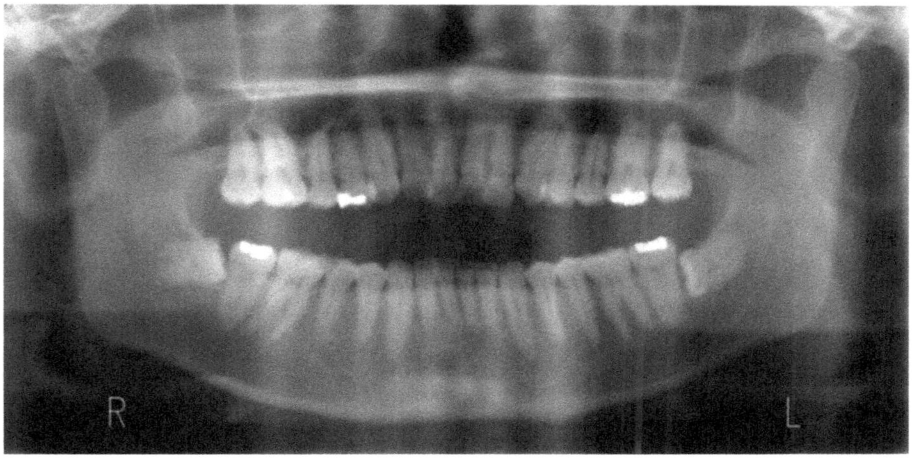

FIGURE 1: A panoramic radiograph obtained before the extraction. The radiograph shows that the right lower third molar was horizontal (Pell and Gregory Class I, position A). There are no prior bone lesions associated with the molar, such as cyst and tumor.

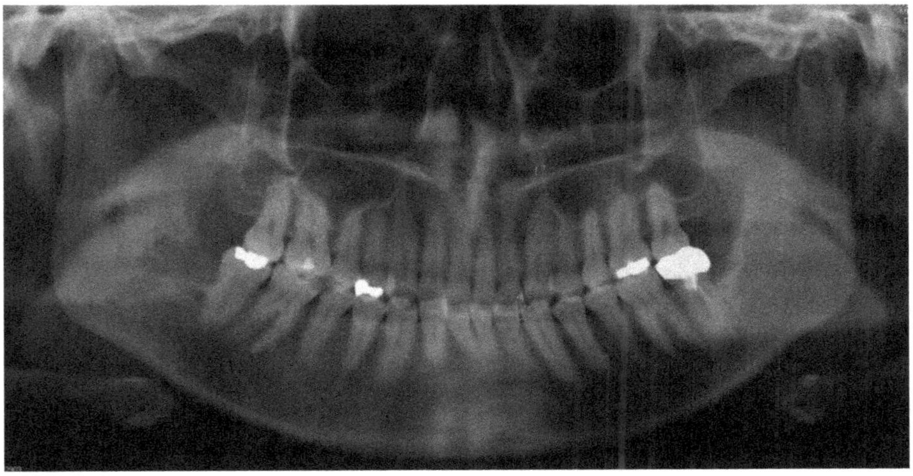

FIGURE 2: A panoramic radiograph obtained during the initial visit. The radiograph shows radiolucency from the extraction socket to the right mandibular angle.

placed on a soft diet; to make matters worse, he had paresthesia of his lower lip and mental region in the right side in addition to worsening of the pain and swelling at 42 days after the procedure. Treatment with mecobalamin and adenosine triphosphate disodium hydrate was initiated, and he was referred to our department for further examination of paresthesia and pain at 55 days after the procedure. Clinical examination at the initial visit showed mild swelling at the right masseteric region, mild paresthesia of his lower lip and mental region in the right side, and trismus (25 mm). Mandibular movements were normal, and there were no observable changes in the dental occlusion. Electric pulp test revealed that mandibular first and second molars of the right side were vital. The alveolar mucosa of mandibular third molar extraction socket was healed, but there was mild tenderness, and the distal periodontal pocket of the second molar was deep and hemorrhagic. Blood tests showed a white blood cell count of 4,900/mL (range, 3,900 to 9,800/mL) and C-reactive protein level of 0.38 mg/dL (range, 0.00 to 0.50 mg/dL). Panoramic radiograph showed a radiolucency from the extraction socket to the right mandibular angle (Figure 2). Computed tomography (CT) showed destruction of the buccal cortical bone from the socket to the right mandibular angle and formation of bone sequestrum. Although the lingual cortical bone was intact, there was periosteal reaction around the buccal bone destruction (Figure 3). Magnetic resonance imaging (MRI) revealed that the mandibular bone marrow from the right ramus to the body had a low signal density on T1-weighted images and a high signal density on short-tau inversion recovery (STIR) images (Figure 4). Bone scintigraphy showed a strong accumulation of technetium medronic acid (99mTc-MDP) in the right mandibular ramus (Figure 5).

After a clinical diagnosis of osteomyelitis of the mandible caused by late fracture following third molar extraction, we performed sequestrectomy and curettage via a mandibular vestibular approach under general anesthesia in April 2018, followed by administration of ampicillin/sulbactam

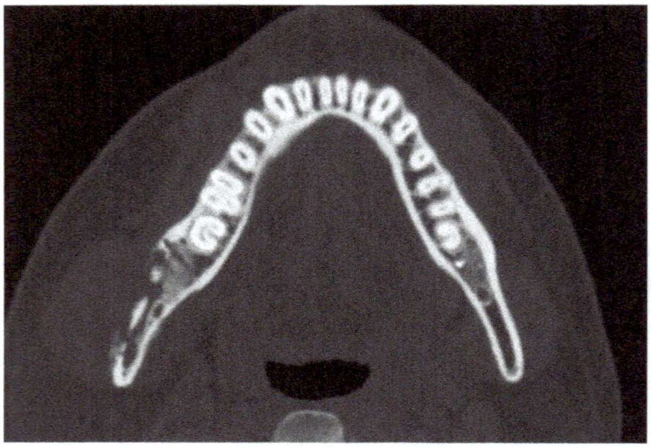

FIGURE 3: Coronal computed tomography (CT) scans obtained during the initial visit. CT shows a destruction of buccal cortical bone from the socket to the right mandibular angle and a formation of bone sequestrum. Although the lingual cortical bone is intact, there is periosteal reaction around the buccal bone destruction.

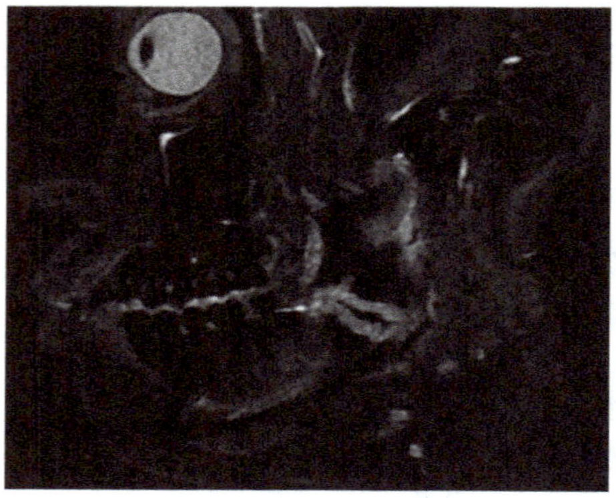

FIGURE 4: Sagittal magnetic resonance imaging (MRI) obtained during the initial visit. MRI shows that the mandibular bone marrow from the right ramus to the body has a high signal density on short-tau inversion recovery (STIR) images and the cortical bone is partially raptured. Moreover, filaments in the low-density area are observed in the high-density area.

for 5 days. After flap elevation, the granulation tissue was eliminated using a sharp curette, and the edges of the remaining bone were rounded off. The sequestrum detected by CT obtained during the initial visit completely disappeared and replaced by immature granulation tissues. The size of the defect of the buccal cortical bone was 25 mm (height) × 8 mm (width) × 6 mm (depth), which reached from the extraction socket to the right mandibular angle (Figure 6). Given that the lingual cortical bone was intact, there was no mobility and an inferior alveolar nerve was not exposed to the surgical field. Pathological findings of the surgical specimen revealed that the granulation tissue had drusen of colonies of *Actinomyces* sp. and gram-positive bacillus (Figures 7(a)–7(c)). The trismus and paresthesia of his lower lip and mental region in the right side disappeared completely, and no relapse occurred during the 6-month follow-up (Figures 8(a)–8(c)).

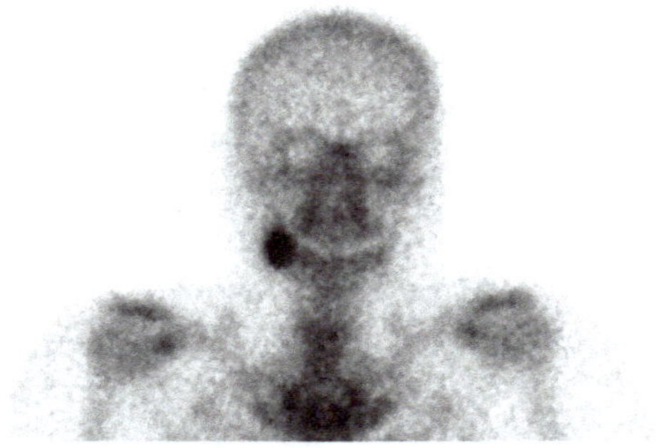

FIGURE 5: Bone scintigraphic findings obtained during the initial visit. Bone scintigraphy shows a strong accumulation of technetium medronic acid (99mTc-MDP) in the right mandibular ramus.

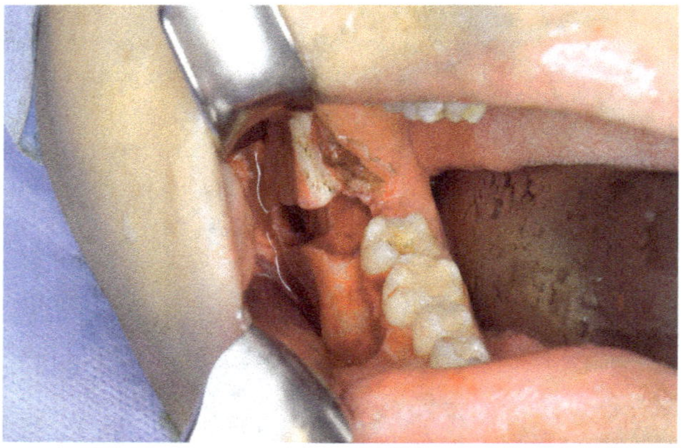

FIGURE 6: An intraoperative photograph. The size of the defect of the buccal cortical bone was 25 mm (height) × 8 mm (width) × 6 mm (depth), which reached from the extraction socket to the right mandibular angle.

3. Discussion

This is a rare and valuable report describing a case of osteomyelitis of the mandible caused by late fracture following third molar extraction. To prevent postoperative mandibular fracture, patients undergoing third molar extraction should maintain a liquid and soft diet and should expect to return to their regular physical activities at four weeks after the procedure [9–14]. Generally, postoperative fractures occurred more common in Class II/III and Type B/C impaction than in Class I and Type A impactions, and patients older than 30-40 years with a full dentition were considered to be a risk group [2, 9, 13, 15, 16]. Moreover, most fractures associated with the extraction of teeth arose postoperatively and usually occurred during second to fourth week [9–12, 14, 17]. Interestingly, a number of fractures occurred during chewing of bagel, nuts, and steak [11]. The masticatory force required to break down food before deglutition can place considerable stress on bone weakened by surgery, which is not yet fully restored [6, 11]. However, preangular courses of fracture have been described as typical for pathological mandibular fractures following third molar removal [2]; Wagner et al. [13] reported two angular courses of fracture.

Early and adequate clinical and radiologic evaluations are required to establish a correct diagnosis of postoperative

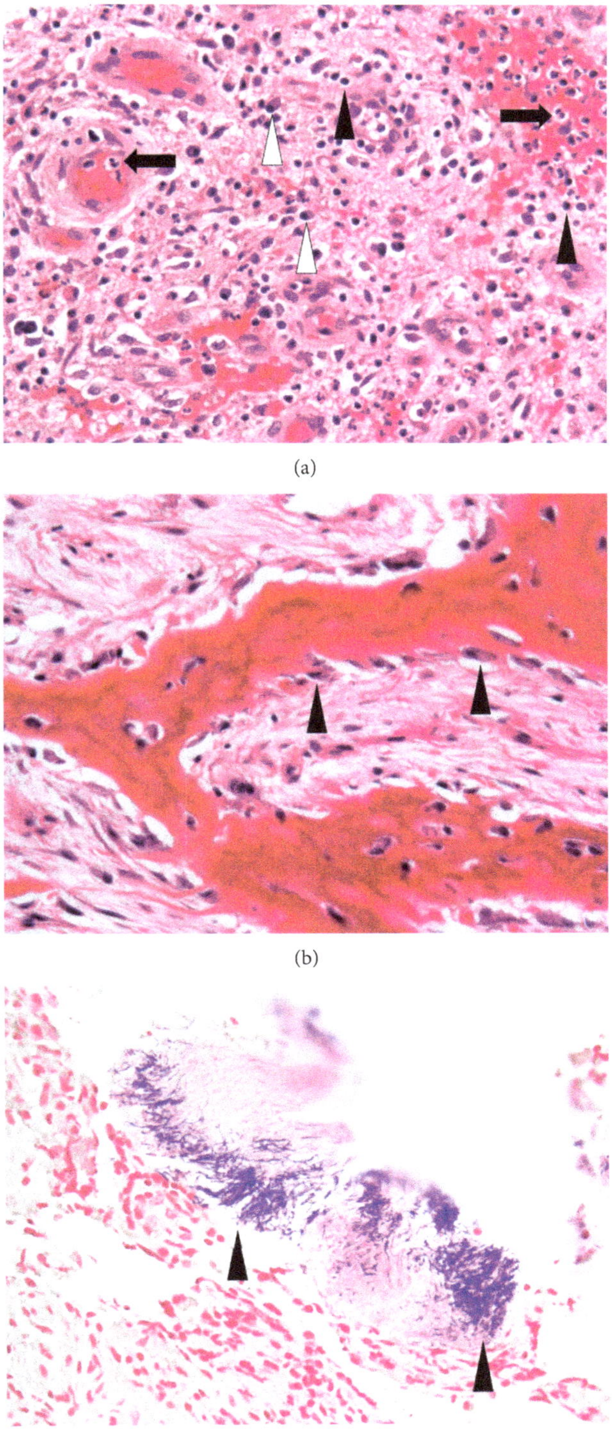

(a)

(b)

(c)

FIGURE 7: Surgical specimen of the granulation tissue. (a) The majority of the surgical specimen is granulation tissue composed of lymphocytes (black arrowheads) and plasma cells (white arrowheads), with neutrophil infiltration (black arrows) (H-E, ×400). (b) The surgical specimen includes neonatal bone accompanied by many osteoblasts (black arrowheads) (H-E, ×400). (c) Colonies of *Actinomyces* sp. (black arrowheads) are recognized in the inflammatory infiltrates (Gram, ×400).

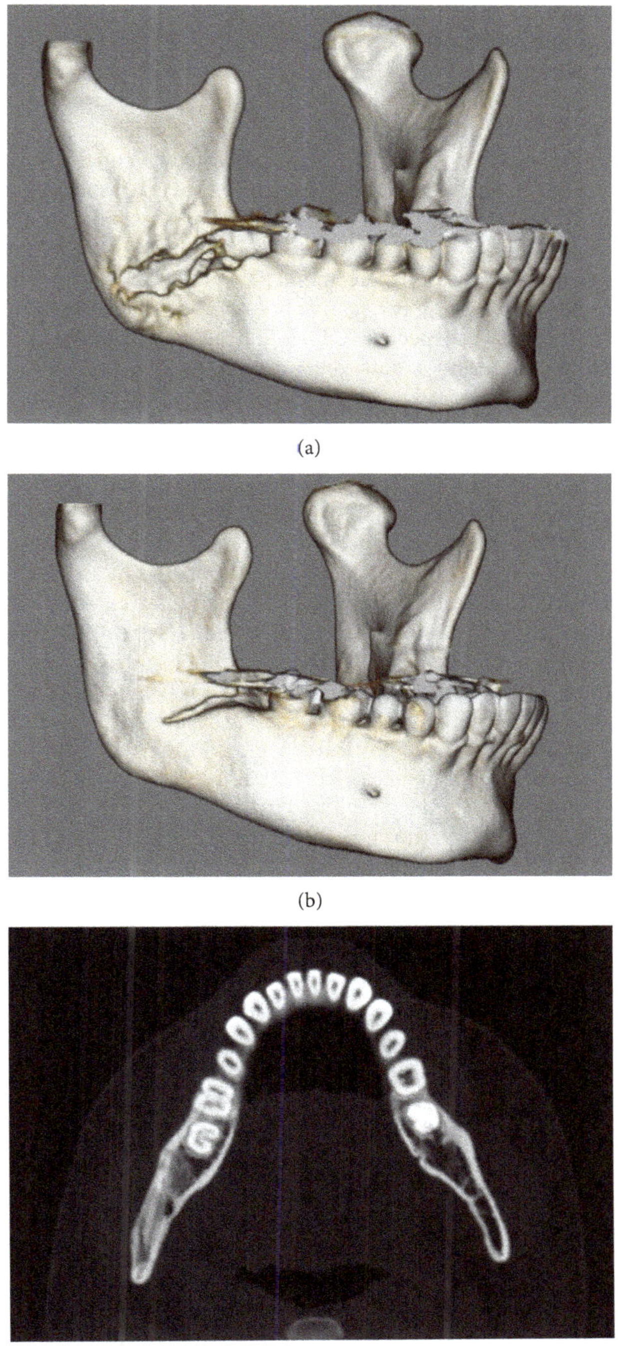

(a)

(b)

(c)

FIGURE 8: Three-dimensional computed tomographic (3D CT) scan obtained during the initial visit (a). 3D CT (b) and coronal CT (c) scans obtained 6 months after sequestrectomy and curettage. Although the CT obtained at the initial visit shows destruction of buccal cortical bone from the socket to the right mandibular angle and formation of bone sequestrum (a), CT obtained at 6 months shows bone healing at the lesion site, except for the remaining slight slit of the buccal cortical bone (b, c).

mandibular fracture. Typically, a cracking sound from the mandible while eating frequently indicated that a fracture had occurred [2, 12, 16]. Then, following the cracking sound, a swelling in the respective mandibular angle was frequently detectable [13]. Given that the course of the patients until this episode had been uneventful, the mandible was considered to have been fractured at the time this cracking sound was heard. On the other hand, initial radiographs may not be able to reveal a fracture, because the majority of patients do not experience occlusal displacement [2, 10]. In cases where the radiographic finding is negative but a nondisplaced mandibular fracture is suspected, CT should be performed [10]. In such a situation, a soft diet should be prescribed, and repeated radiological examinations are indicated several days later for definitive diagnosis [2].

The treatment options for this type of fracture are diverse and include conservative treatment, a postoperative diet of soft food for several months, maxillomandibular fixation with elastics, and open reduction with internal fixation [11, 13]. Particularly, Pires et al. [10] reported in a systemic review that patients with nondisplaced fractures who were prescribed with a soft diet had a successful treatment and achieved bone repair, as observed radiographically. In the present case, the postoperative course was uneventful, but at 23 days after the extraction, when the patient was chewing an innards stew, he heard a cracking sound from the right mandible and began to feel mild pain and swelling in the right masseteric region. Furthermore, he had paresthesia of his lower lip and mental region in the right side in addition to worsening of the pain and swelling at 19 days after the cracking sound. Even in imaging studies, a panoramic radiograph taken immediately after the cracking sound showed no abnormalities, and CT obtained during the initial visit showed buccal cortical bone destruction from the socket to the right mandibular angle and bone sequestrum formation.

From these findings and course, the patient was diagnosed as having osteomyelitis of the mandible caused by late fracture following third molar extraction. First, in brief, fissure fracture of the buccal cortical bone at the right mandibular angle without dislocation occurred when he heard the cracking sound. These results are consistent with previous reports on the common period, typical trigger, and findings of imaging studies. Then, the infection progressed along the fracture line and extended to the mandibular angle, and osteomyelitis occurred. Finally, the paresthesia of his lower lip and mental region in the right side associated with the osteomyelitis occurred 19 days after the cracking sound. In a past report, Iizuka et al. [2] reported a case of mandibular fracture following third molar extraction with an infection at the fracture site during intermaxillary fixation and required removal of granulation tissue. Therefore, it is necessary to recognize the possibility that late fracture following third molar extraction can cause osteomyelitis. In many cases, late fractures are treated with conservative approaches, such as placing the patients on a soft diet. However, regular and strict monitoring should still be performed during the period of conservative therapy to prevent the development of osteomyelitis following a late fracture, as seen in this case.

Second, once osteomyelitis of the mandible caused by late fracture occurred, early and appropriate treatment is necessary because the osteomyelitis develops rapidly, and there is a possibility that it will result in pathological fracture. The bacteria associated with osteomyelitis includes *Staphylococcus* sp., *Peptostreptococcus* sp., *Actinomyces* sp., and *Prevotella* sp. [18–20]. Once seeded, the infections are thought to spread via the medullary marrow space and compromise the blood supply. The affected bone is destroyed at a rapid rate in most suppurative cases with formation of sequestra and involucrum [19]. Necrotic tissue promotes the proliferation of bacteria, which, without an appropriate intervention, will result in incomplete healing and progression of the osteomyelitis [21]. In chronic forms of osteomyelitis, the inflammatory infiltrate is composed of plasma cells, lymphocytes, and macrophages, and reactive bone formation is evident with irregular reversal lines [19]. Given that antibiotics cannot penetrate in the affected bone, an early diagnosis of osteomyelitis and a surgical intervention are essential to avoid serious complications [21, 22]. In the present case, new bone formation by periosteal reaction and mixed infection with *Actinomyces* sp. and gram-positive bacilli occurred. However, CT obtained at 31 days after the cracking sound showed buccal cortical bone destruction from the socket to the right mandibular angle and bone sequestrum formation; the sequestrum was completely replaced by granulation tissues at the time of surgery, which was 41 days after the CT was performed. Given the findings showing the rapid progression of osteomyelitis, if early and appropriate treatment was not performed, there was a possibility that the osteomyelitis may have progressed further and pathological fracture resulting from lingual cortical bone fracture may have occurred.

As a limitation of this case report, we cannot completely rule out the possibility that there was already osteomyelitis of the mandible at the time of the cracking sound and a simple pathological fracture occurred. Thus, further studies on cases of late fracture following third molar extraction are required to confirm whether late fractures can cause osteomyelitis.

4. Conclusion

The course of this patient has two important implications. First, it is necessary to recognize the possibility that late fracture following third molar extraction can cause osteomyelitis. In many cases, late fractures are treated with conservative approaches, such as placing the patients on a soft diet. However, regular and strict monitoring should still be performed during the period of conservative therapy to prevent the development of osteomyelitis following a late fracture, as seen in this case. Second, once osteomyelitis of the mandible caused by late fracture occurred, early and appropriate treatment is necessary because osteomyelitis may progress rapidly and in some cases may result in pathological fracture.

Consent

The patient provided written informed consent for the use of their photographs in this publication.

References

[1] P. Mercier and D. Precious, "Risks and benefits of removal of impacted third molars: a critical review of the literature," *International Journal of Oral and Maxillofacial Surgery*, vol. 21, no. 1, pp. 17–27, 1992.

[2] T. Iizuka, S. Tanner, and H. Berthold, "Mandibular fractures following third molar extraction. A retrospective clinical and radiological study," *International Journal of Oral and Maxillofacial Surgery*, vol. 26, no. 5, pp. 338–343, 1997.

[3] I. R. Blum, "Contemporary views on dry socket (alveolar osteitis): a clinical appraisal of standardization, aetiopathogenesis and management: a critical review," *International Journal of Oral and Maxillofacial Surgery*, vol. 31, no. 3, pp. 309–317, 2002.

[4] C. H. Bui, E. B. Seldin, and T. B. Dodson, "Types, frequencies, and risk factors for complications after third molar extraction," *Journal of Oral and Maxillofacial Surgery*, vol. 61, no. 12, pp. 1379–1389, 2003.

[5] S. K. Chuang, D. H. Perrott, S. M. Susarla, and T. B. Dodson, "Age as a risk factor for third molar surgery complications," *Journal of Oral and Maxillofacial Surgery*, vol. 65, no. 9, pp. 1685–1692, 2007.

[6] G. F. Bouloux, M. B. Steed, and V. J. Perciaccante, "Complications of third molar surgery," *Oral and Maxillofacial Surgery Clinics of North America*, vol. 19, no. 1, pp. 117–128, 2007.

[7] S. K. Chuang, D. H. Perrott, S. M. Susarla, and T. B. Dodson, "Risk factors for inflammatory complications following third molar surgery in adults," *Journal of Oral and Maxillofacial Surgery*, vol. 66, no. 11, pp. 2213–2218, 2008.

[8] B. R. Chrcanovic and A. L. N. Custódio, "Considerations of mandibular angle fractures during and after surgery for removal of third molars: a review of the literature," *Oral and Maxillofacial Surgery*, vol. 14, no. 2, pp. 71–80, 2010.

[9] M. Ethunandan, D. Shanahan, and M. Patel, "Iatrogenic mandibular fractures following removal of impacted third molars: an analysis of 130 cases," *British Dental Journal*, vol. 212, no. 4, pp. 179–184, 2012.

[10] W. R. Pires, J. P. Bonardi, L. P. Faverani et al., "Late mandibular fracture occurring in the postoperative period after third molar removal: systematic review and analysis of 124 cases," *International Journal of Oral and Maxillofacial Surgery*, vol. 46, no. 1, pp. 46–53, 2017.

[11] P. A. Perry and M. H. Goldberg, "Late mandibular fracture after third molar surgery: a survey of Connecticut oral and maxillofacial surgeons," *Journal of Oral and Maxillofacial Surgery*, vol. 58, no. 8, pp. 858–861, 2000.

[12] P. Libersa, D. Roze, T. Cachart, and J. C. Libersa, "Immediate and late mandibular fractures after third molar removal," *Journal of Oral and Maxillofacial Surgery*, vol. 60, no. 2, pp. 163–165, 2002.

[13] K. W. Wagner, J. E. Otten, R. Schoen, and R. Schmelzeisen, "Pathological mandibular fractures following third molar removal," *International Journal of Oral and Maxillofacial Surgery*, vol. 34, no. 7, pp. 722–726, 2005.

[14] V. Grau-Manclús, J. Gargallo-Albiol, N. Almendros-Marqués, and C. Gay-Escoda, "Mandibular fractures related to the surgical extraction of impacted lower third molars: a report of 11 cases," *Journal of Oral and Maxillofacial Surgery*, vol. 69, no. 5, pp. 1286–1290, 2011.

[15] G. J. Pell and B. T. Gregory, "Impacted mandibular third molars: classification and modified techniques for removal," *The Dental Digest*, vol. 39, no. 9, pp. 330–338, 1933.

[16] M. Krimmel and S. Reinert, "Mandibular fracture after third molar removal," *Journal of Oral and Maxillofacial Surgery*, vol. 58, no. 10, pp. 1110–1112, 2000.

[17] L. Bodner, P. A. Brennan, and N. M. McLeod, "Characteristics of iatrogenic mandibular fractures associated with tooth removal: review and analysis of 189 cases," *British Journal of Oral and Maxillofacial Surgery*, vol. 49, no. 7, pp. 567–572, 2011.

[18] Y. Suei, A. Taguchi, and K. Tanimoto, "Diagnosis and classification of mandibular osteomyelitis," *Oral Surgery, Oral Medicine, Oral Pathology, Oral Radiology, and Endodontology*, vol. 100, no. 2, pp. 207–214, 2005.

[19] P. A. Krakowiak, "Alveolar osteitis and osteomyelitis of the jaws," *Oral and Maxillofacial Surgery Clinics of North America*, vol. 23, no. 3, pp. 401–413, 2011.

[20] S. Yamamoto, H. Takegawa, N. Taniike, and T. Takenobu, "Actinomycotic osteomyelitis of the mandible diagnosed using matrix assisted laser desorption ionization-time of flight mass spectrometry: a case report," *Journal of Oral and Maxillofacial Surgery*, vol. 76, no. 10, pp. 2122–2130, 2018.

[21] B. Lorè, M. Gargari, E. Ventucci, A. Cagioli, G. Nicolai, and L. Calabrese, "A complication following tooth extraction: chronic suppurative osteomyelitis," *Oral & Implantology*, vol. 6, no. 2, pp. 43–47, 2013.

[22] B. González-Navarro, C. Arranz-Obispo, R. Albuquerque, E. Jané-Salas, and J. López-López, "Osteomyelitis of the jaw (with pathological fracture) following extraction of an impacted wisdom tooth. A case report," *Journal of Stomatology, Oral and Maxillofacial Surgery*, vol. 118, no. 5, pp. 306–309, 2017.

18

Large Rhinolith Mimicking Atypical Odontogenic Pain: Case Report and Brief Review of the Literature

Zahra Vasegh and Mitra Ghazizadeh Ahsaie

Department of Oral and Maxillofacial Radiology, School of Dentistry, Shahid Beheshti University of Medical Sciences, Tehran, Iran

Correspondence should be addressed to Mitra Ghazizadeh Ahsaie; mitraghazizadeh@gmail.com

Academic Editor: Gavriel Chaushu

Rhinoliths are rare calcified entities in the nasal fossa, frequently originating around a nidus near the midway point in the inferior meatus, where the passage is the narrowest. They can be clinically asymptomatic and undetected for years. In this study, we present a rare case of large rhinolith mimicking atypical odontogenic pain in a 40-year-old Caucasian female in the left nasal cavity. The lesion was detected in the CBCT and removed uneventfully.

1. Introduction

Rhinolith is an uncommon calcification in the nasal fossa. Calcareous concretions that occur in the nose arise from the slow accumulation of inflammatory mineral salts such as calcium phosphate, calcium carbonate, and magnesium, around a nidus [1]. The nidus may be endogenous, mostly in adults, or exogenous (e.g., coins, beads, and seeds), mostly in children [2]. The route of entry of the foreign body into the nasal fossa is usually from the anterior; however, in rare cases, the foreign body enters the nose from posterior following sneezing. Rhinoliths are seen in different shapes and sizes, depending on what the nature of the nidus is [3]. The common signs and symptoms following this entity are pain in the maxillofacial region, toothache, headache, epistaxis, fetid odor sensation, nasal discharge, anosmia, and oral halitosis [4]. However, some cases are completely asymptomatic, and the patient is not aware of the entity unless it is find as an incidental finding in radiography. CBCT is helpful for better detecting the location and extent of the rhinolith three dimensionally, especially if surgery is needed. In addition, CBCT has significantly lower dose in comparison to maxillofacial MDCT [5].

2. Case Presentation

A 40-year-old female was referred to a private oral and maxillofacial radiology clinic with recent two months history of facial and periorbital pain, headache, upper jaw pain, nasal discharge, epistaxis, and fetid odor sensation. The patient had no history of trauma or previous interventions. A medium FOV CBCT scan was acquired from maxilla and paranasal sinuses. The left inferior meatus was completely filled with a well-defined, irregular calcified mass with peripheral mucosal thickening (Figure 1). There was also mucosal thickening in the left maxillary sinus. The initial diagnosis was rhinolith. The patient was further referred to department of the ear, nose, and throat surgery, and the calcified mass was excised endoscopically under general anesthesia. The histopathologic examination confirmed a granulation tissue with nasal lithiasis pattern tissue. The left maxillary sinus also showed inflammatory mucosal thickening compatible with chronic sinusitis. The patient experienced immediate improvement, and postoperative follow-up of patient was uneventful. The area had healed with no complication.

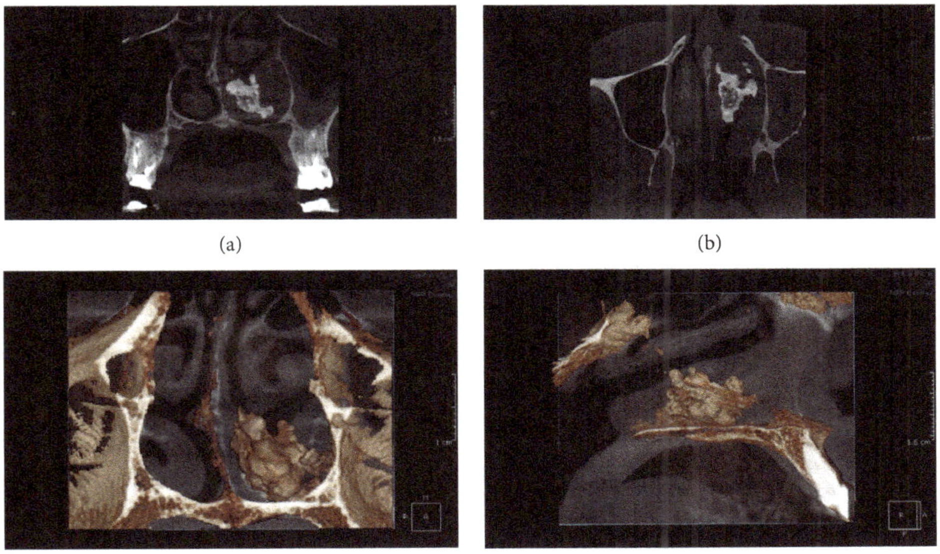

(a) (b) (c) (d)

FIGURE 1: CBCT images of nasal fossa. Coronal (a), axial (b), and multiplanar reformat images show an irregularly large heterogenous calcified mass in the inferior meatus of the left nasal cavity. Note the adjacent mucosal thickening. Coronal (c) and sagittal (d) 3D reformation images better show the space occupying rhinolith and slight deviation of nasal septum to the right side.

3. Discussion

A rhinolith is a calcification around exogenous or endogenous nidus in the nasal cavities. Approximately, 15 years are needed for rhinoliths to form; therefore, they are initially asymptomatic [6]. Further calcification and expansion may impinge on the mucosa leading to pain, congestion, and ulceration. The common complications associated with this entity are nasal obstruction, septal erosion, blood stained rhinorrhea and epistaxis, sinusitis, headache, purulent discharge, and fetid odor sensation [2, 4, 7, 8]. However, the patient may not face any pain or symptoms at all [9]. The patient of this case complained from fetid odor sensation, dental and periorbital pain, and unilateral purulent discharge. Girgis et al. suggested assessment of nasal cavity for rhinoliths in the cases of the anterior maxillary teeth pain in the absence of odontogenic causes [2]. In this case, the ipsilateral maxillary sinus had some mucosal thickening which may be due to partial obstruction of the adjacent nasal cavity. If the rhinolith is large enough, it may cause complete obstruction of maxillary sinus ostium and further results in sinusitis [10].

Previous studies show that rhinolith is usually found in female in their third decade of life. However, it is also detected in younger ages [11, 12]. This case was also found in a 40-year-old female patient, which is consistent with previous studies. Mohiyuddin et al. reported a case of giant rhinolith in a 15-year-old girl [12]. The patient did not suffer from any facial pain or headaches, and the only symptom was mucopurulent nasal discharge.

In this case, the calcified entity was detected in the inferior meatus, where the passage is the narrowest in the nasal cavity. Rare locations for rhinolith have also been detected. Ersozlu et al. reported calcification and presence of rhinolith in a concha bullosa [4]. In this study, the patient suffered from nasal obstruction, snoring, and head ache, but did not have symptoms such as epistaxis. In the study of Kharoubi et al., unusual case of bilateral rhinolithiasis and destruction of the posterior nasal septum was reported [6].

Clinical examination of the patient may include nasal endoscopy, anterior rhinoscopy, and probing of the mass [12]. The clinical differential diagnosis may include chronic rhinosinusitis, especially fungal sinusitis due to the presence of calcification. if the rhinolith is highly calcified, it can be detected by plain radiographs; however, low-density rhinolith requires advanced imaging to be detected [4]. Anthroliths may also be confused with rhinolith in plain radiographic projections such as occlusal or lateral cephalometric view. In the study of Estrela et al., large reactional osteogenesis in the maxillary sinus associated with secondary root canal infection was detected using cone-beam computed tomographic (CBCT) imaging [13]. This reactional osteogenesis presents a radiopaque entity in the maxillary sinus and may also be included in the differential diagnosis. Lesions such as calcifying fibroma, chondroma, and chonrosarcoma and calcified polyps should be included in the possible differential diagnoses [8, 14]. In addition, radiopaque odontogenic lesions such as odontoma, osteoma, and ossifying fibroma should be ruled out. In these cases, three dimensional imaging such as cone-beam computed tomography can easily indicate the location, extension, and probable origin of the lesion.

4. Conclusion

In the absence of obvious clinical dental pathology, sinonasal cavity should be completely assessed for pathology, including the presence of rhinolith [15].

References

[1] O. Dincer Kose, T. E. Kose, M. A. Erdem, and A. B. Cankaya, "Large rhinolith causing nasal obstruction," *Case Reports*, vol. 2015, no. mar10 1, article bcr2014208260, 2015.

[2] S. Girgis, L. Cheng, and D. Gillett, "Rhinolith mimicking a toothache," *International Journal of Surgery Case Reports*, vol. 14, pp. 66–68, 2015.

[3] S. Mallya and E. Lam, *White and Pharoah's Oral radiology E-book: principles and interpretation: Second South Asia Edition E-Book*, Elsevier India, 2019.

[4] T. Ersözlü and E. Gültekin, "Rhinolith in the concha bullosa as a rare location: a case report," *Journal of International Medical Research*, vol. 48, no. 8, article 0300060520951019, 2020.

[5] J. B. Ludlow and M. Ivanovic, "Comparative dosimetry of dental CBCT devices and 64-slice CT for oral and maxillofacial radiology," *Oral Surgery, Oral Medicine, Oral Pathology, Oral Radiology, and Endodontology*, vol. 106, no. 1, pp. 106–114, 2008.

[6] S. Kharoubi, *Revue générale sur les rhinolithiases. in Annales d'Otolaryngologie et de Chirurgie Cervico-faciale*, Elsevier, 2008.

[7] Y. Aziz, J. Chauhan, S. A. Hasan, and S. F. Hashmi, "Staghorn rhinolith in nasopharynx: an unusual case," *Indian Journal of Otolaryngology and Head & Neck Surgery*, vol. 60, no. 1, pp. 91–93, 2008.

[8] D. Brehmer and R. Riemann, "The rhinolith—a possible differential diagnosis of a unilateral nasal obstruction," *Case Reports in Medicine*, vol. 2010, 4 pages, 2010.

[9] A. Chatziavramidis, A. Kondylidou-Sidira, A. Stefanidis, and S. Soldatou, "Longstanding rhinolith leading to anatomical alterations of the ipsilateral inferior nasal meatus and turbinate," *Case Reports*, vol. 2010, no. nov18 1, article bcr0720103155, 2010.

[10] J.-C. Hsiao, C. F. Tai, K. W. Lee, K. Y. Ho, W. R. Kou, and L. F. Wang, "Giant rhinolith: a case report," *The Kaohsiung Journal of Medical Sciences*, vol. 21, no. 12, pp. 582–585, 2005.

[11] A. Yaroko, I. Mohamad, and H. Hashim, "Rhinolith: an important cause of foul-smelling nasal discharge," *Malaysian family physician: the official journal of the Academy of Family Physicians of Malaysia*, vol. 9, no. 1, pp. 30–32, 2014.

[12] M. Ali, "Giant 'staghorn' rhinolith in a 15-year-old girl," *BMJ Case Reports*, vol. 11, no. 1, p. e227587, 2018.

[13] C. Estrela, O. C. L. Porto, N. L. Costa et al., "Large reactional osteogenesis in maxillary sinus associated with secondary root canal infection detected using cone-beam computed tomography," *Journal of Endodontics*, vol. 41, no. 12, pp. 2068–2078, 2015.

[14] K. B. Noh, I. S. Sachlin, N. Gazali, and N. Md Shukri, "Giant rhinolith: a case report," *Egyptian Journal of Ear, Nose, Throat and Allied Sciences*, vol. 18, no. 2, pp. 155–157, 2017.

[15] C. A. Barros, R. R. Martins, J. B. Silva et al., "Rhinolith: a radiographic finding in a dental clinic," *Oral Surgery, Oral Medicine, Oral Pathology, Oral Radiology, and Endodontology*, vol. 100, no. 4, pp. 486–490, 2005.

19

A Case of Buccal Clear Cell Carcinoma Caused by Rare Fusion Gene: *EWSR1-CREM*

Miyako Hoshino,[1] Katsuyuki Inoue,[2] Tomohisa Kaneda,[2] Michiko Nishimura,[1] Kaoru Kusama,[1] Hideaki Sakashita,[2] Yukiko Sato,[3,4] Kengo Takeuchi,[3,4,5] Toshitaka Nagao,[6] and Kentaro Kikuchi[1]

[1]*Division of Pathology, Department of Diagnostic and Therapeutic Sciences, Meikai University School of Dentistry, 1-1 Keyakidai, Sakado, Saitama 350-0283, Japan*
[2]*Second Division of Oral and Maxillofacial Surgery, Department of Diagnostic and Therapeutic Sciences, Meikai University School of Dentistry, 1-1 Keyakidai, Sakado, Saitama 350-0283, Japan*
[3]*Division of Pathology, Cancer Institute, Japanese Foundation for Cancer Research, 3-8-31 Ariake, Koto-ku, Tokyo 135-8550, Japan*
[4]*Department of Pathology, Cancer Institute Hospital, Japanese Foundation for Cancer Research, 3-8-31 Ariake, Koto-ku, Tokyo 135-8550, Japan*
[5]*Pathology Project for Molecular Targets, Cancer Institute, Japanese Foundation for Cancer Research, 3-8-31 Ariake, Koto-ku, Tokyo 135-8550, Japan*
[6]*Department of Anatomic Pathology, Tokyo Medical University, 7-3-1 Hongo, Bunkyo-ku, Tokyo 113-0033, Japan*

Correspondence should be addressed to Miyako Hoshino; miyako-h@dent.meikai.ac.jp

Academic Editor: Mark Darling

Clear cell carcinoma (CCC) is a rare entity in the salivary gland tumor. So far, only 10 cases of primary CCC of the buccal mucosa have been reported. Here, we first report an extremely rare case of buccal CCC with the *EWSR1-CREM* fusion gene. The patient, a 69-year-old woman, presented with a painless mass in the right buccal mucosa. The tumor, which had been present for about 10 years, measured approximately 15 mm in diameter and was pedunculated, elastic hard, smooth, and mobile. Histopathological examination revealed proliferating tumor cells with vacuolated and clear cytoplasm partially surrounded by hyalinized stroma. The tumor was not encapsulated, and no contact with the overlying epithelium was evident. Duct-like structures were occasionally observed in the tumor nests composed of clear cells. The tumor had invaded into surrounding muscle and adipose tissues. Immunohistochemical examination revealed that the clear cells were positive for epithelial cell markers, and myoepithelial markers were negative. Fluorescence in situ hybridization (FISH), performed to search for genetic abnormalities, demonstrated split positivity for *EWSR1*, and fusion with *CREM* was confirmed. These findings suggested a diagnosis of CCC.

1. Introduction

Clear cell carcinoma (CCC) is an epithelial malignant tumor that arises in the salivary glands. CCC in the salivary glands was first reported in 1994 by Milchgrub et al. [1], who described a low-grade salivary gland carcinoma composed of malignant cells with clear cytoplasm, with hyalinization. CCC has a squamoid phenotype and lacks certain features of other clear cell-rich salivary gland carcinomas. It is more common in women, typically presenting in the fifth to eighth decades of life, and rare in children [2]. CCC is rare and accounts for fewer than 1% of all malignant tumors in the salivary glands. It occurs most frequently in the intraoral minor salivary glands, the palate, and the base of the tongue and less frequently in the buccal mucosa [3]. CCC most commonly presents as swelling and may be ulcerated or associated with pain, bone invasion, and soft tissue fixation [2]. Histopathologically, CCC is composed of proliferating

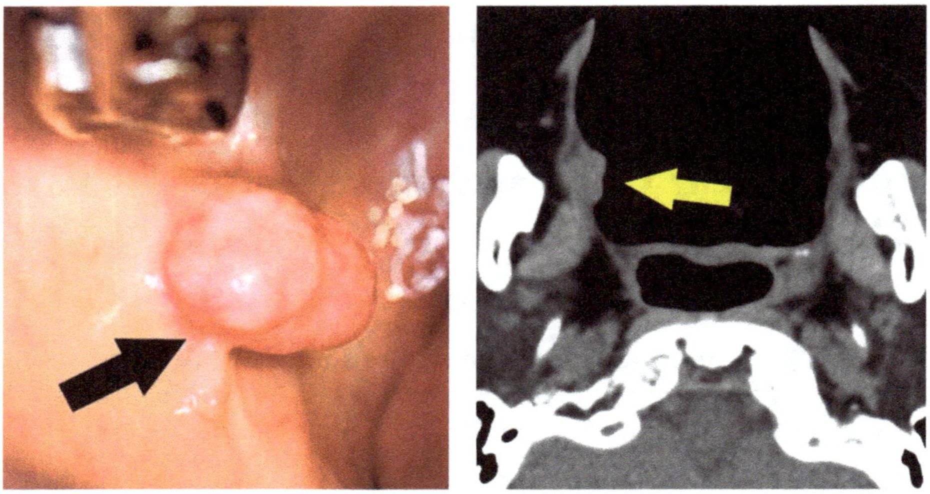

(a) (b)

FIGURE 1: Intraoral appearance of the buccal mucosa and CT image. (a) The mucosal epithelium was normal in color with a smooth surface. There was no induration around the tumor (black arrow). (b) CT (axial view) showed an enhanced lesion on the anterior portion of the right palatoglossal arch (yellow arrow).

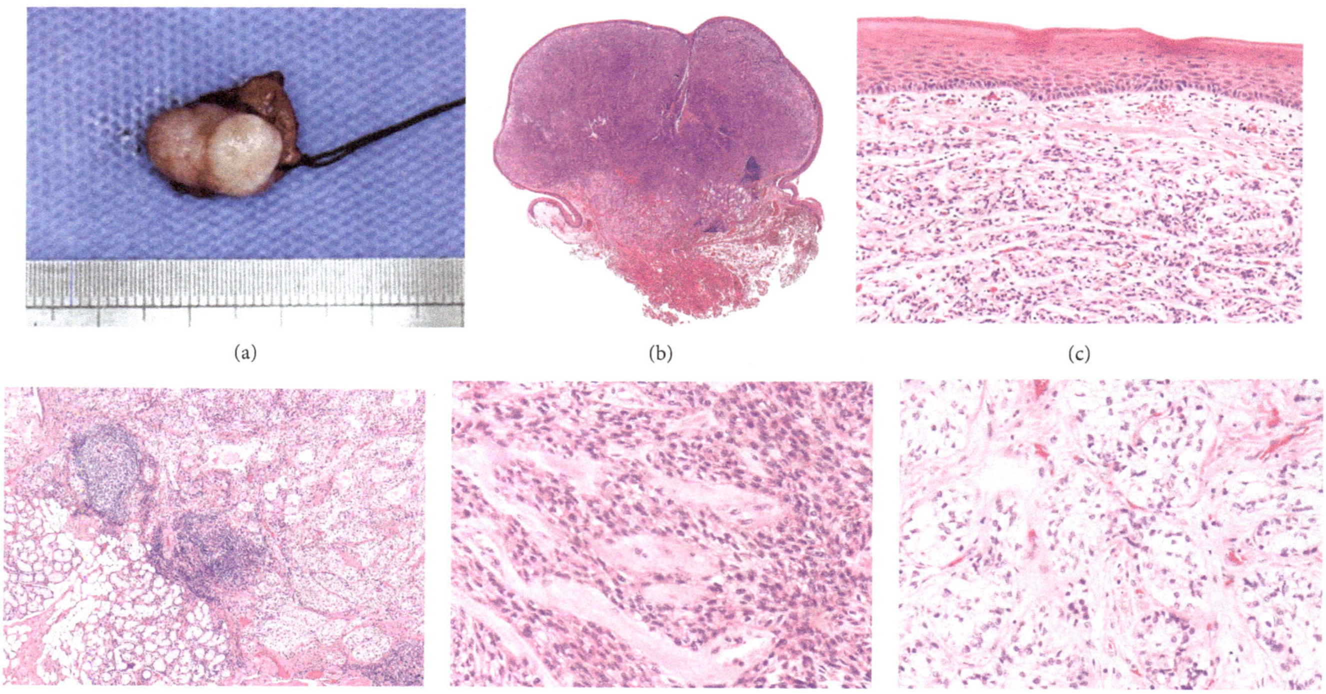

(a) (b) (c)

(d) (e) (f)

FIGURE 2: Microscopic and survey view of the surgical resected specimen. (a) Resected specimen measuring 18 × 12 × 14 mm. (b, c) The tumor demonstrated proliferation of tumor nests with a fibrous stroma. There was no capsule and no contact with the covering epithelium. (d) The tumor had invaded into surrounding muscle and adipose tissues. (e, f) The tumor nests were composed of epithelioid and clear cells partially surrounded by hyalinized stroma. Features suggestive of transition between the two cell types were observed (HE; original magnification: (b) ×1, (c) ×20, (d, f) ×40, and (e) ×100).

epithelial cells with clear cytoplasm organized into trabeculae, cords, or solid nests surrounded by hyalinized stroma [1]. However, differential diagnosis can be difficult because the microscopic features of CCC frequently overlap with those of other salivary gland tumors and metastatic renal cell carcinoma [3]. *EWSR1-ATF1* fusion specific for CCC can be evaluated by RT-PCR as hallmark markers, but in our case, *EWSR1-ATF1* fusion was not detected. To our knowledge

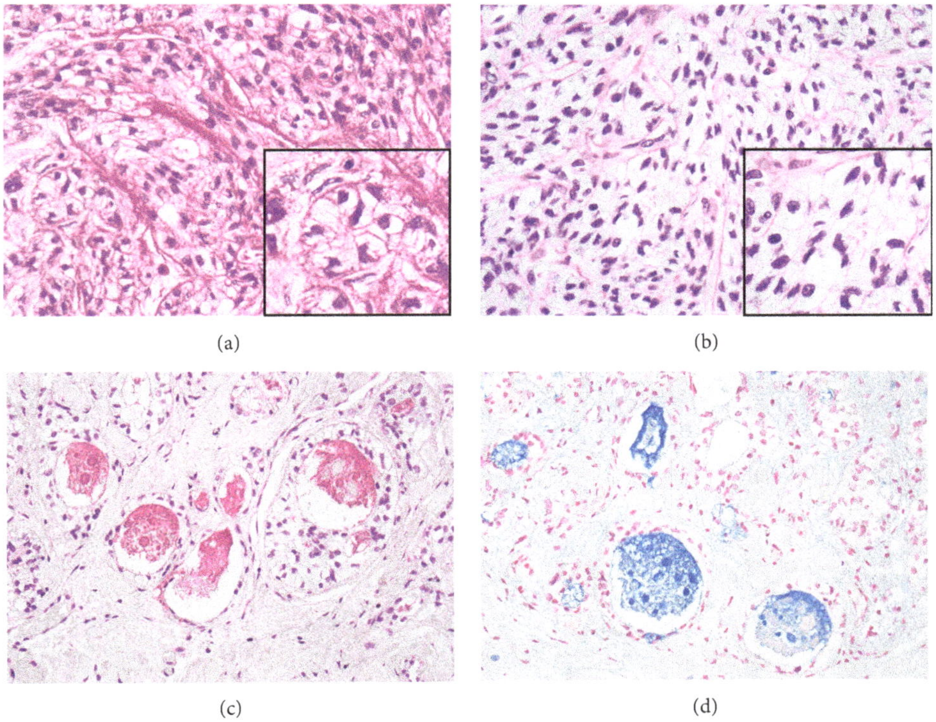

Figure 3: Special stains: (a) PAS, (b) d-PAS, (c) mucicarmine, and (d) Alcian blue. PAS stain shows positive cytoplasmic red material in the clear cells, but PAS with diastase stain was negative, suggesting the presence of glycogen. The contents of duct-like structures were positively stained by mucicarmine and Alcian blue, but mucus-producing cells were not evident in the tumor nests ((a–d) original magnification ×200).

there are previously 3 reported cases of hyalinizing clear cell carcinomas of *EWSR1-CREM* fusion [4]; as an additional case report in the literature, here, we first report a very rare case of buccal CCC with the *EWSR1-CREM* fusion gene.

2. Case Report

A 69-year-old woman presented with a mass in the right buccal mucosa that had been present for about 10 years and untreated because of absence of any pain.

However, as it showed no tendency to improve, and the swelling worsened, she visited a local dentist at first. She was then referred to the Meikai University Hospital for detailed examination and treatment. At the first visit, examination of the oral cavity demonstrated a mass measuring 15×10 mm in the right buccal mucosa on the anterior portion of the lobular polypoid palatoglossal arch (Figure 1(a)). The mucosal epithelium was normal in color with a smooth surface. There was no induration around the tumor. CT showed an enhanced lesion on the anterior portion of the right palatoglossal arch (Figure 1(b)). Surgical excision of the tumor was performed under local anesthesia. The surgical specimen measured $18 \times 12 \times 14$ mm (Figure 2(a)). Histopathologically, the tumor showed proliferation of tumor nests with fibrous stroma. There was no capsule and no contact with the covering epithelium (Figures 2(b) and 2(c)). The tumor invaded surrounding structures such as muscle and adipose tissue (Figure 2(d)).

The tumor nests were composed of epithelioid and clear cells with partially hyalinized stroma (Figures 2(e) and 2(f)). Mitotic figures were rarely evident, and transition between the two cell types was observed in part (data not shown).

Intracytoplasmic fine granules were positive for periodic acid-Schiff (PAS) and were negative for diastase-sensitive PAS (Figures 3(a) and 3(b)). The contents of duct-like structures were positively stained by mucicarmine and Alcian blue, but mucus-producing cells were not evident in the tumor nests (Figures 3(c) and 3(d)). Immunohistochemically, the tumor cells were strongly positive for AE1/AE3 (Figure 4(a)), CK5/6, and p63 (Figure 4(b)), but negative for α-SMA and S100 (Figure 4(c)), and Ki-67-positive cells were rarely found in the tumor nests (Figure 4(d)). The *EWSR1-ATF1* fusion gene could not be detected by reverse transcription polymerase chain reaction (RT-PCR) in the present case. RT-PCR also failed to detect the *CRTC1/3-MAML2* fusion gene, which is specific for mucoepidermoid carcinoma. Using bacterial artificial chromosome clone-derived DNA probes for *EWSR1* and *CREM* (the names of BAC clones used will be provided upon request), fluorescence in situ hybridization (FISH) analysis revealed the presence of *EWSR1-CREM* (Figures 5(a)–5(c)). These findings suggested a diagnosis of CCC with *CREM* fusion instead of *ATF1* fusion.

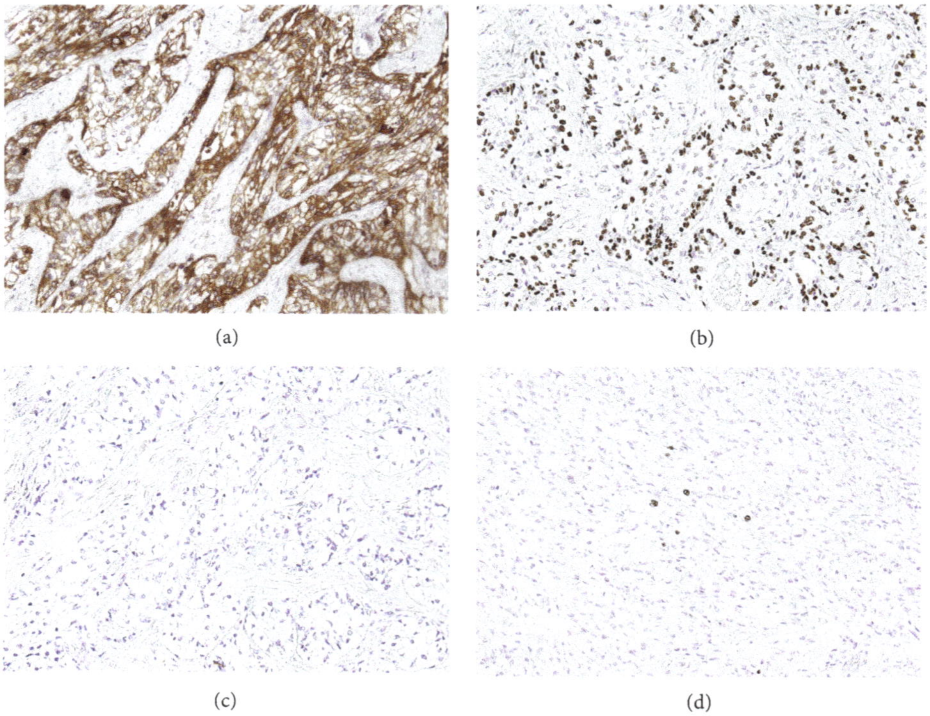

FIGURE 4: Immunohistochemical findings: (a) pancytokeratin (AE1/AE3), (b) p63, (c) S100, and (d) Ki-67. The tumor cells were stained intensely with cytokeratins, but not myoepithelial markers. The nuclei of the clear cells were positive for p63. Ki-67-positive cells were rarely found in the tumor nests ((a–d) original magnification ×200).

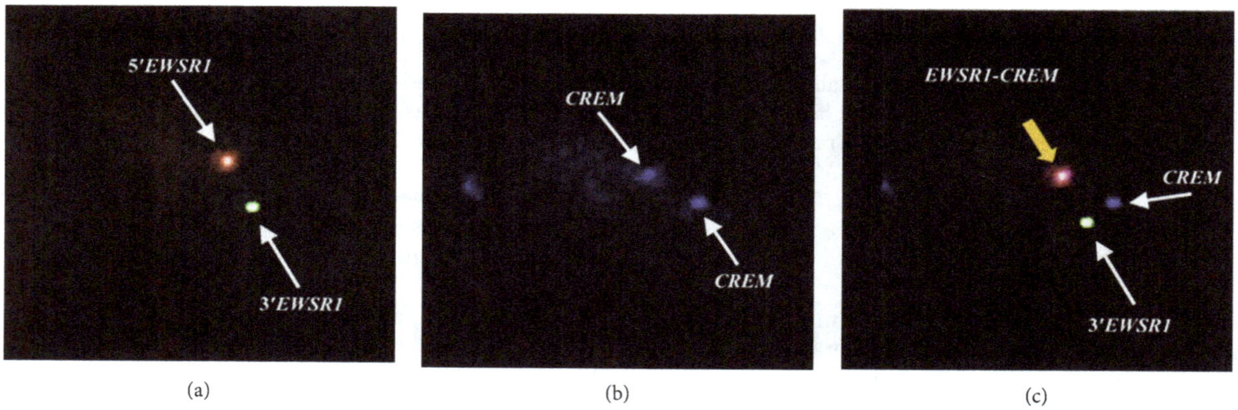

FIGURE 5: FISH analysis: (a) *EWSR1* break-apart; (b) *CREM*; (c) *EWSR1-CREM* gene fusion. *EWSR1* break-apart FISH demonstrate a cell with split red and green signals, indicative of a translocation. This case demonstrated split positivity for *EWSR1*, and fusion with *CREM* was confirmed.

3. Discussion

CCC is a low-grade malignancy with a good prognosis after complete surgical excision. Local recurrence and nodal metastases may occur, but distant metastasis and death due to disease are rare [2]. Clinical features, staining patterns, fusion type, pathological findings, and diagnostic methods reported cases of CCC in the cheek or buccal mucosa are summarized in Tables 1 and 2. The *EWSR1-CREM* fusion gene has not been previously reported in CCC of the buccal mucosa. Differential diagnosis of CCC based on histopathology includes mucoepidermoid carcinoma, acinic cell carcinoma, clear cell oncocytoma, epithelial myoepithelial carcinoma, malignant myoepithelioma, and metastatic renal cell carcinoma, all of which show a significant proportion of clear cells [1, 5]. The clear cell variant of mucoepidermoid carcinoma is positively stained with mucicarmine for tumor cells, which can be very helpful for highlighting the mucous cells and distinguishing them from other clear cell neoplasms [6]. Acinic cell carcinoma contains zymogen granules, which are PAS-positive and diastase resistant [7]. DOG1 and SOX10 are immunopositive in acinar and

TABLE 1: Clinical features and staining patterns of previously reported cheek or buccal mucosa CCC cases.

Authors	Year	Age	Sex	Size (cm)	Metastasis	Immunohistochemical staining						Special staining				Fusion type	Treatment	Recurrence	Follow-up and outcome
						CK	p63	CD10	S100	α-SMA	Ki-67	PAS	d-PAS	MC	ALC				
Simpson et al. [14]	1990	66	M	2.5	—	+	NA	NA	—	NA	NA	NA	NA	NA	NA	NA	Sur	—	NED (11 y)
Hiroki et al. [15]	1999	30	F	3	—	+	NA	NA	—	NA	NA	+	NA	NA	—	NA	Sur	—	NED
Milchgrub et al. [16]	2000	29	F	2	+†	NA	NA	NA	NA	NA	NA	NA	NA	NA	NA	NA	Sur	+	REC (12 mo)
O'Sullivan-Mejia et al. [17]	2009	78	F	1.7	—	+	—	NA	NA	NA	NA	+	NA	—	NA	NA	Sur	—	NED
Solar et al. [9]	2009	49	F	3	NA	+	NA	NA	—	—	NA	+	—	—	NA	NA	Sur	+	REC × 2 (114 mo)
Onoda et al. [11]	2012	59	F	0.8	—	+	—	—	—	—	NA	+	—	NA	—	NA	Sur	—	NED (4 y)
Shah et al. [18]	2013	46	F	NA	+†	+	+	NA	—	—	NA	NA	NA	NA	NA	*EWSR1 re*	Rad, RS	+	NA
	2013	37	F	NA	+†	+	+	NA	—	—	NA	NA	NA	NA	NA	*EWSR1 re*	Sur	+	NA
Yamanishi et al. [3]	2015	52	F	1.5	—	+	+	NA	—	—	NA	NA	NA	—	NA	*EWSR1-ATF1*	Sur	—	NED (11 y)
Albergotti et al. [19]	2016	70	F	4.9	—	NA	NA	NA	NA	NA	NA	NA	NA	NA	NA	*EWSR1 re*	Sur	—	NED (13 mo)
Hernandez-Prera et al. [20]	2017	57	F	2	—	NA	+	NA	—	—	NA	NA	NA	—	NA	*EWSR1-ATF1*	Sur	—	NED (24 mo)
Present study	2020	69	F	1.5	—	+	+	—	—	—	±	+	—	—	—	*EWSR1-CREM*	Sur	—	NED (2 y)

NA: not available or not mentioned; NED: no evidence of disease; REC: recurrence; MC: mucicarmine; ALC: Alcian blue; *re*: rearrangement; Rad: radiotherapy; RS: reduction surgery; Sur: surgery. †Cervical lymph nodes.

TABLE 2: Pathological findings and diagnostic methods of previously reported cheek or buccal mucosa CCC cases.

Authors	Findings						Diagnosis
	Solid sheets	Nests	Cords	Trabeculae	Hyalinizing stroma	Ducts and gland-like spaces	
Simpson et al. [14]	+	+	+	NA	+	NA	IHC, EMS
T Hiroki [15]	+	NA	NA	NA	+	+	IHC, EMS
Milchgrub et al. [16]	NA	+	+	+	+	NA	FNA
O'Sullivan-Mejia et al. [17]	NA	+	+	+	+	NA	IHC
Solar et al. [9]	+	+	+	+	+	NA	IHC
Onoda et al. [11]	+	NA	+	NA	+	NA	IHC
Shah et al. [18]	+	+	NA	+	+	NA	IHC, FISH
	+	+	NA	+	+	NA	IHC, FISH
Yamanishi et al. [3]	+	+	+	+	+	NA	IHC, RT-PCR
Albergotti et al. [19]	NA	+	+	NA	+	NA	FISH
Hernandez-Prera [20]	+	+	NA	+	+	NA	IHC, FISH
Present study	+	+	+	+	+	+	IHC, FISH

intercalated duct cells. Acinic cell carcinoma is usually immunonegative for mammaglobin [8]. Clear cell oncocytoma has a PAS-positive and diastase-PAS-negative cytoplasm. Unlike CCC, it is encapsulated or circumscribed, and the clear cells have a marginal rim of cytoplasm that retains eosinophilic granules. The tumor cells are also positively stained with phosphotungstic acid-hematoxylin and show strong immunohistochemical staining for mitochondria [9]. Epithelial myoepithelial carcinoma and malignant myoepithelioma express S100 protein, α-smooth muscle actin (α-SMA), and SOX10 [6, 10]. SOX10 is positive for myoepithelial carcinoma [10]. Renal cell carcinoma shows immunopositivity for cytokeratins, vimentin, and CD10 [6]. CCC is characterized by trabeculae, cords, or irregular solid nests surrounded by a hyalinized stroma. The tumor cells have clear cytoplasm and circular or polygonal nuclei [11]. Perineural and bone invasion are common, and ducts and gland-like spaces may be evident. CCC is positive for CKs and p63 and negative for other myoepithelial markers. Intracytoplasmic fine granules that give a diastase-sensitive positive PAS reaction are present [2]. The use of special stains and immunohistochemistry, along with careful histological examination of the tumor, in order to identify the typical features found in each of these neoplasms, is helpful for establishing a correct diagnosis [5]. Specific gene fusions have been found to play a definitive role in tumorigenesis. The 2017 WHO classification states that the *EWSR1-ATF1* fusion gene can be identified in CCC [2] and is the most reliable tool for differentiating CCC from other histologically similar tumors. In the present case, however, it could not be detected by RT-PCR. Furthermore, the *CRTC1/3-MAML2* fusion gene characteristic of mucoepidermoid carcinoma was not detected. FISH, performed to search for genetic abnormalities, demonstrated split positivity for *EWSR1*, and fusion with the cAMP response element modulator (*CREM*) was confirmed. Recurrent gene fusions involving *EWSR1* with members of the cAMP response element binding protein (*CREB*) family (*ATF1* and *CREB1*) have been reported in a diverse group of tumors including angiomatoid fibrous histiocytoma, soft tissue and gastrointestinal clear cell sarcoma, primary pulmonary myxoid sarcoma, and hyalinizing clear cell carcinoma of the salivary gland [12]. *CREB* can bind to a few thousand gene promoters that contain *CRE* (cAMP response element), although it remains unknown what fraction of these genes is also functionally regulated upon this binding. *CREM* belongs to the *CREB* family (*ATF1*, *CREB1*, and *CREM*) of transcription factors [12]. The structure and biological functions of both *CREM* and *ATF-1* are similar to *CREB*, which forms heterodimers with *ATF-1* or *CREM* [13]. In the present case, *EWSR1* was fused with one of the *CREB* family members, *CREM*. To our knowledge, there are 3 reported cases of hyalinizing clear cell carcinomas of *EWSR1-CREM* fusion [4], but it has not been reported previously in buccal mucosa. The present case of CCC shows that *CREM* may replace *ATF1* as an *EWSR 1* fusion partner. For future characterization of tumors, molecular diagnostic assays will become increasingly important in addition to the use of special staining and immunohistochemistry.

4. Conclusion

CCC is a rare minor salivary gland tumor exhibiting low-grade malignancy. The diagnosis of clear cells in salivary glands can be challenging and the differential diagnosis being quite broad. However, testing for any *EWSR1* translocation combined with specific histological staining may be a new reliable method for distinguishing CCC from other salivary gland tumors. Here, we have reported an extremely rare case of clear cell-rich salivary gland carcinoma of the buccal mucosa.

Acknowledgments

The authors would like to thank Ms. Satoko Baba at the cancer institute for her technical support.

References

[1] S. Milchgrub, D. R. Gnepp, F. Vuitch, R. Delgado, and J. Albores-Saavedra, "Hyalinizing clear cell carcinoma of salivary gland," *American Journal of Surgical Pathology*, vol. 18, no. 1, pp. 74–82, 1994.

[2] B. M. Wenig, D. Bell, S. Chiosea, H. Inagaki, and R. Seethala, "Clear cell carcinoma," in *World Health Organization Classification of Head and Neck Tumours*, A. K. El-Naggar, J. K. C. Chan, J. R. Grandis, T. Takata, and P. J. Slootweg, Eds., IARC Press, Lyon, 2017.

[3] T. Yamanishi, K. Kutsuma, and K. Masuyama, "A case of hyalinizing clear cell carcinoma, so-called clear cell carcinoma, not otherwise specified, of the minor salivary glands of the buccal mucosa," *Case Reports in Otolaryngology*, vol. 2015, Article ID 471693, 7 pages, 2015.

[4] E. Chapman, A. Skalova, N. Ptakova et al., "Molecular profiling of hyalinizing clear cell carcinomas revealed a subset of tumors harboring a novel *EWSR1-CREM* fusion," *American Journal of Surgical Pathology*, vol. 42, no. 9, pp. 1182–1189, 2018.

[5] T. K. Chao, C. C. Tsai, S. Y. Yeh, and J. E. Teh, "Hyalinizing clear cell carcinoma of the hard palate," *The Journal of Laryngology & Otology*, vol. 118, no. 5, pp. 382–384, 2004.

[6] E. Maiorano, M. Altini, and G. Favia, "Clear cell tumors of the salivary glands, jaws, and oral mucosa," *Seminars Diagnostic Pathology*, vol. 14, no. 3, pp. 201–212, 1997.

[7] K. Pujary, S. Rangarajan, D. R. Nayak, R. Balakrishnan, and V. Ramakrishnan, "Hyalinizing clear cell carcinoma of the base of tongue," *International Journal of Oral and Maxillofacial Surgery*, vol. 37, no. 1, pp. 93–96, 2008.

[8] R. H. W. Simpson, S. Chiosea, N. Katabi, I. Leivo, P. Vielh, and M. D. Williams, "Acinic cell carcinoma," in *World Health Organization Classification of Head and Neck Tumours*, A. K. El-Naggar, J. K. C. Chan, J. R. Grandis, T. Takata, and P. J. Slootweg, Eds., IARC Press, Lyon, France, 2017.

[9] A. A. Solar, B. L. Schmidt, and R. C. K. Jordan, "Hyalinizing clear cell carcinoma," *Cancer*, vol. 115, no. 1, pp. 75–83, 2009.

[10] M. S. Hsieh, Y. H. Lee, and Y. L. Chang, "SOX10-positive salivary gland tumors: a growing list, including mammary analogue secretory carcinoma of the salivary gland, sialoblastoma, low-grade salivary duct carcinoma, basal cell adenoma/adenocarcinoma, and a subgroup of mucoepidermoid carcinoma," *Human Pathology*, vol. 56, pp. 134–142, 2016.

[11] M. Onoda, K. Seki, T. Ikari, W. Kumamaru, T. Sugiura, and K. Shirasuna, "A case of clear cell carcinoma, not otherwise specified (NOS) of the buccal mucosa," *Japanese Journal of Oral and Maxillofacial Surgery*, vol. 58, no. 5, pp. 288–291, 2012.

[12] Y. C. Kao, Y. S. Sung, L. Zhang et al., "*EWSR1* fusions with *CREB* family transcription factors define a novel myxoid mesenchymal tumor with predilection for intracranial location," *American Journal of Surgical Pathology*, vol. 41, no. 4, pp. 482–490, 2017.

[13] X. Wu, C. Spiro, W. G. Owen, and C. T. McMurray, "cAMP Response Element-binding Protein Monomers Cooperatively Assemble to Form Dimers on DNA," *Journal of Biological Chemistry*, vol. 273, no. 33, pp. 20820–20827, 1998.

[14] R. H. W. Simpson, P. T. L. Sarsfield, T. Clarke, and A. V. Babajews, "Clear cell carcinoma of minor salivary glands," *Histopathology*, vol. 17, no. 5, pp. 433–438, 1990.

[15] H. Toyoda, K. Yamaguchi, K. Masumoto, T. Koyama, H. Fukuda, and K. Hashimoto, "A case of hyalinizing clear cell carcinoma of the cheek with thirteen-year delay of the disease," *Journal of the Japanese Stomatological Society*, vol. 48, no. 6, pp. 498–502, 1999.

[16] S. Milchgrub, F. Vuitch, M. Hossein Saboorian, A. Hameed, H. Wu, and J. Albores-Saavedra, "Hyalinizing clear-cell carcinoma of salivary glands in fine-needle aspiration," *Diagnostic Cytopathology*, vol. 23, no. 5, pp. 333–337, 2000.

[17] E. D. O'Sullivan-Mejia, H. D. Massey, W. C. Faquin, and C. N. Powers, "Hyalinizing clear cell carcinoma: report of eight cases and a review of literature," *Head and Neck Pathology*, vol. 3, no. 3, pp. 179–185, 2009.

[18] A. A. Shah, R. D. LeGallo, A. van Zante et al., "*EWSR1* genetic rearrangements in salivary gland tumors," *American Journal of Surgical Pathology*, vol. 37, no. 4, pp. 571–578, 2013.

[19] W. G. Albergotti, E. A. Bilodeau, J. K. Byrd, M. M. Mims, S. Lee, and S. Kim, "Hyalinizing clear cell carcinoma of the head and neck: case series and update," *Head & Neck*, vol. 38, no. 3, pp. 426–433, 2016.

[20] J. C. Hernandez-Prera, R. Kwan, J. Tripodi et al., "Reappraising hyalinizing clear cell carcinoma: a population-based study with molecular confirmation," *Head & Neck*, vol. 39, no. 3, pp. 503–511, 2017.

20

Clear Cell Odontogenic Carcinoma of the Mandible Harboring *EWSR1* Rearrangement: Report of a Massive Jaw Tumor and Review of Diagnostic Considerations

Adepitan A. Owosho[1] **Chukwubuzor Okwuosa,**[2] **Donald I. Obi,**[2] **Robinson O. Okiti,**[3] **and Kurt F. Summersgill**[4]

[1]*Missouri School of Dentistry and Oral Health, A.T. Still University, Kirksville, Missouri, USA*
[2]*University of Nigeria Teaching Hospital, Nsukka, Enugu, Nigeria*
[3]*University College Hospital, Ibadan, Oyo, Nigeria*
[4]*Department of Diagnostic Sciences, School of Dental Medicine, University of Pittsburgh, Pittsburgh, Pennsylvania, USA*

Correspondence should be addressed to Adepitan A. Owosho; adepitanowosho@atsu.edu

Academic Editor: Eugenio Maiorano

Clear cell odontogenic carcinoma (CCOC) is a low-grade malignant neoplasm that affects the jaws. We report an 18 cm massive case of mandibular CCOC in a 43-year-old female. The tumor was composed of nests and cords of round to polygonal monomorphic clear cells separated by prominent stromal hyalinization. Immunohistochemically, the tumor cells showed focal cytokeratin 5/6 positivity and intracytoplasmic PAS-positive granules and were negative for S100 and after diastase treatment (PAS-D). Molecularly, this case was positive for *EWSR1* rearrangement by FISH. The following should be included in the histopathological differential diagnosis: hyalinizing clear cell carcinoma of the salivary gland, clear cell variant of central mucoepidermoid carcinoma, clear cell variant of calcifying epithelial odontogenic tumor, and metastatic renal cell carcinoma. CCOC is a rare entity, with only 79 cases reported in the mandible. This case highlights the propensity for CCOC to exhibit invasiveness, destructive nature, and facial disfigurement if left untreated.

1. Introduction

Clear cell odontogenic carcinoma (CCOC) is a rare malignant odontogenic tumor with less 120 cases reported in the jaws since it was first described by Hansen et al. in 1985 [1]. CCOC was previously known as clear cell odontogenic tumor or clear cell ameloblastoma, when it was classified as a benign neoplasm [1, 2]. However, due to its aggressive clinical characteristics such as invasive growth, regional lymph node involvement, local recurrence, and distant metastasis, the WHO reclassified it as a malignant tumor of odontogenic origin in 2005. CCOC has a preference for females in the 5th decade of life and for the mandible, with 73.8% of reported cases occurring in the mandible [3].

Morphologically, CCOC presents as an infiltrative tumor composed of nests, sheets, or cords of monomorphic round to polygonal clear epithelial cells separated by variable hyalinized stroma [4]. Immunophenotypically, they are positive for cytokeratins, p63, and PAS, are diastase-sensitive (demonstrating intracytoplasmic glycogen), and are negative for mucicarmine and myoepithelial markers such as S100, SMA, and calponin [4, 5]. Molecularly, CCOC has been shown to demonstrate Ewing sarcoma region 1 (*EWSR1*) rearrangement [5]. In this article, we report a massive case of CCOC of the mandible in a Nigerian patient, performing limited immunohistochemical stains (CK5/6 and S100), special stains (PAS and, PAS-D), and FISH molecular analysis for *EWSR1* rearrangement.

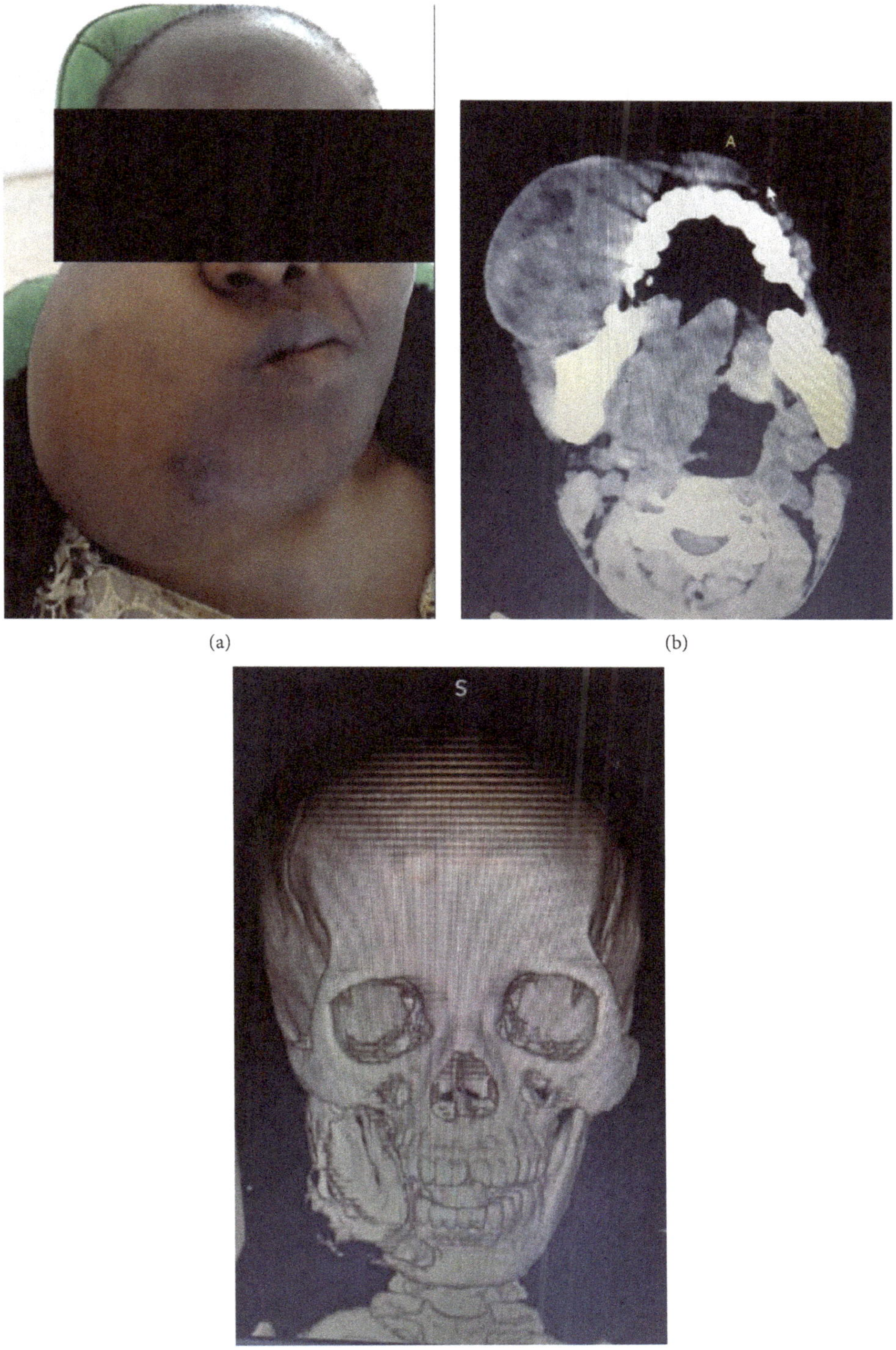

(a) (b)

(c)

FIGURE 1: Clinical image of a 43-year-old female patient diagnosed with a *EWSR1*-rearranged clear cell odontogenic carcinoma of the mandible (a), CT scan axial view (b), and 3D-refomatted CT scan showing an osteolytic destructive mass in the mandible with thinning and perforation of the cortical border of the mandible (c).

2. Case Report

A 43-year-old female patient presented in September 2019 with a 4-year history of a mandibular mass of 18 cm in diameter associated with buccolingual expansion of the mandible (Figure 1(a)) and regional lymph node involvement. Incisional biopsy had been performed 2 years prior, and an initial diagnosis of ameloblastoma was rendered. The mass was reported to have progressively increased in size for the past 2 years prior to presentation. Imaging revealed an osteolytic

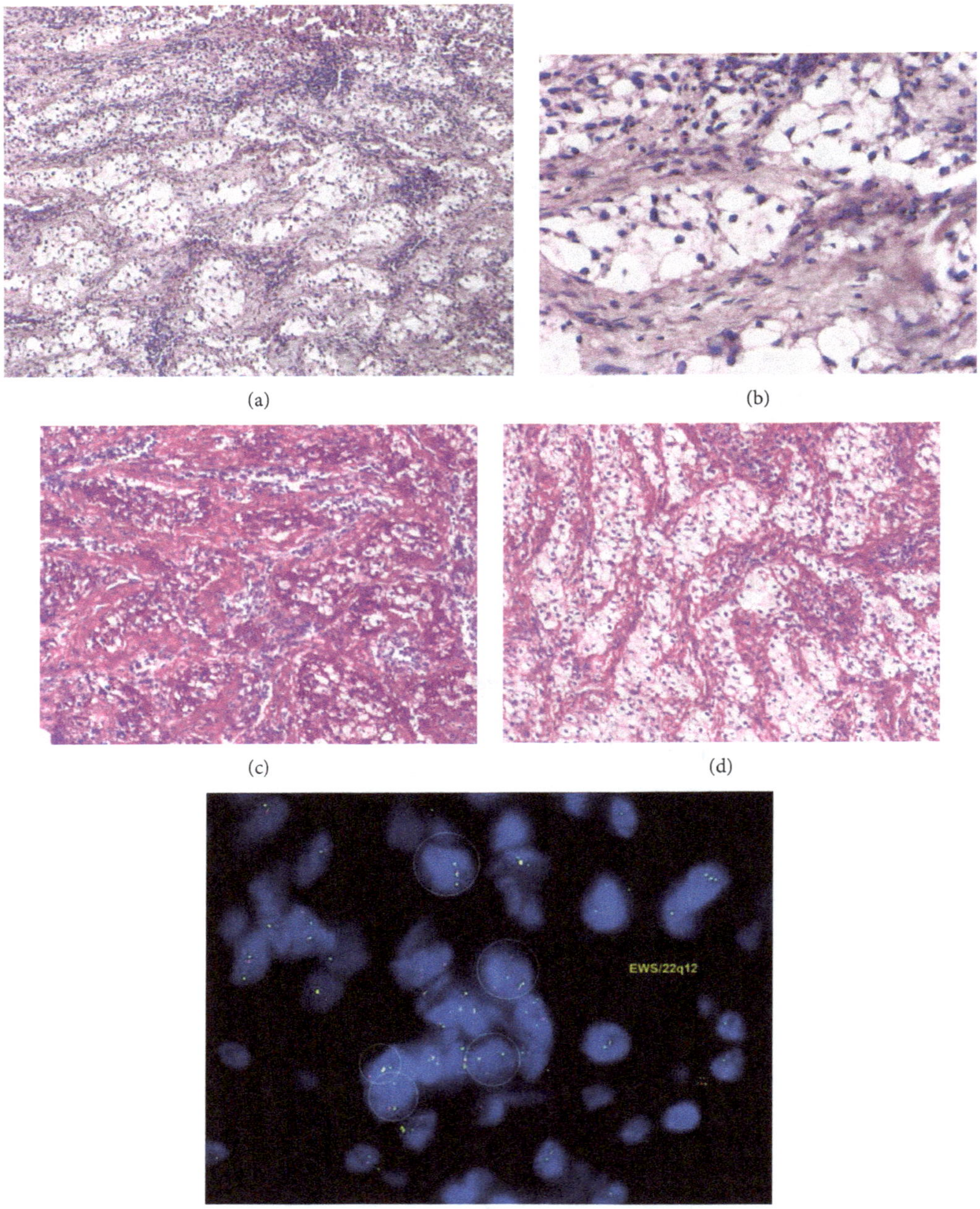

(a) (b) (c) (d) (e)

Figure 2: Histopathology of clear cell odontogenic carcinoma of the mandible in a 43-year-old female patient. (a) Morphology shows nests and cords of round to polygonal monomorphic clear epithelial cells with prominent stromal hyalinization containing lymphocytes (H&E 100x). (b) Higher magnification (H&E 400x). (c) Clear epithelial cells positive for PAS demonstrating intracytoplasmic granules (PAS 200x). (d) Clear epithelial cells are negative after PAS-D (200x). (e) Split of the green signal from the red signal by break-apart FISH demonstrates that the tumor harbors *EWSR1* rearrangement. In contrast, the uninvolved *EWSR1* allele shows a yellow signal (resulting from the fused red and green probes).

destructive mass in the mandible with thinning and perforation of the cortical border of the mandible (Figures 1(b) and 1(c)). A rebiopsy was performed.

Morphologic features of the tumor were of nests and cords of round to polygonal monomorphic clear epithelial cells with prominent stromal hyalinization (Figures 2(a) and 2(b)). The tumor was poorly circumscribed and infiltrative with the presence of lymphocytes in the stroma. The tumor was positive for PAS but negative for PAS-D (demonstrating the presence of intracytoplasmic glycogen) (Figures 2(c) and 2(d)), showed focal expression for CK5/6, and was negative for S100 protein. FISH for *EWSR1* rearrangement was positive with 65% of translocated cells in 60 cells examined (Figure 2(e)). The cut-off for a positive *EWSR1* rearrangement is 12.5% of cells translocated.

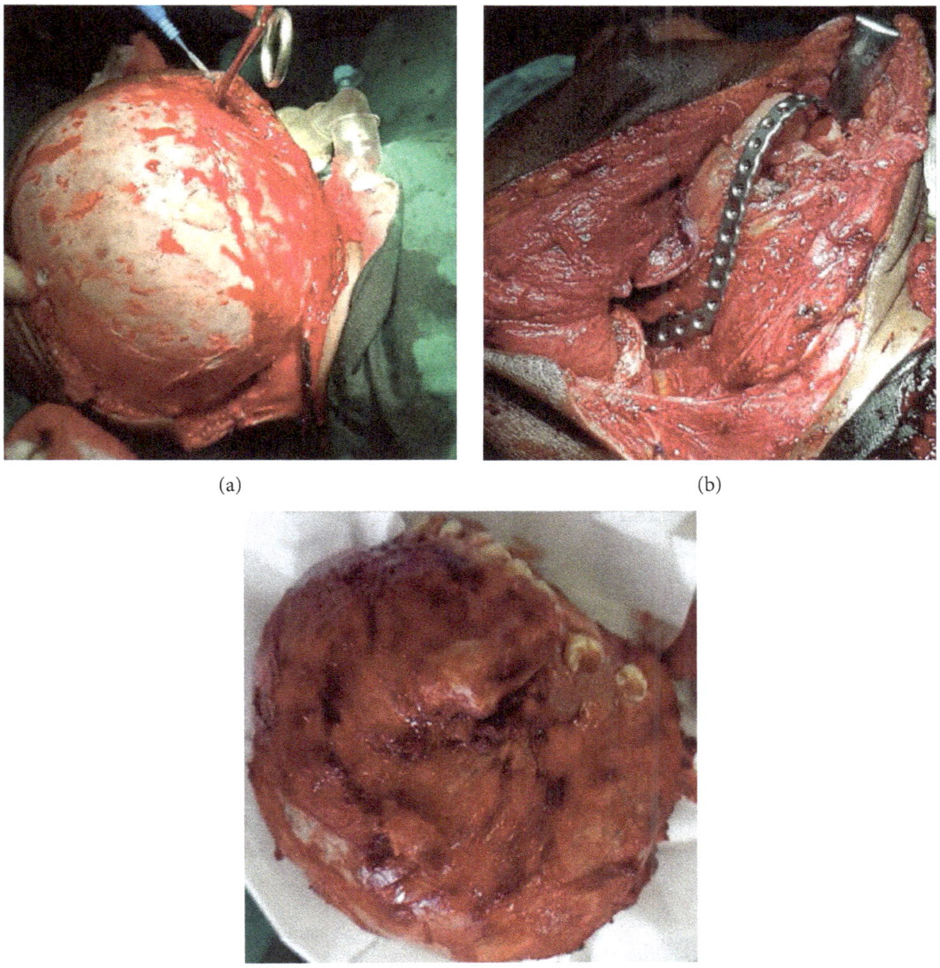

(a) (b) (c)

FIGURE 3: (a) Surgical exposure and resection of the EWSR1-rearranged clear cell odontogenic carcinoma of the mandible. (b) Reconstruction of the surgical defect with a mandibular reconstruction plate. (c) Massive resected *EWSR1*-rearranged clear cell odontogenic carcinoma of the mandible.

Two months after presentation, a subtotal mandibulectomy with neck dissection was performed for the resection of the CCOC (Figures 3(a)–3(c)). The patient is alive without disease and no recurrence at the last follow-up 15 months posttherapy.

3. Discussion

Clear cell odontogenic carcinoma (CCOC) is a rare malignant odontogenic neoplasm characterized by *EWSR1* gene rearrangement. Less than 120 cases have been reported in the literature. A recent review of the literature of 107 patients diagnosed with CCOC showed a predilection for females, the 5th decade of life, and the mandible [3]. In the same review, 13.6% (12/88) of CCOC patients manifested regional nodal involvement, and 11.2% (12/107) of CCOC patients died of disease [3]. In this report, we present a case of CCOC in a 43-year-old female with progressive growing mass, 18 cm in size in its largest diameter, located in the mandible associated with regional lymph node involvement and alive without disease and no recurrence 15 months posttherapy.

EWSR1 rearrangement in CCOC was first described by Bilodeau et al.; the fusion partner identified was the activating transcription factor 1 gene (*ATF1*) on chromosome 12q13 [5]. An alternative fusion partner, *CREB1*, on chromosome 2q34 has been described [6]. *ATF1* and *CREB1* both belong to the cAMP response element-binding protein (CREB) family of transcription factors. *ATF1* remains the most common fusion partner to *EWSR1* identified in CCOC to date. Most cases of CCOC reported in the literature were described before *EWSR1* rearrangement was identified in the tumor. *EWSR1* gene rearrangement has been reported in numerous tumors, such as Ewing sarcoma, extraskeletal myxoid chondrosarcoma, clear cell sarcoma, desmoplastic small round cell tumor, myxoid liposarcoma, angiomatoid fibrous histiocytoma, primary pulmonary myxoid sarcoma, myoepithelial tumors of soft tissue, skin, and salivary glands, and hyalinizing clear cell carcinoma. *EWSR1-ATF1* translocation has been reported in other tumors, such as angiomatoid fibrous histiocytoma, hyalinizing clear cell carcinoma, and clear cell sarcoma [7–9]. Additionally, *EWSR1-CREB1* translocation has been reported in myxoid mesenchymal tumors, angiomatoid fibrous histiocytoma, primary pulmonary myxoid sarcoma, and gastrointestinal-clear cell sarcoma [10–13].

The differential diagnosis of CCOC includes hyalinizing clear cell carcinoma (HCCC) of the salivary gland, clear cell variant of central mucoepidermoid carcinoma (MEC), clear cell variant of calcifying epithelial odontogenic tumor (CEOT), and metastatic renal cell carcinoma. HCCC of the salivary gland is a rare low-grade malignant neoplasm that typically affects the minor salivary glands [14]. It has been argued that CCOC and HCCC are essentially the same analogous tumors with different locations [4, 5]. CCOC occurs centrally in the bone while HCCC occurs peripherally in the submucosa. CCOC and HCCC share similar morphologic, immunophenotypic, and molecular features [5].

MEC is the most common malignant salivary gland tumor that needs to be differentiated from CCOC, despite the presence of intercellular bridging of true epidermoid areas. MEC is composed of epidermoid, mucinous, and intermediate cells in variable proportion depending on its grade, forming solid and cystic patterns. MEC has been described in the jaw bone [15]. Clear cells have been described in MEC, and when predominant, they are called the clear cell variant of MEC. Immunohistochemical stains are not helpful in differentiating MEC from CCOC. However, PAS-D shows positive intracytoplasmic globules in MEC, which are negative in CCOC [4, 16]. MEC is negative for *EWSR1* rearrangement but may be positive for *CRTC1/CRTC3-MAML2* fusion [17].

CEOT is a rare invasive epithelial odontogenic tumor also known as Pindborg tumor. CEOT is composed of sheets, nests, and/or cords of polygonal eosinophilic epithelial cells with a prominent stroma [18]. These epithelial cells may present with clear cytoplasm, making it challenging to differentiate it from CCOC. However, cellular pleomorphism and the presence of amyloid and Liesegang calcified rings in the stroma that define CEOT are absent in CCOC. The eosinophilic amyloid material can be highlighted with Congo red stain, showing the classic apple-green birefringence with polarized light.

Metastasis of renal cell carcinoma to jaw should also be considered in the differential diagnosis of CCOC. These patients may have a history of a renal mass, or the metastasis to the oral cavity may be the first indication of a malignancy [19]. The metastatic renal cell carcinoma will be positive for PAX8, CD10, and CAIX in contrast to CCOC and negative for *EWSR1* rearrangement.

The case described here originated from the jaw, negative for PAS-D, and positive for PAS and *EWSR1* rearrangement, ruling out the aforementioned differential diagnoses. In conclusion, we report a rare form of jaw neoplasm "clear cell odontogenic carcinoma" with a propensity for invasiveness, destructive nature, and facial disfigurement if left untreated in a Nigerian patient harboring *EWSR1* rearrangement.

Authors' Contributions

Adepitan A. Owosho and Chukwubuzor Okwuosa are coequal first authors.

References

[1] L. S. Hansen, L. R. Eversole, T. L. Green, and N. B. Powell, "Clear cell odontogenic tumor–a new histologic variant with aggressive potential," *Head & Neck Surgery*, vol. 8, no. 2, pp. 115–123, 1985.

[2] C. A. Waldron, I. A. Small, and H. Silverman, "Clear cell ameloblastoma–an odontogenic carcinoma," *Journal of Oral and Maxillofacial Surgery*, vol. 43, no. 9, pp. 707–717, 1985.

[3] F. P. S. Guastaldi, W. C. Faquin, F. Gootkind et al., "Clear cell odontogenic carcinoma: a rare jaw tumor. A summary of 107 reported cases," *International Journal of Oral and Maxillofacial Surgery*, vol. 48, no. 11, pp. 1405–1410, 2019.

[4] E. A. Bilodeau, A. P. Hoschar, E. L. Barnes, J. L. Hunt, and R. R. Seethala, "Clear cell carcinoma and clear cell odontogenic carcinoma: a comparative clinicopathologic and immunohistochemical study," *Head and Neck Pathology*, vol. 5, no. 2, pp. 101–107, 2011.

[5] E. A. Bilodeau, I. Weinreb, C. R. Antonescu et al., "Clear cell odontogenic carcinomas show EWSR1 rearrangements," *The American Journal of Surgical Pathology*, vol. 37, no. 7, pp. 1001–1005, 2013.

[6] R. Vogels, D. Baumhoer, J. van Gorp et al., "Clear cell odontogenic carcinoma: occurrence of EWSR1-CREB1 as alternative fusion gene to EWSR1-ATF1," *Head and Neck Pathology*, vol. 13, no. 2, pp. 225–230, 2019.

[7] K. H. Hallor, F. Mertens, Y. Jin et al., "Fusion of the EWSR1 and ATF1 genes without expression of the MITF-M transcript in angiomatoid fibrous histiocytoma," *Genes, Chromosomes & Cancer*, vol. 44, no. 1, pp. 97–102, 2005.

[8] C. R. Antonescu, N. Katabi, L. Zhang et al., "EWSR1-ATF1 fusion is a novel and consistent finding in hyalinizing clear-cell carcinoma of salivary gland," *Genes, Chromosomes & Cancer*, vol. 50, no. 7, pp. 559–570, 2011.

[9] I. Panagopoulos, F. Mertens, M. Dêbiec-Rychter et al., "Molecular genetic characterization of the EWS/ATF1 fusion gene in clear cell sarcoma of tendons and aponeuroses," *International Journal of Cancer*, vol. 99, no. 4, pp. 560–567, 2002.

[10] Y. C. Kao, Y. S. Sung, L. Zhang et al., "EWSR1 fusions with CREB family transcription factors define a novel myxoid mesenchymal tumor with predilection for intracranial location," *The American Journal of Surgical Pathology*, vol. 41, no. 4, pp. 482–490, 2017.

[11] C. R. Antonescu, P. Dal Cin, K. Nafa et al., "EWSR1-CREB1 is the predominant gene fusion in angiomatoid fibrous histiocytoma," *Genes, Chromosomes & Cancer*, vol. 46, no. 12, pp. 1051–1060, 2007.

[12] C. R. Antonescu, K. Nafa, N. H. Segal, P. Dal Cin, and M. Ladanyi, "EWS-CREB1: a recurrent variant fusion in clear cell sarcoma–association with gastrointestinal location and absence of melanocytic differentiation," *Clinical Cancer Research*, vol. 12, no. 18, pp. 5356–5362, 2006.

[13] K. Thway, A. G. Nicholson, K. Lawson et al., "Primary pulmonary myxoid sarcoma with EWSR1-CREB1 fusion: a new tumor entity," *The American Journal of Surgical Pathology*, vol. 35, no. 11, pp. 1722–1732, 2011.

[14] X. H. Yang, L. Liu, Y. Y. Shi, Y. J. Hu, Q. G. Hu, and P. Zhang, "Hyalinizing clear cell carcinoma of salivary gland origin in the head and neck: clinical and histopathological analysis," *International Journal of Oral and Maxillofacial Surgery*, vol. 47, no. 6, pp. 692–698, 2018.

[15] C. A. Waldron and M. L. Koh, "Central mucoepidermoid carcinoma of the jaws: report of four cases with analysis of the literature and discussion of the relationship to mucoepidermoid, sialodontogenic, and glandular odontogenic cysts," *Journal of Oral and Maxillofacial Surgery*, vol. 48, no. 8, pp. 871–877, 1990.

[16] A. C. Buch, P. H. Jariwala, N. K. Panicker, and M. Joshi, "The utility of periodic acid schiff with diastase and alcian blue stains on fine needle aspirates of breast and salivary gland neoplasms," *Journal of Cytology*, vol. 29, no. 4, pp. 221–225, 2012.

[17] G. Tonon, S. Modi, L. Wu et al., "T(11;19)(q21;p13) translocation in mucoepidermoid carcinoma creates a novel fusion product that disrupts a notch signaling pathway," *Nature Genetics*, vol. 33, no. 2, pp. 208–213, 2003.

[18] C. D. Franklin and J. J. Pindborg, "The calcifying epithelial odontogenic tumor: a review and analysis of 113 cases," *Oral Surgery, Oral Medicine, and Oral Pathology*, vol. 42, no. 6, pp. 753–765, 1976.

[19] A. A. Owosho, B. Xu, A. Kadempour et al., "Metastatic solid tumors to the jaw and oral soft tissue: a retrospective clinical analysis of 44 patients from a single institution," *Journal of Cranio-Maxillo-Facial Surgery*, vol. 44, no. 8, pp. 1047–1053, 2016.

21

Step-by-Step Esthetic Rehabilitation with Chairside System

Rim Kallala,[1,2,3] Mohamed Habib Chaouch,[1] Karim Nasr,[4] and Teva Courset[4]

[1]*Dental Faculty of Monastir, Tunisia*
[2]*University of Monastir, Research Laboratory of Occlusodontics and Ceramic Prostheses LR16ES15, 5000 Monastir, Tunisia*
[3]*Department of Dental Faculty at the Dental Faculty of Monastir, Tunisia*
[4]*Faculty of Dental Surgery and University Hospital, Toulouse, France*

Correspondence should be addressed to Rim Kallala; dr.kallalarim@gmail.com

Academic Editor: Andrea Scribante

In modern dentistry, Computer-Aided Design and Manufacturing (CAD/CAM) is a promising technology that allows fabrication of prosthetic restorations through milling procedures. Over years, with the continuous improvement of technology, direct CAD/CAM or "chairside" technology is becoming a widespread approach which offers immediate rehabilitation with long-term rates reported by several studies compared to conventional techniques. All steps are generally carried out in the dental office during the same treatment session. The present paper is about a healthy female patient with a decayed 36 tooth which was restored by ceramic onlay using Planmeca's PlanCAD system. Through the present clinical case, a detailed protocol of chairside technology would be presented from the digital impression to the milling process. It would detail impression steps. It would also highlight especially the virtual design confection of prosthetic restoration using a biogeneric model included in the software. It also illustrated tools which could be used by the dentist to perform the design. Also, some useful tips would be presented in order to perform the confection. On this subject, various studies showed the viability of such technology. To summarize, referring to previous studies, this promising technology allows especially time-saving and patient's comfort compared to the indirect one.

1. Introduction

In modern dentistry, Computer-Aided Design and Manufacturing (CAD/CAM) is a promising technology that allows fabrication of the prosthetic restorations through milling procedures [1]. Over years, with the continuous improvement of technology, direct CAD/CAM or "chairside" technology is becoming a widespread approach which offers immediate rehabilitation. The first one was introduced by the CEREC system [1, 2]. Due to this technology, all steps are generally carried out in the dental office during the same treatment session. CAD/CAM systems registered a constantly increasing use in many fields of dentistry and allow a completely digital workflow, from impression to the final framework, with good clinical reliability [2, 3] and excellent patient feedback [4]. The purpose of this paper was to detail the protocol of chairside system and provide a useful evaluation tool, through a clinical case carried out in the dental clinic of the Faculty of Dental Surgery Paul Sabatier Toulouse. The direct CAD/CAM system used was Planmeca's PlanCAD.

2. Clinical Presentation

It was a 34-year healthy female patient who consulted for rehabilitation of the left first lower molar (Figure 1). She had high esthetic expectations. The clinical examination showed good oral hygiene and a decayed and nonvital 36 tooth. Radiological examination confirmed a good quality of root canal filling.

In accordance with the therapeutic gradient and taking into consideration residual dental tissue, it was decided to

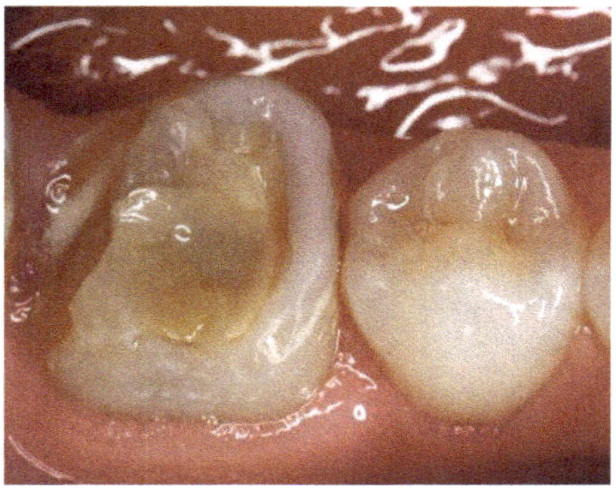

Figure 1: Initial situation.

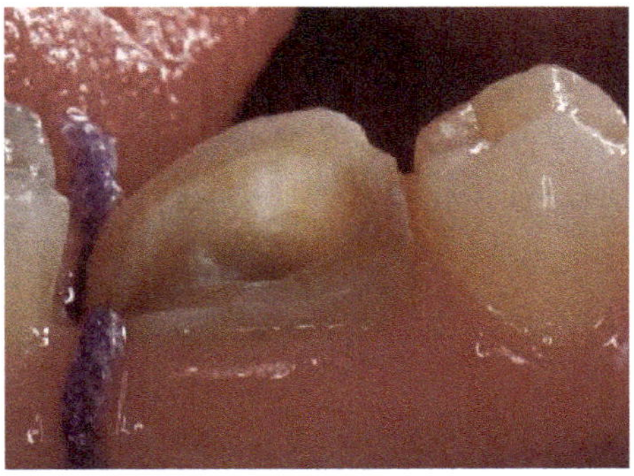

Figure 2: After preparation with placed retractor cord before impression.

place a ceramic onlay using the direct CAD/CAM technique. The first step was the removal of decayed tissue. Dictated by caries morphology, preparation was done while preserving the maximum of enamel tissue and avoiding sharp angles and wide shoulders. After preparation, dental residual tissue was mainly supragingival which would facilitate optical impression and future bonding (Figure 2). All the workflow is summarized in Figure 3.

2.1. Computer-Aided Design and Manufacturing Steps

2.1.1. Administrative File (Figure 4). At the software level (Romexis, Planmeca Oy 4.0, Helsinki, Finland), the concerned tooth, restoration type, and material were selected.

2.1.2. Digital Impression (Figure 5). Before the digital impression, a retraction cord (Pro Retract, FGM, Jovinile Brasil) was placed in the sulcus and the tooth was air-dried. Then, intraoral scanning was carefully performed using the Planmeca Emerald camera which is a powder-free technology. It was a true-color high-resolution procedure. Three sectoral impressions were necessary: concerned and antagonist sectors (intraoral scan), as well as recording of the occlusion (buccal scan). At this stage, it was possible to switch the models to the monochrome mode in order to visualize the accuracy of the recording. Likewise, it was easy to check the available prosthetic thicknesses and whether there are any gaps in the impression. If necessary, the impression could be retouched and completed. Also, unnecessary areas could be cleaned using an eraser tool.

2.1.3. Design Confection of the Prosthetic Restoration Figures 6 and 7. The virtual cast orientation was the first step. Determination of the insertion path and the model axis was then necessary. After that, the finishing line was rigorously drawn. This operation was semiautomatic and should be controlled by the practitioner. The software, thus, after analyzing the neighboring teeth, proposed a design of the future restoration. It could be modified through variable tools: displacement, fine retouching, and adjustments of the contact zones (occlusal and proximal). The color code indicated the intensity of these contact zones. An analysis of the material thicknesses could also be done in order to avoid areas of extreme thinness which may cause fractures. Before the milling process, the virtual onlay would be visualized.

2.1.4. Manufacturing or Milling Process. Leucite-reinforced glass ceramics was chosen for the present case. The operator, then, inserted the appropriate ingot (material and size) inside the machine. Via wireless, data were sent to the computer-controlled milling unit. The milling machine (PlanMill 40S, Planmeca, Helsinki, Finland) uses dual spindles and could mill simultaneously two sides of restoration according to customized and calculated milling paths. Finally, the milling process was rapidly performed and took 12 min. At the end of machining, the block was removed from the machine and then separated from the machining lug.

After intraoral checking, only minor adjustments were done using diamond instruments. Modified zones were then polished. The restoration underwent a finishing phase (coloring, glazing, and polishing) before the bonding.

The patient was happy with the final result (Figure 8).

3. Discussion

Today, chairside or direct CAD/CAM systems are a promising technology saving time with total independence from the laboratory technician and better communication with the patient [4–6]. The indirect CAD/CAM systems or classical methods usually require conventional impression [1, 7]. On obtained gypsum casts, digital acquisition would be done and the milling process would be performed in the dental laboratory [7–12]. The major flaw of conventional impression is the risk of errors due to material dependence especially the dimensional deformations during polymerization. According to Boitelle and Fromentin [13, 14], there is a physical dispersion which could drive to errors and spoil the precision and the quality of the dentoprosthetic joint. Lima et al. [15] reported statistically significant differences by comparing the marginal adaptation of prosthetic restorations milled through both direct and indirect CAD/CAM systems in favor of the direct one. The study of Carvalho et al. [16] confirmed the

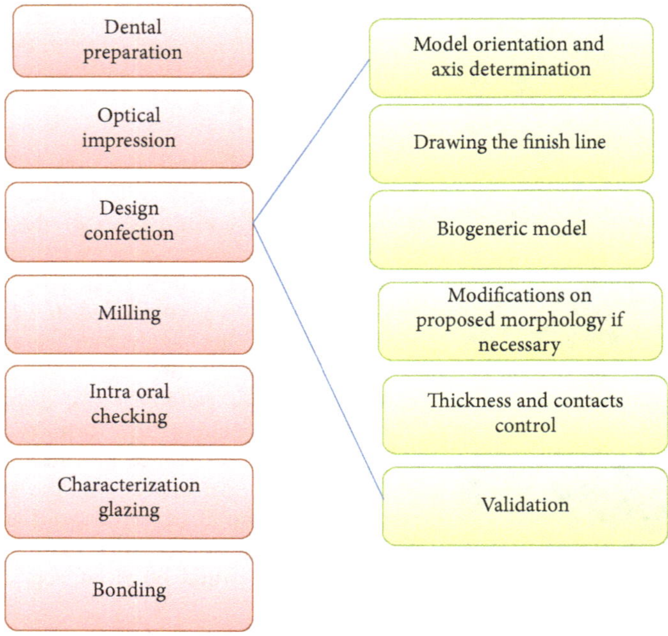

FIGURE 3: Chairside workflow.

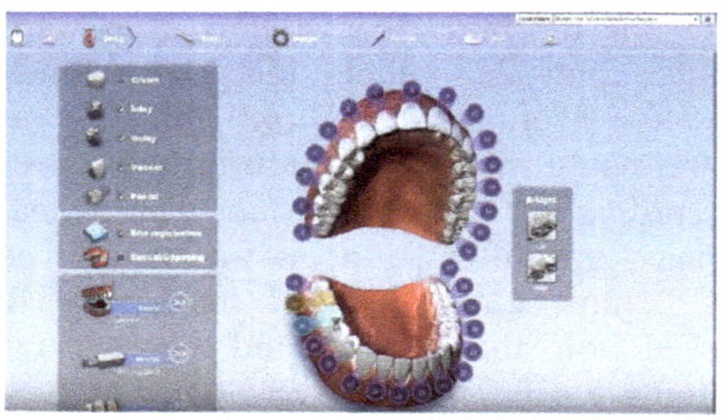

FIGURE 4: The administrative file.

superiority of digital techniques in comparison with conventional methods. However, the systematic review of Goujat et al. [17] reported that the marginal adaptation obtained was satisfactory without statistically significant differences between the two techniques. The meta-analysis could not be performed as findings were heterogeneous. For Aswani et al. [18], variable results were reported depending on the systems used. According to Ender and Mehl [19], optical impressions provided levels of accuracy in the same order as those of conventional impressions. Some studies [19–21] reported statistically not significant differences between the impression techniques. Indeed, Boitelle and Fromentin [13] reported that physical dispersion exists also for the direct CAD/CAM technique. It could be linked to different interactions of the light beam and dental tissues. Besides, errors could be due to the oral environment, to external environments (brightness of the treatment room), and to the manipulation also [13]. The study of Kuhr et al. [21] pointed out that conventional casts seem to be similar to digital impression models. But secondary areas, such as grooves and pits, were better reproduced in gypsum models. To sum up, chairside technology allows especially saving time [16] as digital scanning is easy and rapid. Besides, there is no need to disinfect and clean dental impressions either waiting cast pouring.

On the other hand, the restoration occlusal design is considered among the most important conditions for an optimal outcome, through harmonic relation to adjacent teeth and interference-free occlusal contacts [22]. In CAD/CAM technology, it is adjusted thanks to an algorithmic equation which involves a library of intact tooth morphology integrated into the software called the biogeneric model [6, 23]. In this regard, several studies have been carried out comparing the morphologies of natural teeth and those given by the biogeneric models and have concluded with similar morphologies [7, 24, 25]. Ender et al. concluded that according to experts, obtained morphologies were natural looking [24]. Others compared the morphology of natural teeth and those of wax-ups made by laboratory technicians in favor of the biogeneric model [26, 27].

Otherwise, in the present clinical situation, the tooth could be reconstructed with a fiber post and core followed by a crown.

Nevertheless, this promising technology has some limitations: The first is the high cost which requires huge investment. Then, as it provides monolithic restorations, the esthetic outcome would be better using a stratification technique which allows characterization in the framework depending on the laboratory technician's skills and performances [26]. Tuncel reported statistically significant differences in terms of translucency between monolithic zirconia and framework zirconia [29].

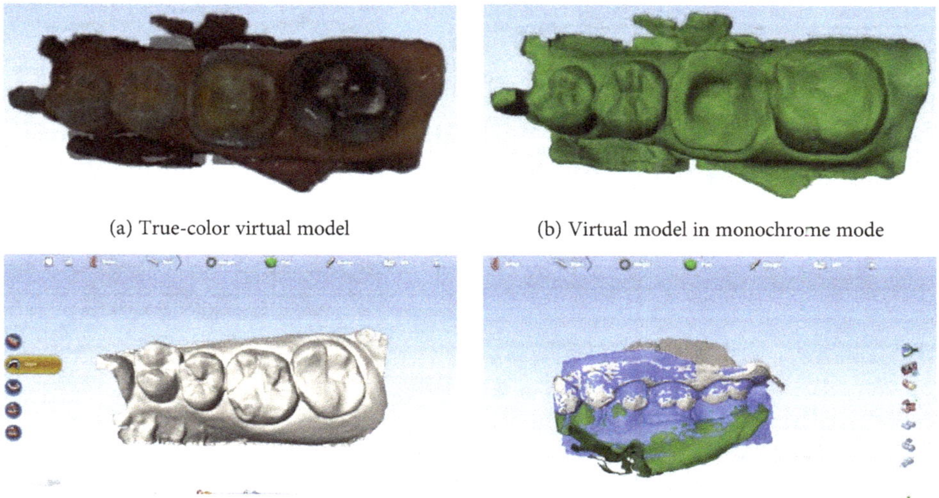

(a) True-color virtual model

(b) Virtual model in monochrome mode

(c) Virtual antagonist model

(d) Confronted virtual models

FIGURE 5: Virtual models obtained after digital impression.

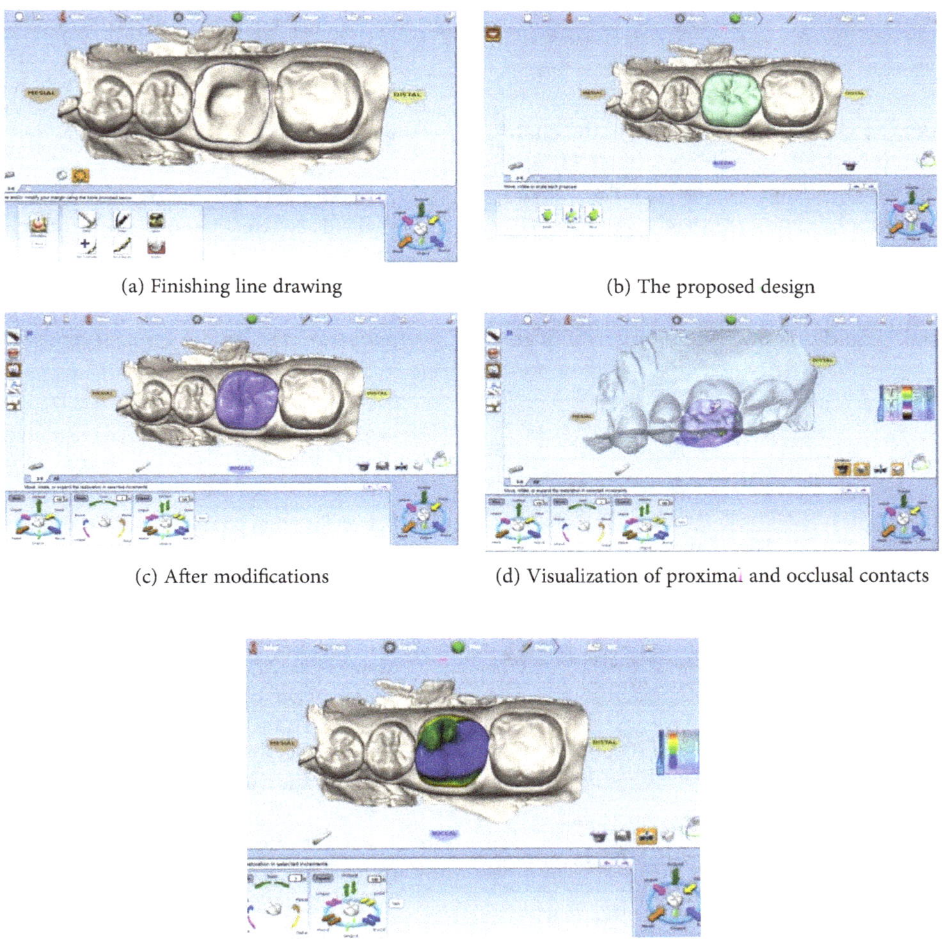

(a) Finishing line drawing

(b) The proposed design

(c) After modifications

(d) Visualization of proximal and occlusal contacts

(e) Color codes for the material thickness

FIGURE 6: Design confection of the future restoration.

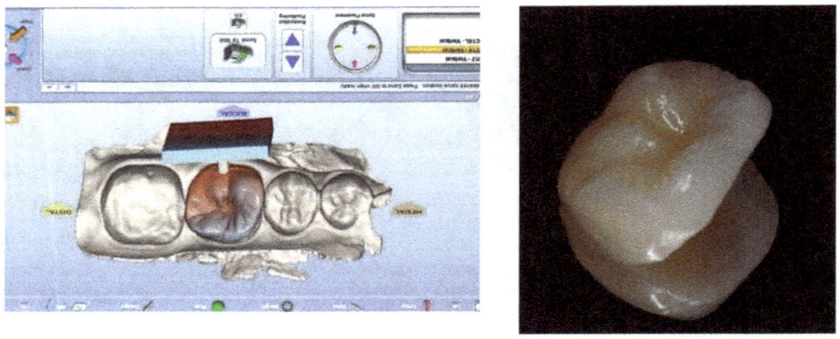

(a) Virtual milled onlay (b) Ceramic milled onlay after glazing

FIGURE 7: Milled onlay.

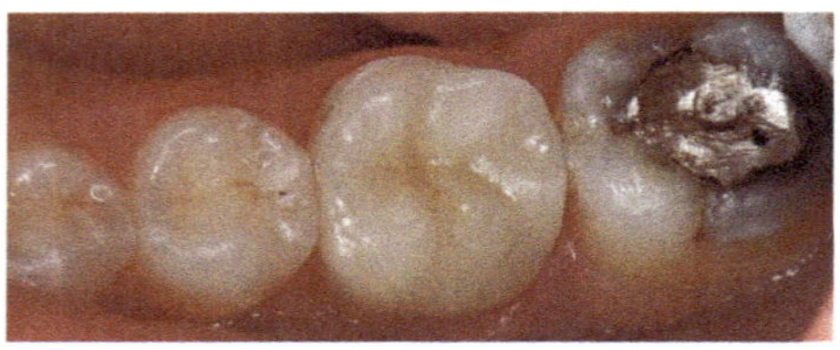

FIGURE 8: Final outcome after bonding.

4. Conclusion

The arrival of CAD/CAM technology, particularly the chairside system, has revolutionized dental prostheses. It is a promising technique which allowed especially time-saving and comfort for the patient. The appropriate use of corresponding software, as well as the adjustment method, is required for successful restorations. Also, an appropriate occlusal context and adequate bonding, respecting the properties of each material, would guarantee the longevity of the future restoration.

References

[1] G. Sannino, S. Germano, L. Arcuri, E. Bigelli, C. Arcuri, and A. Barlattani, "CEREC CAD/CAM chairside system," *Oral Implantology*, vol. 7, no. 3, pp. 57–70, 2014.

[2] S. Rinke, A.-K. Pabel, M. Rödiger, and D. Ziebolz, "Chairside Fabrication of an All-Ceramic Partial Crown Using a Zirconia-Reinforced Lithium Silicate Ceramic," *Case Reports in Dentistry*, vol. 2016, Article ID 1354186, 7 pages, 2016.

[3] R. Alessandretti, M. Borba, P. Benetti, P. H. Corazza, R. Ribeiro, and A. Della Bona, "Reliability and mode of failure of bonded monolithic and multilayer ceramics," *Dental Materials*, vol. 33, no. 2, pp. 191–197, 2017.

[4] M. F. Sfondrini, P. Gandini, M. Malfatto, F. Di Corato, F. Trovati, and A. Scribante, "Computerized casts for orthodontic purpose using powder-free intraoral scanners: accuracy, execution time, and patient feedback," *BioMed Research International*, vol. 2018, Article ID 4103232, 8 pages, 2018.

[5] G. Akgungor, D. Sen, E. Bal, and M. Ozcan, "Simultaneous replacement of maxillary central incisors with CEREC biogeneric reference technique: a case report," *Journal of dental research, dental clinics, dental prospects*, vol. 7, no. 2, pp. 112–118, 2013.

[6] F. Wang, Q. Tang, S. Xi, R. Liu, and L. Niu, "Comparison and evaluation of the morphology of crowns generated by biogeneric design technique with CEREC chairside system," *PLoS One*, vol. 15, no. 1, article e0227050, 2020.

[7] M. Kollmuss, S. Kist, J. E. Goeke, R. Hickel, and K. C. Huth, "Comparison of chairside and laboratory CAD/CAM to conventional produced all-ceramic crowns regarding morphology, occlusion, and aesthetics," *Clinical Oral Investigations*, vol. 20, no. 4, pp. 791–797, 2016.

[8] T. Miyazaki, Y. Hotta, J. Kunii, S. Kuriyama, and T. Yc, "A review of dental CAD/CAM: current status and future perspectives from 20 years of experience," *Dental Materials Journal*, vol. 28, no. 1, pp. 44–56, 2009.

[9] G. C. Santos Jr., M. J. M. C. Santos Jr., A. S. Rizkalla, D. A. Madani, and O. El-Mowafy, "Overview of CEREC CAD/CAM chairside system," *General Dentistry*, vol. 61, pp. 36–40, 2013.

[10] M. Andreiotelli, P. Kamposiora, and G. Papavasiliou, "Digital data management for CAD/CAM technology. An update of current systems," *The European journal of prosthodontics and restorative dentistry*, vol. 21, pp. 9–15, 2013.

[11] R. Van Noort, "The future of dental devices is digital," *Dental Materials*, vol. 28, no. 1, pp. 3–12, 2012.

[12] D. J. Fasbinder, "Computerized technology for restorative dentistry," *American Journal of Dentistry*, vol. 26, no. 3, pp. 115–120, 2013.

[13] P. Boitelle and O. Fromentin, "Lesdispersions de données dans les chaînes DE CFAO Partie1- Dispersions physiques," *Biomatériaux Cliniques*, vol. 3, p. 7, 2018.

[14] S. Quaas, H. Rudolph, and R. G. Luthardt, "Direct mechanical data acquisition of dental impressions for the manufacturing of CAD/CAM restorations," *Journal of Dentistry*, vol. 35, no. 12, pp. 903–908, 2007.

[15] F. F. Lima, C. F. Neto, J. H. Rubo, G. C. Santos, and M. J. M. C. Santos, "Marginal adaptation of CAD-CAM onlays: influence of preparation design and impression technique," *The Journal of Prosthetic Dentistry*, vol. 120, no. 3, pp. 396–402, 2018.

[16] T. F. Carvalho, J. F. M. Lima, J. D. M. De-Matos et al., "Evaluation of the accuracy of conventional and digital methods of obtaining dental impressions," *International journal of odontostomatology*, vol. 12, no. 4, pp. 368–375, 2018.

[17] A. Goujat, H. Abouelleil, P. Colon et al., "Marginal and internal fit of CAD-CAM inlay/onlay restorations: a systematic review of in vitro studies," *The Journal of Prosthetic Dentistry*, vol. 121, no. 4, pp. 590–597.e3, 2019.

[18] K. Aswani, S. Wankhade, A. Khalikar, and S. Deogade, "Accu-

racy of an intraoral digital impression: a review," *The Journal of Indian Prosthodontic Society*, vol. 20, no. 1, pp. 27–37, 2020.

[19] A. Ender and A. Mehl, "Full arch scans: conventional versus digital impressions-an in-vitro study," *International Journal of Computerized Dentistry*, vol. 14, no. 1, pp. 11–21, 2011.

[20] T. Abdel-Azim, K. Rogers, E. Elathamna, A. Zandinejad, M. Metz, and D. Morton, "Comparison of the marginal fit of lithium disilicate crowns fabricated with CAD/CAM technology by using conventional impressions and two intraoral digital scanners," *The Journal of Prosthetic Dentistry*, vol. 114, no. 4, pp. 554–559, 2015.

[21] F. Kuhr, A. Schmidt, P. Rehmann, and B. Wöstmann, "A new method for assessing the accuracy of full arch impressions in patients," *Journal of Dentistry*, vol. 55, pp. 68–74, 2016.

[22] Y. Arslan, S. K. Nemli, M. B. Güngör, E. Tamam, and H. Yılmaz, "Evaluation of biogeneric design techniques with CEREC CAD/CAM system," *The Journal of Advanced Prosthodontics*, vol. 7, no. 6, pp. 431–436, 2015.

[23] A. Mehl, V. Blanz, and R. Hickel, "Biogeneric tooth: a new mathematical representation for tooth morphology in lower first molars," *European Journal of Oral Sciences*, vol. 113, no. 4, pp. 333–340, 2005.

[24] A. Ender, W. H. Mörmann, and A. Mehl, "Efficiency of a mathematical model in generating CAD/CAM-partial crowns with natural tooth morphology," *Clinical Oral Investigations*, vol. 15, no. 2, pp. 283–289, 2011.

[25] R. Zhang, Q. Ding, Y. Sun, L. Zhang, and Q. Xie, "Assessment of CAD-CAM zirconia crowns designed with 2 different methods: a self-controlled clinical trial," *The Journal of Prosthetic Dentistry*, vol. 120, no. 5, pp. 686–692, 2018.

[26] C. Ellerbrock and B. Kordass, "Comparison of computer generated occlusal surfaces with functionally waxed-on surfaces," *International Journal of Computerized Dentistry*, vol. 14, no. 1, pp. 23–31, 2011.

[27] M. Kollmuss, F.-M. Jakob, H.-G. Kirchner, N. Ilie, R. Hickel, and K. C. Huth, "Comparison of biogenerically reconstructed and waxed-up complete occlusal surfaces with respect to the original tooth morphology," *Clinical Oral Investigations*, vol. 17, no. 3, pp. 851–857, 2013.

[28] J. Carames, L. T. Suinaga, Y. C. P. Yu, A. Pérez, and M. Kang, "Clinical advantages and limitations of monolithic zirconia restorations full arch implant supported reconstruction: case series," *International Journal of Dentistry*, vol. 2015, Article ID 392496, 7 pages, 2015.

[29] "Evaluation of translucency of monolithic zirconia and framework zirconia materials," *The Journal of Advanced Prosthodontics*, vol. 8, no. 3, pp. 181–186, 2016.

22

Minimal Invasive Surgical Management of Familial Arteriovenous Malformation

Mokhtar Mamdouh Abdel-Latif[1] and Shankargouda Patil[2]

[1]*Maxillofacial Surgery and Diagnostic Sciences, Division of Oral Surgery, College of Dentistry, Jazan University, Jazan, Saudi Arabia*
[2]*Maxillofacial Surgery and Diagnostic Sciences, Division of Oral Pathology, College of Dentistry, Jazan University, Jazan, Saudi Arabia*

Correspondence should be addressed to Shankargouda Patil; dr.ravipatil@gmail.com

Academic Editor: Pia L. Jornet

Introduction. Familial arteriovenous malformations are exceedingly rare. They are often noted at birth. They can also present during childhood or adolescence. Sclerotherapy has proven to have a favorable outcome. *Case Presentation.* The present case report describes the treatment of arteriovenous malformations on the tongue, labial mucosa, and vermilion border in siblings treated with boiling saline injections. *Conclusion.* Sclerotherapy using boiling saline had shown to effectively treat arteriovenous malformations in the oral region without any significant morbidity.

1. Introduction

"Vascular malformation" is a generalized term used for the description of a set of congenital errors during vascular development, due to anomalous proliferation of vascular (angio/lympho) structures. This condition occurs in about one percent of births and is often very mild and does not require therapy [1]. Currently, Mulliken and Glowacki's 1982 classification system is still held as a standard for vascular anomalies. The classification system is based on the parameters that include the clinical, histopathological presentation, and biological behavior [2, 3]. Arteriovenous malformations (AVMs) are categorized as malformations with a high-flow capability as they involve arterovenous communications without the intermediate capillary network [4]. Also, the proliferation of AVM is induced by several other factors such as ischemia secondary to thrombosis, puberty, changes in hormonal levels, trauma, and ectasia. In the case of trauma, only a single vessel is involved in AVM; however, when the condition is familial, multiple vessels are involved [5, 6].

The head and neck are one of the most common sites (nearly 60% cases) for AVM [7]. 4 to 5% of all craniofacial AVMs occur in the gnathic bones. AVMs of the gnathic bones are relatively harder to treat [4]. Familial AVMs are exceedingly rare. RASA1 gene mutation expressing p120-Ras GAP, on chromosome 5q, has been reported to be associated with familial congenital AVM [8]. Most cases of familial AVMs are noted at birth although childhood or adolescence manifestations are not uncommon. Rarely, AVMs can associate with high output cardiac failure and cardiomegaly. The lesions progress gradually and have can potentially manifest in any body part including the oral cavity. Within the oral cavity, the tongue (anterior two-thirds), gingival, palate, and buccal mucosa are the most frequently reported sites of occurrence [9]. Kohout et al. has reported the largest case series of 81 cases of AVM that manifested in the oral cavity. In their case series, 31% occurred in the cheek (31%), 16% in the ears, 10% in the nose and forehead each, 7% in the upper labial mucosa, 5% each in the mandible and neck, and 4% each in the scalp and maxilla [5].

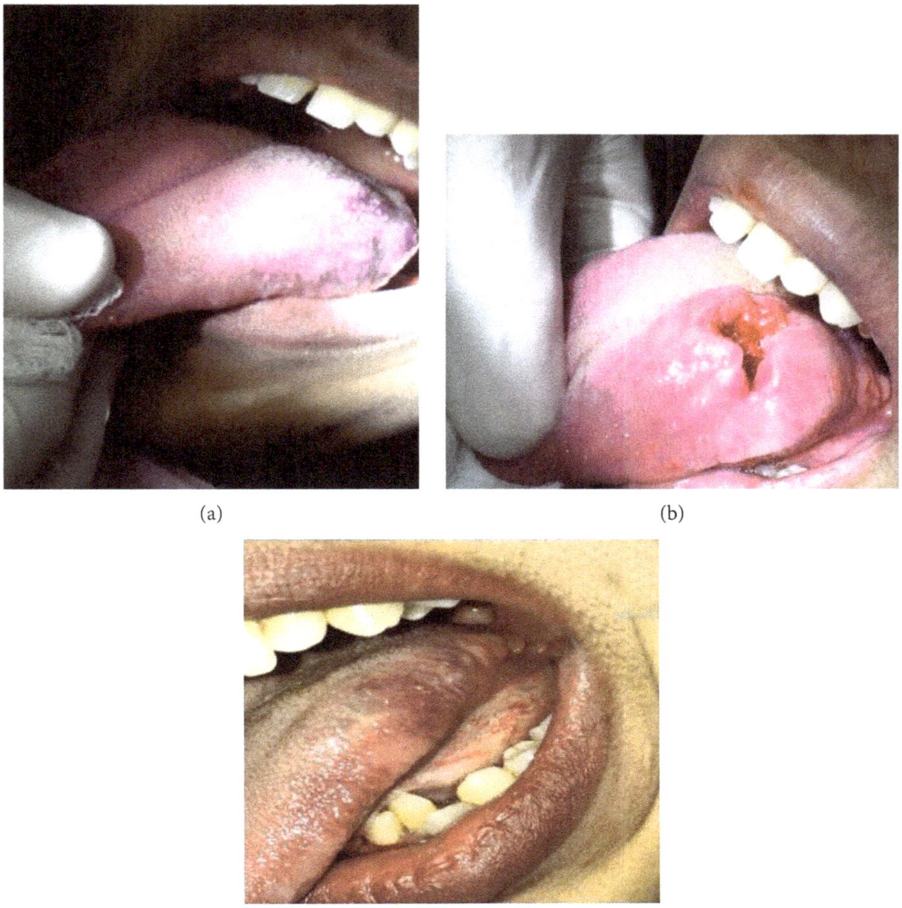

(a) (b)

(c)

Figure 1: (a) Preoperative AVM primary lesion of the left posterior region of the tongue; (b) AVM primary lesion opened after being injected 2 times; (c) follow-up after complete resolution of the primary AVM lesion by 3 years.

Clinically, these lesions occur as a pulsatile mass with a thrill, bruit, and rarely local hyperthermia with bleeding. There is a decreased vascularity leading to decreased nutrition supply resulting in necrosis, ulceration, bleeding, and impairment of function. The skin over the lesions is seen to have a reddish or true port-wine hue [10, 11].

Considering the diagnosis of the condition, the most common diagnostic modalities include radiography, CT (computed tomography scans), MRI (magnetic resonance imaging), and angiography [12]. Given the complex anatomical pathology, the treatment strategy for an AVM often involves multispecialties. The most common conventional therapeutic modalities suggested for AVM are a combination of surgical resection, sclerotherapy, and endovascular embolization techniques [12]. Ramakrishnan et al. in their systematic review have reported that the management of various vascular malformations included AVM. In their review, 6 articles reported various management techniques of AVM [13]. Deng et al. had reported Superselective Intra-Arterial Embolization (SIAE) followed by curettage (CT) or surgical resection (SR) for the management of AVM with complete involution and favorable prognosis [14].

SIAE and CT followed by sclerotherapy with complete involution and absence of recurrence was reported by Chen et al. [15]. Chen et al. reported 60.7% involution with recurrence and complications associated with sclerotherapy and fractionated radiotherapy [16]. Fan et al. reported 80% involution associated with complications in direct puncture embolization [17], and Zhao et al. reported 100% involution and nil recurrence with sclerotherapy alone [18]. Behnia et al. reported that curettage via proximal osteotomy without complete resection is an effective and less invasive method with more esthetics and better function in comparison with surgical resection [19].

Recently, LASERs, especially CO_2 and Er, Cr:YSGG, have been reported to be a successful tool for the treatment of AVM cases [20]. In the present paper, we present the minimally invasive surgical management of familial soft tissue AVM of the oral cavity reported in siblings.

2. Case Reports

2.1. 1st Case. A female patient 16 years of age reported to the Department of Oral and Maxillofacial Surgery of the College of Dentistry, Jazan University, Jazan, Saudi Arabia. The patient's medical history did not reveal any significant findings. The primary complaint of the patient was a persistent

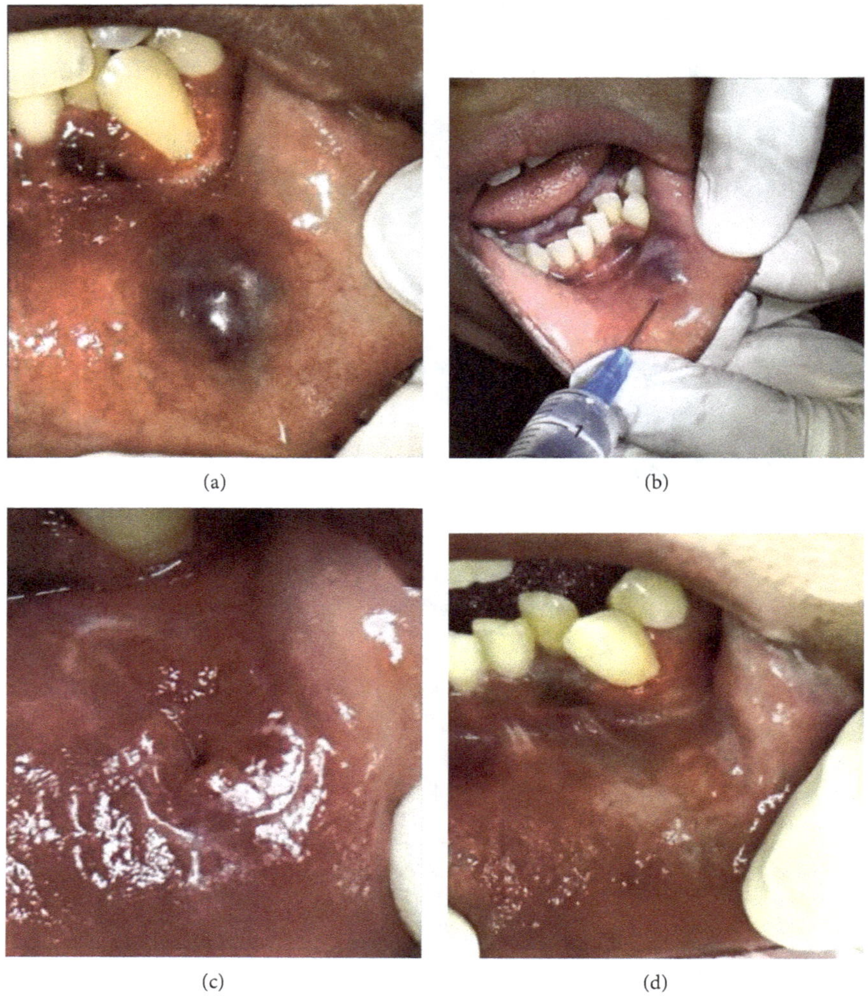

Figure 2: (a) Second lesion which appeared after the tongue lesion had resolved by 2 years; (b) boiling saline injection of the second AVM lesion; (c) second AVM lesion on the way to healing after 3 boiling saline injections; (d) second AVM lesion after 1 year of complete healing.

swelling of 10-year duration in the tongue. The swelling was not associated with pain and had been increasing in size gradually. There were no other symptoms associated with the swelling. On examination, the lesion was multilobulated and bluish with intact overlying mucosa and was present along the left lateral border and dorsum of the tongue opposite the mandibular left second molar. The lesion measured 4 cm by 6 cm by 0.7 cm (Figure 1(a)).

The consistency of the swelling was soft. Palpation did not reveal any tenderness. On compression, the swelling blanched. The swelling did not have any significant pulsation. All hematological parameters were within the physiological limit. Potential bone involvement was ruled out with the aid of plain radiographs. The AVM diagnosis was inferred using the findings from the MRI.

The patient was advised conservative surgical management using boiling saline injection. The procedure and possible complications were explained to the patient, and written informed consent was obtained. The patient was injected with 5 ccs of boiling saline after she was given a lingual nerve block, then the pressure was applied to the lesion to control bleeding. The patient was given postoperative instructions and recalled after two weeks. The same procedure was repeated at the recall appointment. One week later, the lesion was examined, and fibrosis was observed along with an open wound on the surface at the center of the lesion (Figure 1(b)). The patient was prescribed Levofloxacin Tab 500 mg (Sanofi Winthrop industries, 56, route de Choisy au Bac, 60205 Compiegne, France), one tablet a day for 5 days, and Ibuprofen Tab 200 mg (Wyeth Pharmaceuticals Company, Guayama, PR, USA), 2 tablets twice a day for 5 days. The lesion had healed uneventfully three months after the first injection (Figure 1(c)). The patient was followed up for three years, and the tongue lesion was free from any symptoms or recurrence. However, two years into the treatment of the tongue lesion, another arteriovenous malformation at the labial mucosa on the left side opposite the left lower canine tooth was noticed. The lesion was about 4 × 3 cm in size and about 0.5 cm in height (Figure 2(a)). The patient was administered the first boiling saline injection after giving her a mental nerve block (Figure 2(b)).

The saline (4 ccs) was injected around the lesion from different aspects while pointing the needle towards the depth of

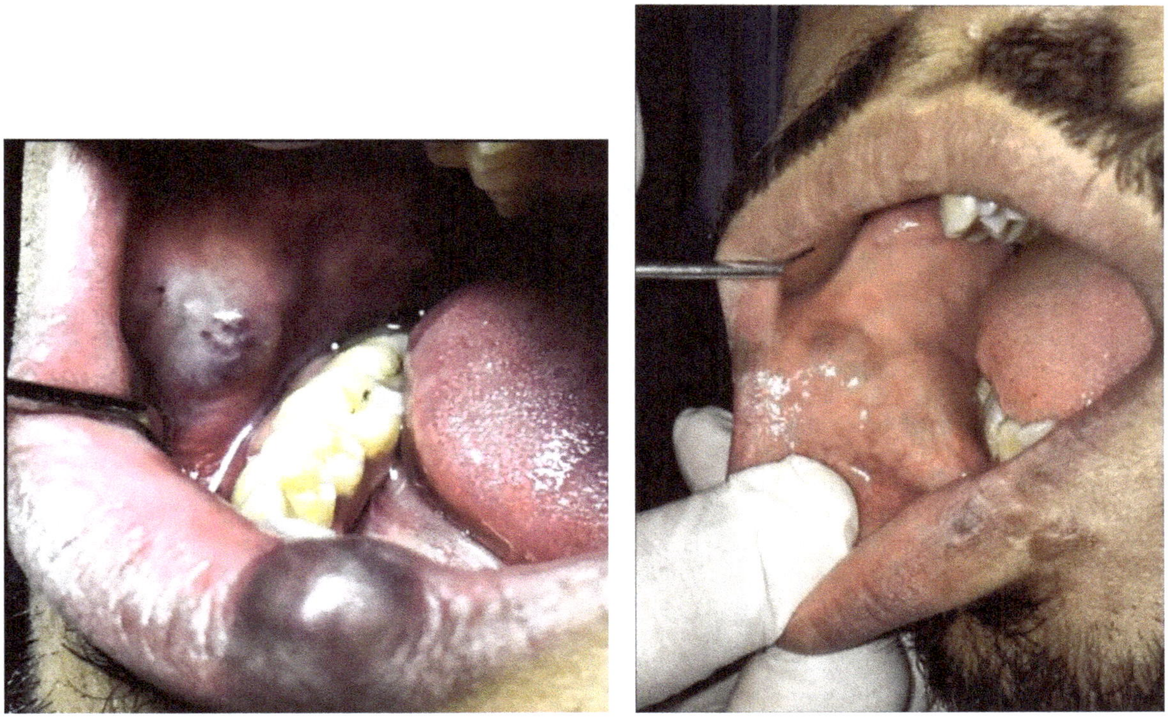

(a) (b)

FIGURE 3: (a) Preoperative photograph of both lip and cheek AVM lesions; (b) postoperative photograph of both lip and cheek AVM lesions.

the lesion. For this lesion, the patient was injected with boiling saline on two other occasions that are two and three months after the first injection. The lip lesion started healing uneventfully four months after the first appointment (Figure 2(c)). There were no signs of any complications or recurrence at the six-month and one-year follow-up (Figure 2(d)).

2.2. 2nd Case. The brother of the patient in case 1 was a 23-year-old who used to visit the department with his sister for her appointments. The patient had two AVMs. The first lesion was on the lower vermillion border on the left side and measured 2.5 cm by 1.5 cm. The lesion led to the visible asymmetry of the lower lip. The second lesion was present on the right buccal mucosa opposite to the first lower right molar and extending to the canine tooth, measuring about 4 × 3 cm (Figure 3(a)). The lesions were not associated with pain and had been increasing in size gradually. On examination, the lesion was multilobulated and bluish. The examination did not reveal any discontinuity in the surface mucosa. As reported for the 1st case, palpation revealed that the lesion was soft and nontender and on compression exhibited blanching. No significant pulsation was noted. Hematological parameters were all within the physiological limit. Bone involvement was ruled out with plain radiographs. AVM diagnosis was inferred with the findings from the MRI. Citing cosmetic concerns, treatment was sought for the lesion. After obtaining informed consent, the same treatment plan as used for the sister was advised to the patient. He was injected with 4 ccs of boiling saline around the lip lesion and at different depths under the mental nerve block. The pressure was applied to the lesion to control bleeding. The patient was given postoperative instructions and recalled after two weeks.

The patient was given three additional injections at one week, four weeks, and six weeks after the first injection. Additionally, the patient was prescribed Panthenol 10% gel (Pamex Pharmaceuticals, Germany) for application on the skin of the lip. The healing was uneventful with no complication or recurrence at the three-month and six-month appointments (Figure 3(b)).

3. Discussion

AVMs frequently noted at birth can manifest in childhood/adolescence [1, 9]. In the present cases, the patients had a history of the AVMs for about ten years and have been constantly growing in size. Kohout et al. reported the location of 81 AVMs in the head and neck. The cheek (31%) was the most common site followed by the ear (16%), nose (10%), upper lip (7%), mandible (5%), neck (5%), scalp (5%), and maxilla (4%) [8]. Within the oral cavity, the AVM's most frequent site is the tongue as in the present case. The lesser-known sites for intraoral AVM include the gingiva, palate, and buccal mucosa. AVM can be a major hurdle during speech, mastication, and deglutition and often get traumatized resulting in ulceration and secondary infection [21, 22]. In our cases, one lesion was on the tongue and two were on the lip (one on the labial mucosa and one on the vermillion border). The patients did not report any symptoms associated with the lesions and decided to undergo treatment for aesthetic reasons only.

Management of AVMs has always posed a challenge among clinicians because of their unpredictable behavior and high recurrence rate [23, 24]. Over the years, a plethora of approaches, including surgical excision, irradiation, electrocoagulation, cryotherapy, intravascular magnesium or copper needles, systemic corticosteroids, interferon-α, embolization, lasers, and sclerotherapy, has been tried for the management of these lesions. However, there is no universally accepted model of treatment for AVMs [25–27]. Moreover; each method has its limitations and disadvantages. Surgical excision, owing to the complicated anatomy of the face and neck, may result in significant loss of function, aesthetic issues, hemorrhage, or nerve damage [28]. Laser therapy is expensive. Additionally, it may lead to scarring and hyperpigmentation. Similar issues have also been noted with cryotherapy [29, 30]. Corticosteroids have systemic effects like adrenal suppression and weight gain [31].

Sclerotherapy is a conservative and low-cost technique for the effective treatment of vascular lesions of benign nature, including AVMs. It is particularly advantageous in surgically inaccessible areas. Sclerotherapy causes minimal scarring and has relatively fewer complications as compared to surgical excision [32]. Many sclerosing agents, for example, 5% sodium morrhuate, 5% ethanolamine oleate, sodium phyllite, 1% polidocanol, sodium tetradecyl sulfate, quinine urethane, hypertonic saline, and absolute ethanol, alone or in combination, have been used with varying results [24, 27].

In the present cases, boiling saline was used as the sclerosing agent for the treatment. The heat released from the boiling saline dehydrates the endothelial and red blood corpuscles, causing necrosis-induced vessel lumen obliteration, which in turn augments blood coagulation and vessel death. Additionally, it is readily available, acceptable to the patients as it is not a chemical, hypoallergenic, and inexpensive [33–35].

Sclerotherapy has certain potential complications like ulcerations, swelling, infection, transient nerve damage, hemorrhage, and anaphylaxis [35]. However, none of the aforementioned complications were observed in our patients. Eltohami and Abuaffan used hot saline for the treatment of a venous malformation in the tongue with success [33]. Water and hypertonic saline have also been used as means for sclerotherapy in venous malformations by Obuekwe et al. [36] and Oji et al. [37].

4. Conclusion

Arteriovenous malformations of the oral cavity might be associated with several complications apart from being an aesthetic concern. Therefore, prompt diagnosis and treatment are warranted for such lesions. Sclerotherapy with boiling saline provides an effectively safe therapeutic modality for intraoral AVMs. This method resulted in complete remission and alleviation of their symptoms, with no complications. No recurrence of the lesions was observed during the follow-up period.

Consent

Consent for publication was obtained for every individual person's data included in the study. Informed consent was obtained from all individual participants included in the study.

Authors' Contributions

Mokhtar Mamdouh Abdel-Latif performed treatment of the cases and contributed to writing the manuscript. Shankargouda Patil diagnosed the case and contributed to writing the manuscript. All the authors approved the final manuscript being submitted here.

References

[1] F. Martines and V. Immordino, "Arteriovenous malformation of the base of tongue in pregnancy: case report," *Acta Otorhinolaryngologica Italica*, vol. 29, no. 5, pp. 274–278, 2009.

[2] G. T. Richter and A. B. Friedman, "Hemangiomas and vascular malformations: current theory and management," *International Journal Of Pediatrics*, vol. 2012, Article ID 645678, 10 pages, 2012.

[3] J. B. Mulliken and J. Glowacki, "Hemangiomas and vascular malformations in infants and children: a classification based on endothelial characteristics," *Plastic and Reconstructive Surgery*, vol. 69, no. 3, pp. 412–420, 1982.

[4] M. N. Pandhare, D. B. Jyoti, M. S. Mandale, and R. B. Suresh, "Acquired arteriovenous malformation of lip occurring as an occupational hazard: a case report with review of literature," *Journal of Oral and Maxillofacial Pathology*, vol. 22, no. 2, p. 287, 2018.

[5] M. P. Kohout, M. Hansen, J. J. Pribaz, and J. B. Mulliken, "Arteriovenous malformations of the head and neck: natural history and management," *Plastic and Reconstructive Surgery*, vol. 102, no. 3, pp. 643–654, 1998.

[6] J. B. Boyd, J. B. Mulliken, L. B. Kaban, J. Upton, and J. E. Murray, "Skeletal changes associated with vascular malformations," *Plastic and Reconstructive Surgery*, vol. 74, no. 6, pp. 789–795, 1984.

[7] N. Syed, "Vascular lesions of head and neck: a literature review," *Indian Journal of Dental Sciences*, vol. 8, no. 3, p. 176, 2016.

[8] M. Pujari, S. Bahirwani, B. P, R. Kaul, B. Shah, and D. Daryani, "Arteriovenous malformation of tongue: a case report and review of literature," *Journal of Indian Academy of Oral Medicine and Radiology*, vol. 23, pp. 139–142, 2011.

[9] S. M. Manjunath, S. Shetty, N. J. Moon et al., "Arteriovenous malformation of the oral cavity," *Case Reports in Dentistry*, vol. 2014, Article ID 353580, 5 pages, 2014.

[10] Y. W. Chiu, H. T. Wu, Y. W. Chan, M. T. Lui, and S. Y. L. W. Kao, "A giant venous malformation of face and neck—a case report," *Taiwan Journal of Oral and Maxillofacial Surgery*, vol. 22, no. 2, pp. 110–117, 2011.

[11] I. C. Duncan and P. A. Fourie, "Vascular malformations part 2- current classification of vascular malformations," *South African Journal of Radiology*, vol. 8, no. 1, p. 23, 2004.

[12] G. Noreau, P. P. Landry, and D. Morais, "Arteriovenous malformation of the mandible: review of literature and case his-

tory," *Journal of the Canadian Dental Association*, vol. 67, no. 11, pp. 646–651, 2001.

[13] K. Ramakrishnan, I. Palanivel, V. Narayanan, S. Chandran, and P. Gurram, "Management of vascular malformations in the oral and maxillofacial region: a systematic review," *Journal of Stomatology, Oral and Maxillofacial Surgery*, vol. 20, 2021.

[14] W. Deng, D. Huang, S. Chen et al., "Management of high-flow arteriovenous malformation in the maxillofacial region," *The Journal of Craniofacial Surgery*, vol. 21, no. 3, pp. 916–919, 2010.

[15] W. Chen, J. Ye, L. Xu, Z. Huang, and D. Zhang, "A multidisciplinary approach to treating maxillofacial arteriovenous malformations in children," *Oral Surgery, Oral Medicine, Oral Pathology, Oral Radiology, and Endodontics*, vol. 108, no. 1, pp. 41–47, 2009.

[16] W. Chen, J. Wang, J. Li, and L. Xu, "Comprehensive treatment of arteriovenous malformations in the oral and maxillofacial region," *Journal of Oral and Maxillofacial Surgery*, vol. 63, no. 10, pp. 1484–1488, 2005.

[17] X. Fan, Z. Zhang, C. Zhang et al., "Direct-puncture embolization of intraosseous arteriovenous malformation of jaws," *Journal of Oral and Maxillofacial Surgery*, vol. 60, no. 8, pp. 890–896, 2002, discussion 896-7.

[18] X. Zhao, Z. Huang, W. Chen, Y. Wang, and Z. Lin, "Percutaneous sclerotherapy of arteriovenous malformations of the face using fibrin glue combined with OK-432 and bleomycin after embolisation," *The British Journal of Oral & Maxillofacial Surgery*, vol. 54, no. 2, pp. 187–191, 2016.

[19] H. Behnia, I. Ghodoosi, M. H. K. Motamedi, A. Khojasteh, and A. Masjedi, "Treatment of arteriovenous malformations: assessment of 2 techniques – transmandibular curettage versus resection and immediate replantation," *Journal of Oral and Maxillofacial Surgery*, vol. 66, no. 12, pp. 2557–2565, 2008.

[20] U. Romeo, A. del Vecchio, C. Russo et al., "Laser treatment of 13 benign oral vascular lesions by three different surgical techniques," *Medicina Oral, Patología Oral y Cirugía Bucal*, vol. 18, no. 2, pp. e279–e284, 2013.

[21] M. C. Garzon, J. T. Huang, O. Enjolras, and I. J. Frieden, "Vascular malformations: part I," *Journal of the American Academy of Dermatology*, vol. 56, no. 3, pp. 353–370, 2007, quiz 371-374.

[22] R. Modak, R. Modak, A. Mhapuskar, D. Hiremutt, and M. G. S. Hebbale, "Arteriovenous malformation of the oral cavity: a case report," *Journal of Pharmaceutical and Biomedical Sciences*, vol. 6, no. 9, pp. 514–517, 2016.

[23] D. Kademani, B. J. Costello, D. Ditty, and P. Quinn, "An alternative approach to maxillofacial arteriovenous malformations with transosseous direct puncture embolization," *Oral Surgery, Oral Medicine, Oral Pathology, Oral Radiology, and Endodontology*, vol. 97, no. 6, pp. 701–706, 2004.

[24] I. El-Hakim and A. Alyamani, "Management of palatal vascular malformation using absolute ethanol sclerotherapy," *Clinics and Practice*, vol. 1, no. 4, pp. 182–184, 2011.

[25] J. S. Lewin, E. M. Merkle, J. L. Duerk, and R. W. Tarr, "Low-flow vascular malformations in the head and neck: safety and feasibility of MR imaging-guided percutaneous sclerotherapy–preliminary experience with 14 procedures in three patients," *Radiology*, vol. 211, no. 2, pp. 566–570, 1999.

[26] Z. P. Li, "Therapeutic coagulation induced in cavernous hemangioma by use of percutaneous copper needles," *Plastic and Reconstructive Surgery*, vol. 89, no. 4, pp. 613–622, 1992.

[27] A. C. B. R. Johann, M. C. F. Aguiar, M. A. V. do Carmo, R. S. Gomez, W. H. Castro, and R. A. Mesquita, "Sclerotherapy of benign oral vascular lesion with ethanolamine oleate: an open clinical trial with 30 lesions," *Oral Surgery, Oral Med Oral Pathol Oral Radiol Endodontology*, vol. 100, no. 5, pp. 579–584, 2005.

[28] T. Yamaki, M. Nozaki, and K. Sasaki, "Color duplex-guided sclerotherapy for the treatment of venous malformations," *Dermatologic Surgery*, vol. 26, no. 4, pp. 323–328, 2000.

[29] B. A. Drolet, N. B. Esterly, and I. J. Frieden, "Hemangiomas in children," *The New England Journal of Medicine*, vol. 341, no. 3, pp. 173–181, 1999.

[30] L. Van Doorne, M. De Maeseneer, C. Stricker, R. Vanrensbergen, and M. Stricker, "Diagnosis and treatment of vascular lesions of the lip," *The British Journal of Oral & Maxillofacial Surgery*, vol. 40, no. 6, pp. 497–503, 2002.

[31] S. J. Fishman and J. B. Mulliken, "Hemangiomas and vascular malformations of infancy and childhood," *Pediatric Clinics of North America*, vol. 40, no. 6, pp. 1177–1200, 1993.

[32] J. L. Orlando, J. G. Mendes Pereira Caldas, H. G. do Amaral Campos, K. Nishinari, and N. Wolosker, "Ethanol sclerotherapy of superficial venous malformation: a new procedure," *Dermatology*, vol. 220, no. 4, pp. 376–380, 2010.

[33] Y. I. Eltohami and A. H. Abuaffan, "Venous malformation case report," *Journal of Hospital & Medical Management*, vol. 2, no. 2, pp. 1–3, 2016.

[34] S. Wiegand, B. Eivazi, A. P. Zimmermann, A. M. Sesterhenn, and J. A. Werner, "Sclerotherapy of lymphangiomas of the head and neck," *Head & Neck*, vol. 33, no. 11, pp. 1649–1655, 2011.

[35] C. L. Dietzek, "Sclerotherapy: introduction to solutions and techniques," *Perspectives in Vascular Surgery and Endovascular Therapy*, vol. 19, no. 3, pp. 317–324, 2007.

[36] O. N. Obuekwe, M. A. Ojo, O. Akpata, and B. D. Saheeb, "Haemangiomas of the maxillofacial region in Benin city, Nigeria," *Annals of Biomedical Sciences*, vol. 1, no. 1, 2008.

[37] C. Oji, F. Chukwuneke, and N. Mgbor, "Tobacco-pouch suture technique for the treatment of vascular lesions of the lip in Enugu, Nigeria," *British Journal of Oral and Maxillofacial Surgery*, vol. 44, no. 3, pp. 245–247, 2006.

23

Management of a Rare Case of Geminated and Fused Central Incisors in the Same Maxillary Dental Arch

Anas Alyahya, Humam Karkoutly, and Hussam Milly

Department of Conservative Dentistry and Endodontics, Dental Institute, Damascus University, Damascus, Syria

Correspondence should be addressed to Hussam Milly; milly.hussam@gmail.com

Academic Editor: Andrea Scribante

A 27-year-old man presented with developmental disorders in the maxillary incisors and asymmetric smile. Differential diagnosis between geminated and fused maxillary central incisors was conducted using cone-beam computed tomography (CBCT). The complexities of root canal system was handled using suitable shaping instruments and ultrasonic activation tips. Root apexes were sealed with mineral trioxide aggregate plugs. The anterior maxillary gingiva was surgically recontoured, and CAD/CAM Zirconia crowns were placed after the gingival healing phase. The combination of the 3D radiological examination, the clinical screening, and the use of a diagnostic wax-up presented a successful approach to manage this rare clinical case.

1. Introduction

Gemination is a malformation of a single tooth during its development to form a completely or partially separated crown with a single root [1]. The union of two or more teeth that normally develops separately is referred as fusion [2]. Gemination exhibits a normal number of teeth, whilst fusion presents a reduced number within the dental arch [3]. The clinical management of teeth with gemination or fusion may present difficulties since the size/shape of the crown deteriorates the aesthetic appearance, and the root canal morphology complicates the endodontic treatment [4].

Visualizing the internal anatomy of roots to obtain sufficient details about their surroundings is critical to achieve successful endodontic treatment [5]. The use of the standard two-dimensional radiographic technologies exhibits a limitation for the localization and characterization of complex root canal systems [6]. The application of cone-beam computed tomography (CBCT) has been revealed to be beneficial for endodontic treatment, particularly in understanding the complicated root canal morphology of fused/geminated teeth [7–9]. The flowing report describes multidisciplinary approach to restore the function and the esthetics appearance of both fused and geminated maxillary central incisors with the aid of CBCT.

2. Case Presentation

A 27-year-old male patient was referred to the Department of Conservative Dentistry and Endodontics with developmental disorders in the maxillary incisors and asymmetric smile. The clinical examination revealed an abnormal morphology of teeth #11 and #21. The absence of #12 and the presence of tooth #22 suggested the probability of fusion between #11 and #12 and a gemination in #21 (Figure 1). All vital signs were found to be normal. The teeth were not sensitive to palpation or percussion. The mobility of the teeth was within the normal limits. Periodontal probing using PCP-UNC 15 probe (Hu-Friedy, Leimen, Germany) showed no periodontal pocketing around the teeth. The two-dimensional radiographic examination (Figure 2) showed a complex pulp structure with no periodontal ligament space around the teeth. CBCT images were obtained using Vatech Pax-Duo3D Pano/CBCT (Vatech™, Seoul, South Korea) unit. CBCT images were reconstructed in three dimensions (3D) using Ez3D-I software (Vatech™, Seoul, South Korea). The CBCT images (Figure 3) revealed separated pulp chambers in the coronal third of #21, then a fusion of both root canals. The teeth #11 and #12 showed a separation under 1 mm of the cemento-enamel junction in the CBCT images (Figure 4).

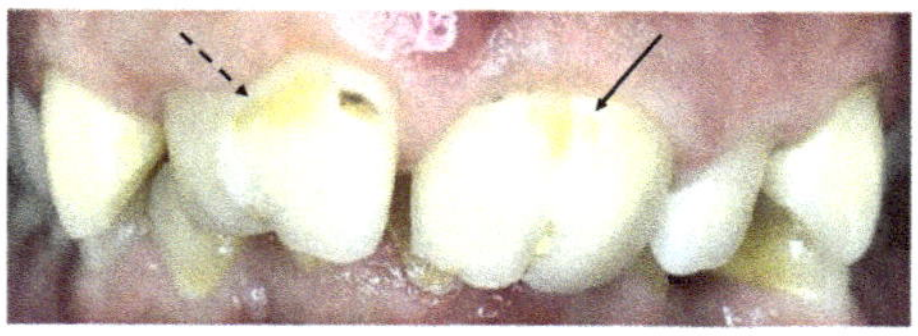

Figure 1: Preoperative image presenting geminated (arrow) and fused maxillary central incisors (dashed arrow).

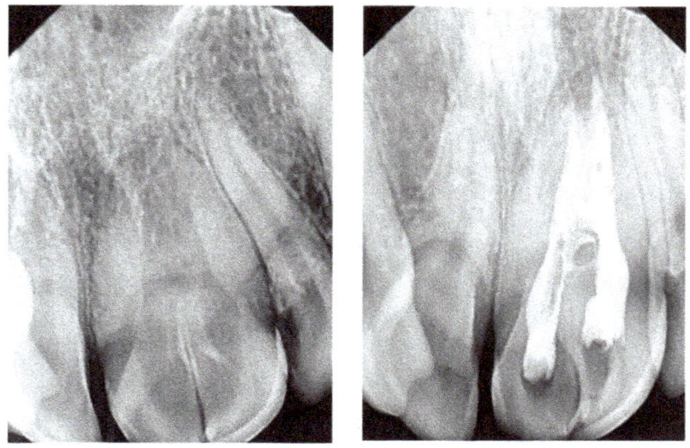

(a) (b)

Figure 2: (a) Initial radiograph of tooth #21 before the endodontic intervention. (b) Radiograph of tooth #21 after the endodontic treatment, with the set of the 3 mm apical plugs of MTA.

In this case, the correction of the shape/size of the anterior maxillary teeth would be conducted using fixed prosthesis after crown sectioning and preparation. The potential exposure of pulp chamber of both central incisors indicated the need for root canal treatment, which was conducted before crown preparation and restoration. A diagnostic waxed-up was made (Figure 5), and a mock-up was tried *in vivo*. The treatment plan was discussed thoroughly with the patient, and a written informed consent was obtained.

Anesthesia was administrated, and a rubber dam was applied. Root canals were prepared and shaped using XP-endo Shaper (FKG Dentaire, La Chaux-de-Fonds, Switzerland). Root canals were fully irrigated with 2.5% sodium hypochlorite (NaOCl) and activated using Sonofile K-file tips #25 (Satelec Acteon, Merignac Cedex, France) mounted in a P5 Booster ultrasonic scaler (Satelec Acteon). Apexes were sealed with 3 mm apical MTA (mineral trioxide aggregate) plugs (Dentsply Tulsa Dental, Tulsa, OK, USA). After 24 hours, resin-based sealer (Tgadeal, Technical, and General LTD London) was used with warm gutta-percha (BeeFill 2 in 1, VDW, Munich, Germany) for back-filling (Figure 2). Then, GIC restoration (Fuji IX, GC, Tokyo, Japan) was placed.

A session was set after 2 weeks of the endodontic obturation to recontour the anterior maxillary gingiva. The gingival pocket was 3.5 mm when measured; thus, there was no need for bone crest modification, and the cutting was within 1 mm. The patient returned for the next session after 2 weeks with a completely healed gingiva. The crowns of the anterior maxillary teeth from tooth #13 to tooth #23 were prepared for reshaping and smile correcting according to the cast module analysis. Crown cores were fabricated from zirconia blocks (Vita Zahnfabrik, Bad Säckingen, Germany) using CAD-CAM (computer-aided design and computer-aided manufacturing) system (Roland DWX-52® 5-Axis, California, USA), then gingival color modifiers were added to mimic the surrounding gingiva. The posttreatment photograph with final result is presented in Figure 6.

3. Discussion and Conclusion

Dental fusion is the union of two or more dental germs [10]. The fusion maybe a complete or incomplete depending upon stage of teeth development at the time of merging [10]. Such abnormality might be confused with gemination, since gemination is an abnormal development of a tooth separating the crown into two, while sharing a common root [11]. Gemination is the result of a single tooth bud division attempt [12]. Fusion can be differentiated from gemination by the count of teeth within a dental arch and have the number being reduced in fusion whilst remaining normal in gemination [4, 13–15]. In this report, a case of a partially fused central incisor to lateral incisor is presented in the upper right arch. In the upper left arch, however, the number of teeth is normal, and differentiation from gemination is impossible. The differentiation between gemination and fusion may not be critically significant for the clinical treatment [16].

In the dental literature, different clinical approaches are advocated to manage fused/geminated teeth. Those approaches include orthodontic treatment, tooth extraction, reduction of crown size followed by restoration, sectioning of the fused teeth, and no treatment [17].

The developmental anomaly in this clinical case was associated with appearance disapproval and social apprehension, reported by the patient. Therefore, a significant alternation in the teeth shape, size, and proportion was required to achieve a satisfied outcome.

The diagnosis/treatment of fused teeth is intractable. High-resolution 3-dimensional imaging has been demonstrated to be superior to periapical radiography in vitro and in vivo, particularly for canal identification and characterization of internal and external root morphology [18, 19]. In this report, the CBCT images helped in having a 3-dimensional view of the root systems, establishing the fact of having a partial or complete fusion, thus offering the best protocol for endodontic treatment. Wax-up and mock-up revealed the best treatment choices available and enabled the patient to see the expected results before initiating the treatment.

Endodontic treatment was conducted in this case as a significant modification in the incisors' shape was required for esthetic reason. Periodic clinical follow-up

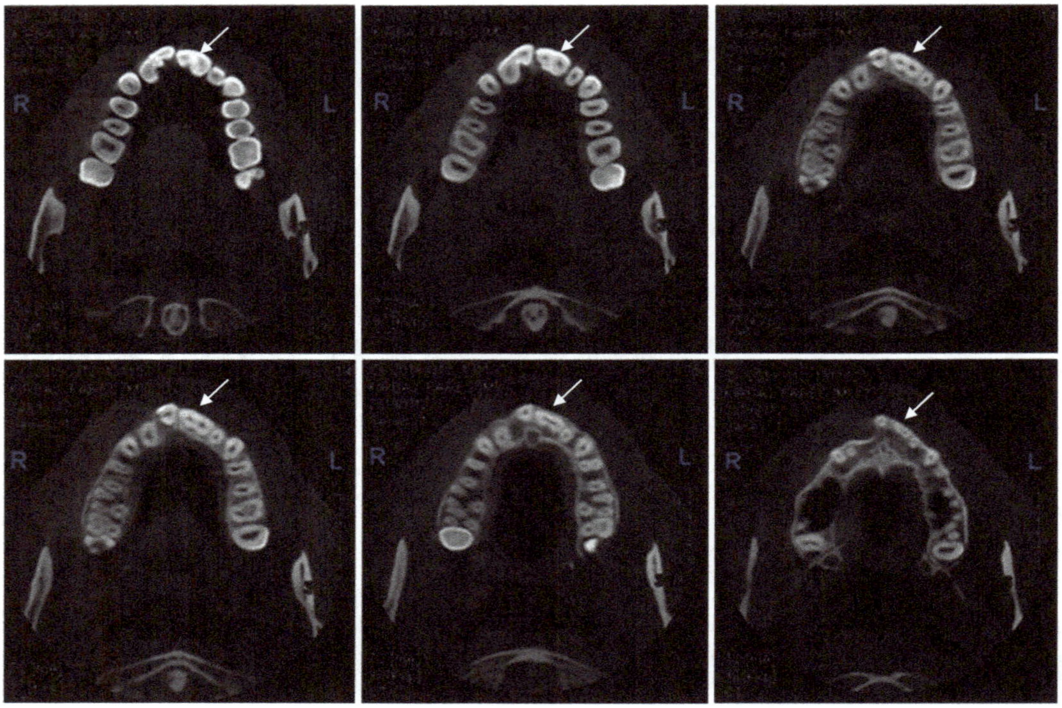

Figure 3: Plane of axial CBCT sections of maxillary showing fusion between #11 and #12 and a gemination in #21. The gemination presents a separated pulp chambers and merging root canals (arrow).

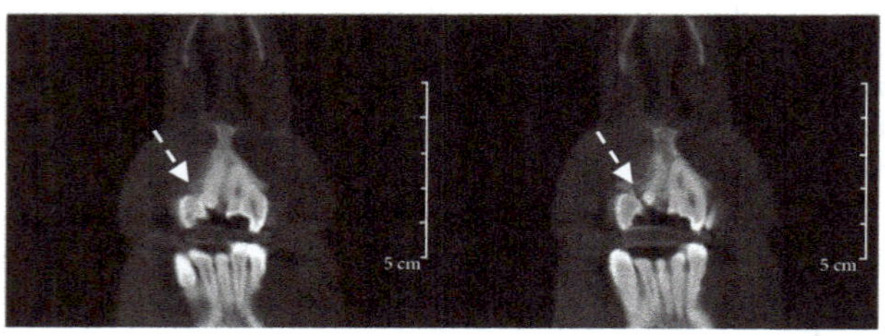

Figure 4: Plane of coronal CBCT sections of maxillary showing the separation level of the fused #11 and #12 (arrow).

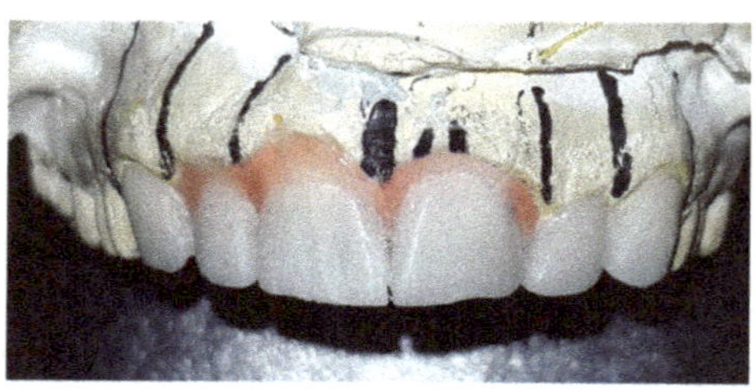

Figure 5: Initial wax-up showing the size/shape of the teeth. A new gingival level was placed.

is of utmost importance to ascertain the long-term success of the endodontic therapy [20]. The main limitation of the technique used in the management of the present

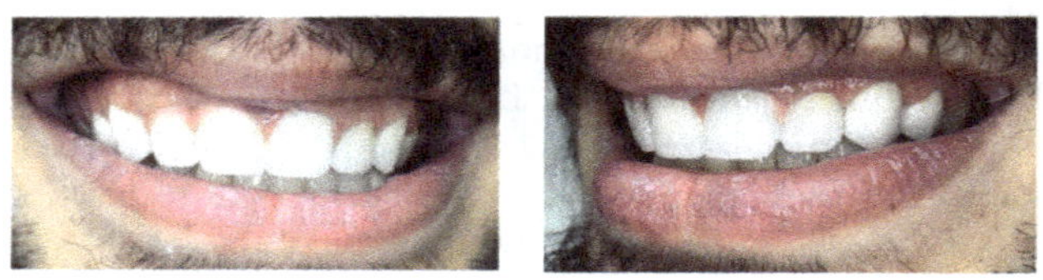

(a) (b)

Figure 6: Posttreatment photograph with final result.

case is that it was not minimally invasive. Esthetic reshaping of anterior teeth required a considerable removal of tooth substance. However, the selection of monolithic zirconia helped in reducing tooth structure loss [21].

Periodic periodontal assessment and treatment are essential for the success of indirect fixed dental prostheses [22]. Different variables affect significantly the prognosis of the treated teeth including oral rinsing solutions, toothbrushing technique, and motivation in self-performed plaque control [23–25].

In conclusion, careful case diagnosis and a precise treatment plan are obligated for the successful management of such rare case. A three-dimensional CBCT introduced valuable information about root canal systems and their surroundings which contributed substantially to the success of the endodontic therapy and case management.

Consent

Informed consent was obtained from the patient. Written informed consent was obtained from the patient before the study.

References

[1] A. Braun, T. Appel, and M. Frentzen, "Endodontic and surgical treatment of a geminated maxillary incisor," *International Endodontic Journal*, vol. 36, no. 5, pp. 380–386, 2003.

[2] S. Bernardi, S. Bianchi, G. Bernardi et al., "Clinical management of fusion in primary mandibular incisors: a systematic literature review," *Acta Odontologica Scandinavica*, vol. 78, no. 6, pp. 417–424, 2020.

[3] E. Grammatopoulos, "Gemination or fusion?," *British Dental Journal*, vol. 203, no. 3, pp. 119-120, 2007.

[4] I. Tsesis, N. Steinbock, E. Rosenberg, and A. Y. Kaufman, "Endodontic treatment of developmental anomalies in posterior teeth: treatment of geminated/fused teeth–report of two cases," *International Endodontic Journal*, vol. 36, no. 5, pp. 372–379, 2003.

[5] F. J. Vertucci, "Root canal morphology and its relationship to endodontic procedures," *Endodontic Topics*, vol. 10, no. 1, pp. 3–29, 2005.

[6] S. Patel, A. Dawood, T. P. Ford, and E. Whaites, "The potential applications of cone beam computed tomography in the management of endodontic problems," *International Endodontic Journal*, vol. 40, no. 10, pp. 818–830, 2007.

[7] S. Hegde, V. Ajila, J. S. Kamath, S. Babu, D. S. Pillai, and S. M. Nair, "Importance of cone-beam computed tomography in dentistry: an update," *SRM J Res Dent Sci.*, vol. 9, no. 4, p. 186, 2018.

[8] H. Rabiee, N. J. McDonald, R. Jacobs, A. Aminlari, and M. R. Inglehart, "Endodontics program directors', residents', and endodontists' considerations about CBCT-related graduate education," *Journal of Dental Education*, vol. 82, no. 9, pp. 989–999, 2018.

[9] K. Mensch, L. Simonffy, C. Dombi et al., "Endodontic and microsurgical treatments of maxillary lateral incisor dens invaginatus in combination with cone-beam-computed tomography fusion imaging," *Oral Radiology*, vol. 33, no. 2, pp. 147–152, 2017.

[10] S. Ballal, G. S. Sachdeva, and D. Kandaswamy, "Endodontic management of a fused mandibular second molar and paramolar with the aid of spiral computed tomography: a case report," *Journal of Endodontia*, vol. 33, no. 10, pp. 1247–1251, 2007.

[11] S. Gupta, M. Goel, and S. Dutta, "Synodontia between permanent maxillary lateral incisor and a supernumerary tooth: surgical treatment perspective," *Journal of Oral Health and Community Dentistry*, vol. 1, no. 3, pp. 52–55, 2007.

[12] C. Gadimli and Z. Sari, "Interdisciplinary treatment of a fused lower premolar with supernumerary tooth," *Eur J Dent.*, vol. 5, no. 3, pp. 349–353, 2011.

[13] S. S. Miri, H. Ghorbani, and A. R. Mohassel, "Endodontic treatment of fused teeth with talon cusp," *Case Reports in Dentistry*, vol. 2014, Article ID 738185, 4 pages, 2014.

[14] R. Rajendran, "Developmental disturbances of oral and para-oral structures," *Shafer's textbook of oral pathology*, vol. 5, pp. 3–112, 2006.

[15] B. W. Neville, D. D. Damm. C. M. Allen, and A. C. Chi, *Oral and Maxillofacial Pathology*, Elsevier Health Sciences, 2015.

[16] E. KIM and Y. JOU, "A supernumerary tooth fused to the facial surface of a maxillary permanent central incisor: case report," *Journal of Endodontia*, vol. 26, no. 1, pp. 45–48, 2000.

[17] K. Kremeier and M. Hülsmann, "Fusion and gemination of teeth: review of the literature, treatment considerations, and report of cases," *ENDO*, vol. 1, no. 2, pp. 111–123, 2007.

[18] M. Mashyakhy, H. R. Chourasia, A. Jabali, A. Almutairi, and G. Gambarini, "Analysis of fused rooted maxillary first and second molars with merged and C-shaped canal configurations: prevalence, characteristics, and correlations in a Saudi Arabian population," *Journal of Endodontia*, vol. 45, no. 10, pp. 1209–1218, 2019.

[19] L. Wu, B. Shi, R. Zhang, and J. Liu, "Case report root canal therapy of a supernumerary tooth fused with maxillary second molar: a case report," *International Journal of Clinical and Experimental Medicine*, vol. 12, no. 4, pp. 4422–4427, 2019.

[20] I. Sailer, N. A. Makarov, D. S. Thoma, M. Zwahlen, and B. E. Pjetursson, "All-ceramic or metal-ceramic tooth-supported fixed dental prostheses (FDPs)? A systematic review of the survival and complication rates. Part I: single crowns (SCs)," *Dental Materials*, vol. 31, no. 6, pp. 603–623, 2015.

[21] F. S. Schwindling, M. Waldecker, P. Rammelsberg, S. Rues, and W. Bömicke, "Tooth substance removal for ceramic single crown materials—an in vitro comparison," *Clinical Oral Investigations*, vol. 23, no. 8, pp. 3359–3366, 2019.

[22] C. Ercoli and J. G. Caton, "Dental prostheses and tooth-related factors," *Journal of Periodontology*, vol. 89, no. S, pp. 223–236, 2018.

[23] A. Butera, S. Gallo, C. Maiorani et al., "Probiotic alternative to chlorhexidine in periodontal therapy: evaluation of clinical and microbiological parameters," *Microorganisms*, vol. 9, no. 1, p. 69, 2021.

[24] F. W. M. G. Muniz, J. Cavagni, G. P. J. Langa, B. Stewart, Z. Malheiros, and C. K. Rösing, "A systematic review of the effect of oral rinsing with H2O2 on clinical and microbiological parameters related to plaque, gingivitis, and microbes," *International Journal of Dentistry*, vol. 2020, Article ID 8841722, 18 pages, 2020.

[25] M. Yamada, S. Hino, S. Nakamura, Y. Iijima, T. Kaneko, and N. Horie, "Accidental oral injuries by electric toothbrush: a report of three cases," *Case Reports in Dentistry*, vol. 2020, 4 pages, 2020.

24

A Conservative Management Approach for Unusual Presentation of Oral Actinomycosis

Qamar Hashem

Clinical Dental Sciences Department/Endodontic Division College of Dentistry, Princes Noura Bint Abdulrahman University, Riyadh, Saudi Arabia

Correspondence should be addressed to Qamar Hashem; qmhashem@pnu.edu.sa

Academic Editor: Giuseppe Alessandro Scardina

Actinomycosis is gram-positive saprophytic infection that is characterized by chronic suppurative and granulomatous lesion. It could be found in the oral cavity, lungs, colon, and genital area. In the oral cavity, it is commonly associated with infected root canals presented as persistent infections. This case reports demonstrate an atypical presentation of actinomycosis in the lower left mandibular canine/premolar area showing painless soft tissue lesion associated with bone sequestration. Nonsurgical curettage of the lesion followed by nonsurgical root canal treatment and retreatment to the offended teeth was determined as the treatment modality for this case.

1. Introduction

Actinomycosis is saprophytic infection that is characterized by chronic suppurative and granulomatous lesion by endogenous flora of the mouth [1]. Actinomycosis is caused by microaerophilic or anaerobic types of bacteria that usually colonize in the oral cavity and other areas of the body like the lungs, the female genital tract, and the gastrointestinal tract [2]. It belongs to the nonacid fast gram-positive bacteria, and most of the species identified from the actinomycosis lesion are *Actinomymyces israelii*, *Actinomymyces odontolyticus*, *Actinomymyces viscosus*, *Actinomymyces naeslundii*, or *Actinomymyces meyeri* [3].

Intraorally, the infection could present in chronic, acute, or subacute forms. Involving both the bone and soft tissue together or one of them solely, the infection spreads in atypical form in to the surrounding organs or tissues leading for sinus tracked production [4].

Cervicofacial actinomycosis rarely involves the bone; nevertheless, it affects the soft tissues more frequently. The incident differs depending on the location, the temporomandibular joint, chin, cheek, and the maxilla that are the less common affected locations. However, more than 50% of the cases are found in the mandible [5].

Periapical actinomycosis is believed to be a nonresolving periapical lesion associated with actinomycotic infection and has been suggested as a contributing factor in the perpetuation of periapical radiolucencies after root canal treatment. Actinomycotic osteomyelitis of the mandible is an uncommon consequence of odontogenic infections [6]. Diagnosis is especially difficult and usually made by identifying the typical actinomycotic colonies in a surgical specimen [4]. Periapical actinomycosis is thought to be rare, and the data reported the frequency of periapical actinomycosis and the possibilities of it that is correlation between such condition and cervicofacial actinomycosis is limited [7].

Typically, a disruption in the integrity of the mucous membrane due to injury, infection, or surgical intervention may allow microorganisms to access deeper structure and disease progression. In some conditions, microorganisms emerging from the canal can conquer the protective barriers and produce an extraradicular contamination, thus giving the clinical presentation of a periapical lesion with a bone fragment of osteomyelitis in the mandible [6].

In this case report, we are presenting a lesion in the mandibular left side related to a poor endodontically treated tooth having both a periapical lesion and a segment of the necrotic bone.

2. Case Presentation

A 56-year-old male complains from a white patch on his facial gingiva of his lower teeth that causes him discomfort and pain that started few weeks ago. The patient with no knowing allergies reported a medical history of myocardial infarction two years ago, hypothyroidism and dyslipedimia. In addition, he is a heavy smoker for more than 20 years. As a result, he is under multiple medications in order to manage his general health like bisoprolol fumarate (Concor), perindopril arginine (Coversyl), and clopidogrel bisulfate (Plavix).

The patient reported localizes swelling in the lower left area few months ago. The patient was giving an antibiotic course and pain medication by their local doctors and referred the patients to the ENT. Then, nystatin was prescribed as antifungal medication, but no improvement was noted, and the complaint persists. Following that, the patient was referred to the dental department for proper management and long-term planning.

The intraoral examination revealed a soft tissue lesion associated with bone sequestration on buccal mucosa relative to tooth number #33 and #34 (Figure 1).

Tooth #33 is sound, but tooth #34 had previous root canal treatment (RCT) with apical transportation and was restored with temporary filling few years ago. However, no pus discharged or any lymphadenopathy was noted. The general practitioner few weeks before endodontic appointment did a sinus tract tracing using gutta-percha point size 30.

A provisional diagnosis of chronic infection lesion made based of the provided history and clinical findings. These finding were more investigated through radiographical examination, an orthopantomogram (OPG) (Figure 3) and periapical radiograph for tooth #34 (Figure 2) were taken. Finding includes generalized periodontitis, and missing teeth #26 and #27 and periapical radiolucency extended from tooth #32 to tooth #34.

In order to exclude malignancies as a differential diagnosis, routine blood examination, excisional biopsy, and culture sample from the lesion were performed. Regarding the routine blood test, apart from elevated neutrophils and lymphocytes, no abnormalities were detected. The pathological report of the biopsy revealed fragments of the necrotic bone and bacteria. In addition, trabecular surface and bone sequestrum of the necrotic bone were showing actinomycosis colonies (Figure 4). Therefore, a definitive diagnosis of actinomycosis was made. No histological sampling of the periapical root structure was performed at the time, as was not seen as necessary since the root structure has been curettage with the surrounding area.

The treatment plan will include patient education and motivation, nonsurgical curettage of the lesion, and nonsurgical root canal retreatment for tooth #34. Prior to removal of lesion, vitality testing of the adjacent teeth (#32, #33, #35, and #36) was assessed and gives vital normal response except for tooth # 33 which gives negative response. Accordingly, RCT for tooth #33 added to the treatment plan.

Removal of the bony sequestration ($0.5 \times 0.5 \times 0.15$ cm) and placed in formalin was carried out and submitted for histopathological analysis as well as swap from the exposed area (Figure 5).

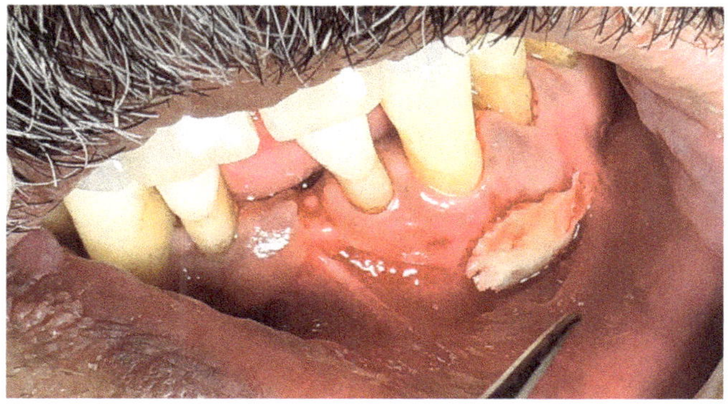

FIGURE 1: Intraoral picture of lesion in buccal vestibule of the mandibular left side.

Lastly, curettage of the area and irrigation with saline done, augmentin 1 g twice/day (bid) for one week, was prescribed and patient schedule for treatment. In the subsequent visit, local anesthesia (LA) as xylocaine with epinephrine 2% administered a rubber dam (RD) isolation for both #33 and #34. Tooth #34 previous root canal filling was removed and access done, working length determination, cleaning and shaping done using the rotary system (crown down technique), and 5.25% NaOCl used for irrigation. Due to previous treatment misshape of an open apex and failure to achieve apical stop, mineral trioxide aggregate (MTA) plug placed at the apical 1/3. Obturation of the remaining canal with gutta-percha and AH 26 sealer, with continuous wave compaction, temporized with cavit and silver glass ionomer (Ketac) as temporary (Figure 6). Tooth #33, a conventional RCT, carried out following the same steps of tooth #34 but obturation was made using gutta-percha and AH 26 sealer (Figure 6), and then the tooth was restored with temporary filling. The slight amount of extruded MTA will not affect the healing due to its compatibility [8].

Patient referred for periodontist in order to manage the generalize periodontitis and then for prosthodontist for final restorations for #33 and #34. The patient was followed up at six months and one year period with no evidence of lesion recurrence (Figure 7).

3. Discussion

Actinomycosis is one of the infectious diseases that affect both humans and animals in a chronic, granulomatous form. The contribution factors for endodontic treatment failures are many; however, with it is low prevalence among all periapical lesions (less than 5%), actinomycosis cannot be consider as a common cause leading for RCT failure. Cervicofacial actinomycosis is classified into two subtypes, peripheral and central [7]. While the central type is considered very rare, actinomycosis falls under central type which itself is very uncommon among central varieties [9]. Early diagnosis of actinomycosis combined with proper intervention has an excellent prognosis. Cure rates are high, and neither deformity nor death is common.

Knowing that extraradicular infection can be dependent or independent of the intraradicular infections, *Actinomyces*

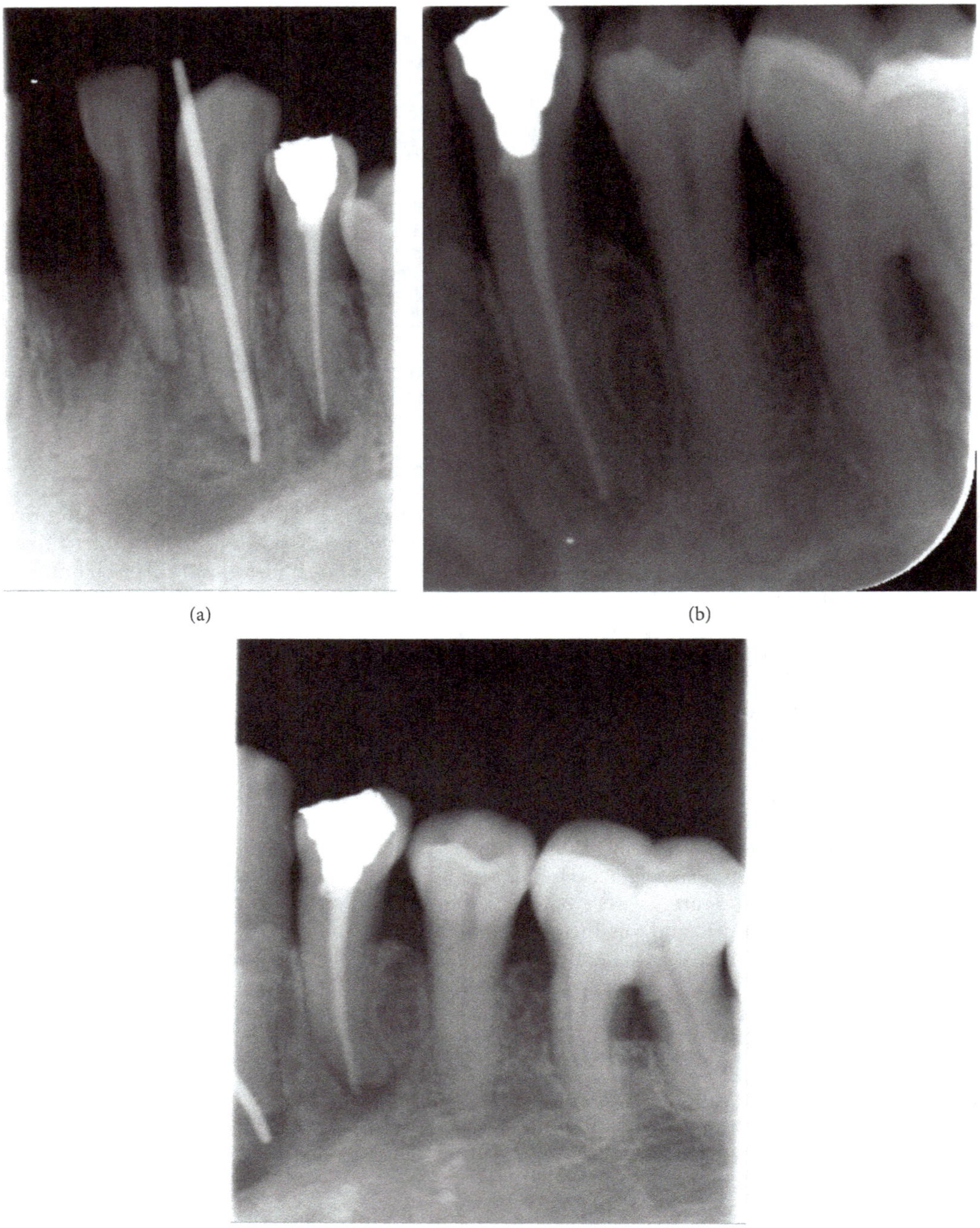

(a) (b) (c)

FIGURE 2: Intraoral preoperative periapical radiograph showing an irregular periapical radiolucency involving both #33 and #34. (a) Tracing was made using gutta-percha point done. (b, c) Other periapical angles.

and *Propionibacterium propionicu* species are the only species capable of forming an independent extraradicular infection in pathological entity named apical actinomycosis. In this case, the endodontic failure may be due to both the previous substandard endodontic treatment and the presence of the *Actinomyces* species in the periapical area [10, 11].

Many local (oral) and general health factors contribute to the physiopathological pathways of cervicofacial actinomycosis. Poor oral hygiene, dental caries, gingival inflammation or trauma, traumatic dental extraction, and cervicofacial surgery are among the oral factors. On the other hand, general health factors include immunocompromise and diabetic patients, male gender, and steroids [12]. In our presented case, the patient had many of these risk factors like age, medical conditions, and poor oral health.

Most of the publications on apical actinomycosis are case reports. Many treatment approaches were done that depend on the case. Alhezami in 2010 did incision and drainage of the lesion. Two weeks later, endodontic apical surgery was done [13]. On the other hand, extraction of the involved teeth

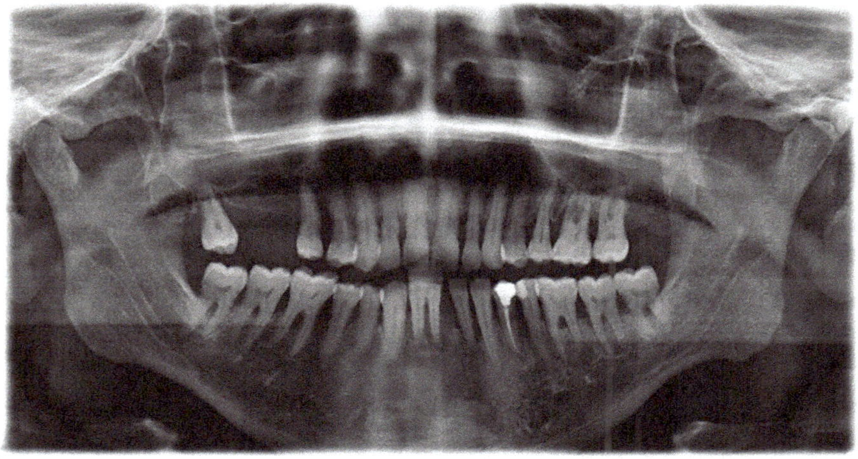

Figure 3: Orthopantomogram showing multiple missing teeth and endodontic treatment of tooth #34.

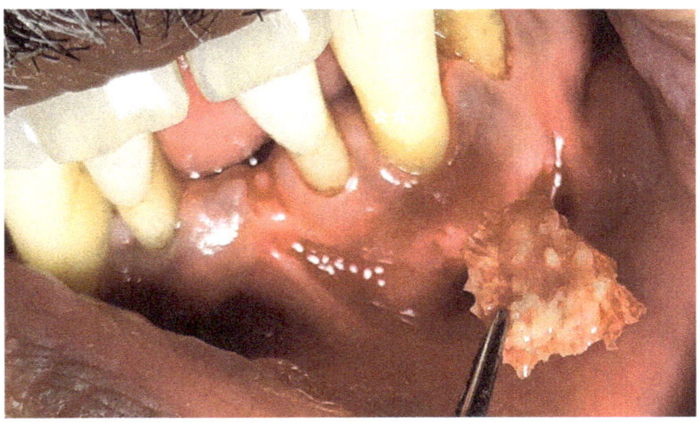

(a)

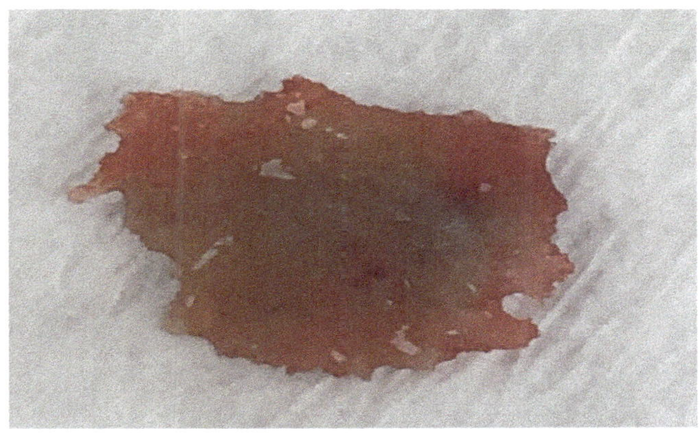

(b)

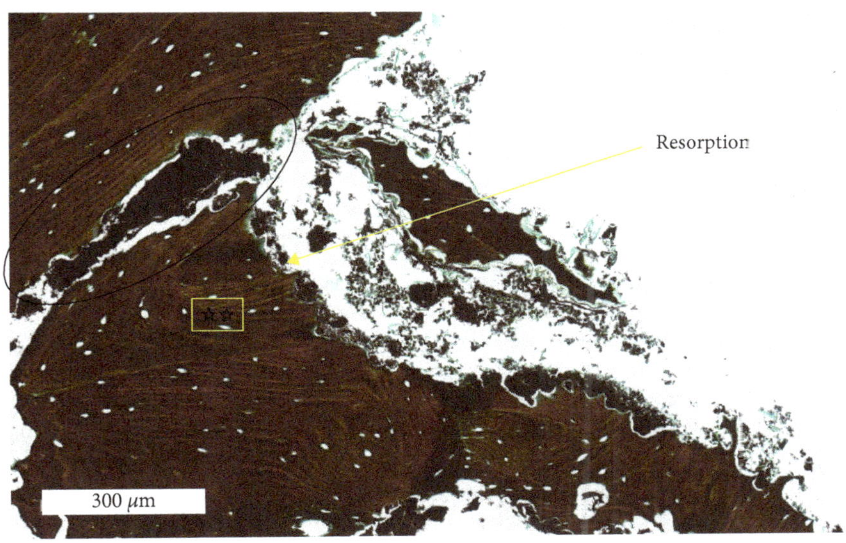

(c)

Figure 4: (a, b) Intraoral photograph after bone removal. (c) Necrotic bony trabeculae with actinomycosis filaments on the trabecular surface (black circle) and extensive sclerosis of bone showing prominent resting and reversal lines (**).

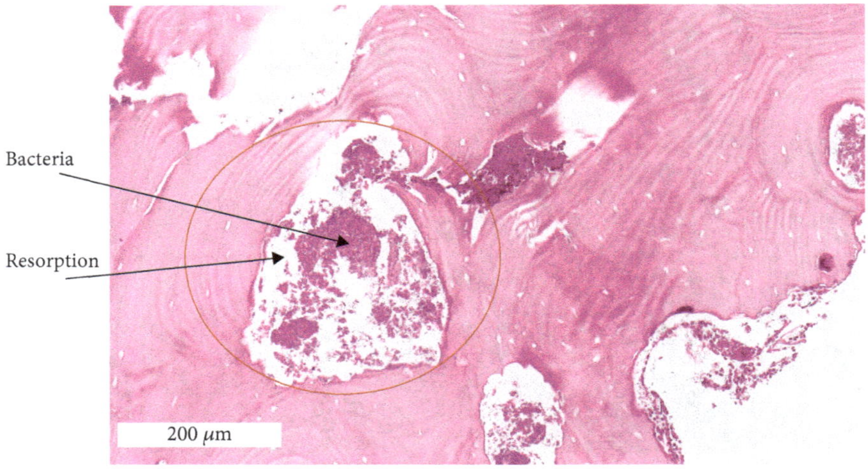

FIGURE 5: H&E stain showing bacterial invasion in the bone causing resorption. Bacteria (black arrow) and resorption of bone (black stars).

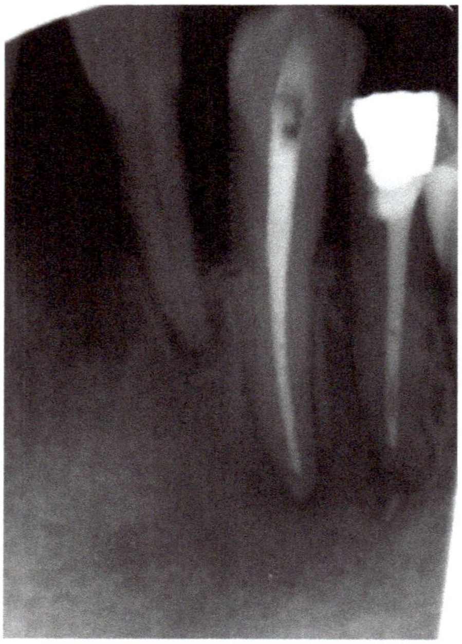

FIGURE 6: Postoperative periapical radiograph showing endodontic treatment of both teeth #33 and #34.

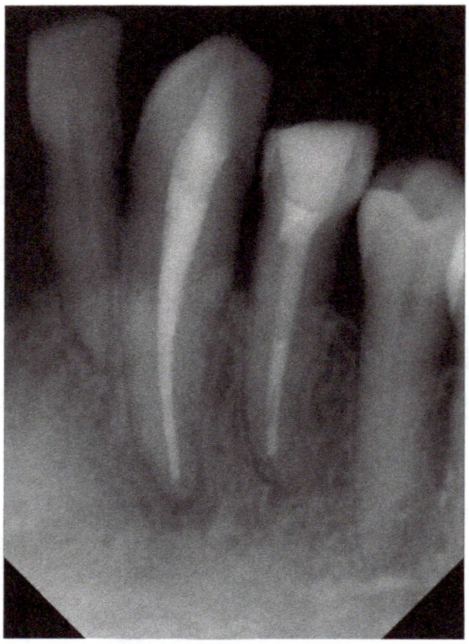

FIGURE 7: 1-year recall periapical radiograph showing healing of the lesion.

in order to evaluate the deeper tissue and relief the pain considered to manage actinmycosis. This was done by Gannepalli et al., and few teeth were extracted followed by debridement of the area. In our case, the infection pathway was extremely irregular leading for osteomyelitis and hard texture alongside free gingiva and buccal vestibule location [5]. As a result, a conservative surgical approach by excisional biopsy and root canal retreatment was ending to symptom relief and proper healing. In addition, avoiding extraction when possible will lead for better oral health and improve the patient quality of life.

MTA used apically for 5 mm for RCT retreatment for #34. A 5 mm barrier demonstrated significantly greater microhardness than the 2 mm barrier MTA used after root canal preparation favored the occurrence of the apexification and periapical healing. The initial use of Ca $(OH)_2$ paste was not necessary for apexification to occur and has shown to be strongly related to the extrusion of MTA and formation of barriers beyond the limits of the root canal walls [14]. Low cytotoxicity and the induction of mineralization are 2 desirable properties of MTA that may explain the bioregenerative and the biocompatibility of this biomaterial. The extrusion of the MTA root canal filling biomaterial from an open apex tooth into a periradicular lesion does not produce any complications [15].

Apart from the periapical type of actinomycosis, long-term systemic antibiotic therapy has been the treatment of choice for all the other types of actinomycosis. With duration ranging usually from 3 months to 1 year, the penicillin is the first drug of choice, and erythromycin and tetracyclines are alternative options [16]. In long-standing infections, fibrosis can reach in to advance level of sclerosis that inhibits the antibiotic penetration as a result of the poor vascularity. In addition, the sulfur granule has a protective nature, making high doses needed for effective therapy following RCT, extraction, or surgical intervention [16]. In our case, the previous oral antibiotic taken by the patient was ineffective. However, after lesion removal and RCT, antibiotic was prescribed as shown by some reported cases and considering patient medical history.

4. Conclusion

Oral periapical actinomycosis is a long-standing infection presents in unusual ways in the mouth. With its benign potential, educating the health care providers and general dental practitioner will result in better transfer of the case for proper diagnosis and management. Using cultures and histopathology to reach the definitive diagnosis, a conservative approach that avoids extraction should be considered if possible specially when it reliefs the patient symptoms and provides good prognosis.

References

[1] M. M. Rubin and B. S. Krost, "Actinomycosis presenting as a midline palatal defect," *Journal of Oral and Maxillofacial Surgery*, vol. 53, no. 6, pp. 701–703, 1995.

[2] T. A. Russo, "Agents of actinomycosis," in *Principles and Practice of Infectious Diseases*, G. L. Mandel and J. E. Bennett, Eds., pp. 2646–2654, Churchill Livingstone, London, 5th ed. edition, 2000.

[3] M. Miller and A. J. Haddad, "Cervicofacial actinomycosis," *Oral Surgery, Oral Medicine, Oral Pathology, Oral Radiology, and Endodontology*, vol. 85, no. 5, pp. 496–508, 1998.

[4] R. E. Marx and D. Stern, "Inflammatory, Reactive, and infectious Diseases," in *in oral and maxillofacial pathology—a rational for diagnosis and treatment*, pp. 57–67, Quintessence Publishing, Batavia, Illinois, 2003.

[5] A. Gannepalli, B. K. Ayinampudi, P. V. Baghirath, and G. V. Reddy, "Actinomycotic Osteomyelitis of Maxilla Presenting as Oroantral Fistula: A Rare Case Report," *Case Reports in Dentistry*, vol. 2015, Article ID 689240, 5 pages, 2015.

[6] S. S. Simre, A. A. Jadhav, and C. S. Patil, "Actinomycotic osteomyelitis of the mandible - A rare case report," *Annals of Maxillofacial Surgery*, vol. 10, no. 2, p. 525, 2020.

[7] A. Hirshberg, I. Tsesis, Z. Metzger, and I. Kaplan, "Periapical actinomycosis: A clinicopathologic study," *Oral Surgery, Oral Medicine, Oral Pathology, Oral Radiology, and Endodontology*, vol. 95, no. 5, pp. 614–620, 2003.

[8] P. N. R. Nair, "Pathology of apical periodontitis," in *Essential endodontology*, D. Orstavik and T. R. Pitt ford, Eds., pp. 68–104, Blackwell Science, London, 1st edition, 1998.

[9] S. P. Pasupathy, D. Chakravarthy, S. Chanmougananda, and P. P. Nair, "Periapical actinomycosis," *Case Reports*, vol. 2012, no. jul31 1, pp. bcr2012006218–bcr2012006218, 2012.

[10] Y. Noiri, A. Ehara, T. Kawahara, N. Takemura, and S. Ebisu, "Participation of Bacterial Biofilms in Refractory and Chronic Periapical Periodontitis," *Journal of Endodontia*, vol. 28, no. 10, pp. 679–683, 2002.

[11] J. F. Siqueira Jr., "Reaction of periradicular tissues to root canal treatment: benefits and drawbacks," *Endodontic Topics*, vol. 10, pp. 123–147, 2005.

[12] V. K. Wong, T. D. Turmezei, and V. C. Weston, "Actinomycosis," *BMJ*, vol. 343, no. oct11 3, pp. d6099–d6099, 2011.

[13] K. Al-Hezaimi, "Apical actinomycosis: case report," *Journal of the Canadian Dental Association*, vol. 76, p. a113, 2010.

[14] G. D. Matt, J. R. Thorpe, J. M. Strother, and S. B. McClanahan, "Comparative Study of White and Gray Mineral Trioxide Aggregate (MTA) Simulating a One- or Two-Step Apical Barrier Technique," *Journal of Endodontics*, vol. 30, no. 12, pp. 876–879, 2004.

[15] E. Tahan, D. Çelik, K. Er, and T. Taşdemir, "Effect of unintentionally extruded mineral trioxide aggregate in treatment of tooth with periradicular lesion: a case report," *Journal of Endodontics*, vol. 36, no. 4, pp. 760–763, 2010.

[16] A. B. M. Moniruddin, H. Begum, and K. Nahar, "Actinomycosis: An Update," *Medicine Today*, vol. 22, no. 1, pp. 43–47, 2010.

25

Oral Squamous Cell Carcinoma in a Patient with Fanconi Anemia

Milla Huuhka[1] **and Aaro Turunen**[1,2]

[1]*Department of Oral and Maxillofacial Diseases, Turku University Hospital, Turku, Finland*
[2]*Department of Oral and Maxillofacial Surgery, Institute of Dentistry, University of Turku, Turku, Finland*

Correspondence should be addressed to Milla Huuhka; milla.huuhka@tyks.fi

Academic Editor: Giuseppe Alessandro Scardina

Fanconi anemia (FA) is a rare autosomal recessive genetic disorder characterized by different types of malformations, skin lesions, bone marrow failure, and increased risk for both hematological malignancies and solid tumors, especially head and neck squamous cell carcinomas (HNSCC). FA patients may also display a low tolerance to oncologic treatments. The authors present a case of mandibular squamous cell carcinoma in a young FA patient. Because of the aggressive nature of the SCC and complex treatment options, we recommend a strict lifelong follow-up for all FA patients to detect early changes in the oral mucosa.

1. Introduction

Fanconi anemia (FA) is a rare genetic disorder with an estimated prevalence of 1 : 160 000 at birth. It is inherited mainly via an autosomal recessive pathway [1]. The disease is characterized by progressive bone marrow failure, hyperpigmentation, pancytopenia, predisposition to both solid tumors and hematological malignancies (i.e., acute myeloid leukemia), and different kinds of congenital malformations [1–3]. Pathogenesis of FA involves biallelic mutations in at least one of the 23 genes responsible for chromosome stability and DNA repair via the FA/BRCA pathway [3].

On most patients, the diagnosis of FA is first suspected in childhood based on hematological abnormalities, growth retardation, and/or congenital malformations. Laboratory analysis by choromosome exposure to cross-linking agents such as diepoxybutane (DEB) or mitomycin C (MMC) reveals complex metaphasic chromatid exchange patterns in the peripheral blood sample, usually leading to FA diagnosis [2]. Because of the progressive nature of FA, the only curative treatment for bone marrow failure is hematopoietic stem cell transplantation (HSCT). After HSCT, patients are susceptible to developing acute or chronic graft versus host disease (GVHD). Chronic GVHD is a known risk factor for malignancies such as OSCC.

FA leads to a 200- to 800-fold increased risk for head and neck squamous cell carcinomas. Majority of the tumors are oral squamous cell carcinomas (OSCC), and the patients are unusually young at disease presentation [3]. As the overall outcome of HSCT has improved during the last decade, the patients with FA live longer lives. Thus, considering the cumulative risk of carcinoma development and increased survival in FA, frequency of OSCCs associated with this rare disorder can be expected to increase in the future [3–5].

2. Case Presentation

A 28-year-old female with FA was referred to consultation by a local dentist due to an asymptomatic tumor in the lingual side of the patient's left mandibular gingiva (Figure 1). According to the patient, she had noticed the mass 3-4 weeks prior to the visit. The patient did not have a history of smoking, and her alcohol use was minimal. She had undergone a hematopoietic stem cell transplant (HSCT) 14 years prior and had suffered a mild GVHD mainly affecting the skin and lungs. At presentation, her only regular medication was estrogen replacement. Histological examination confirmed squamous cell carcinoma grade 1. A CT scan of the tumor revealed invasion of the mandibular bone and two pathologic lymph nodes in the ipsilateral submandibular space (Figures 2

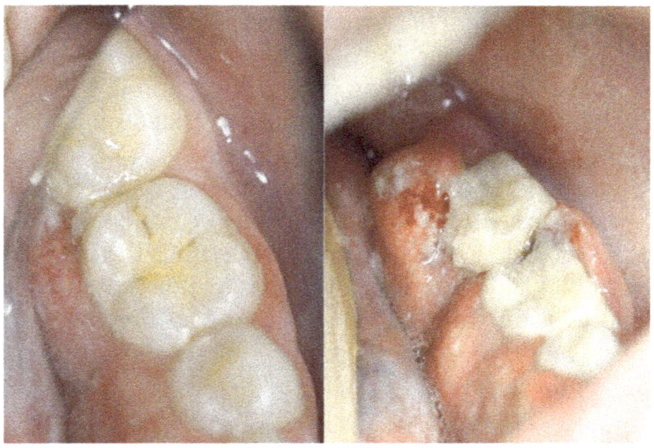

FIGURE 1: The patient at presentation/biopsy appointment (a) and one month later, before surgery (b). A marked enlargement of the tumor area is shown, with extension to the buccal side of the molar teeth. Plaque accumulation is also detected, owing to pain during brushing. Clinical photography proved difficult due to pain and discomfort affecting the area.

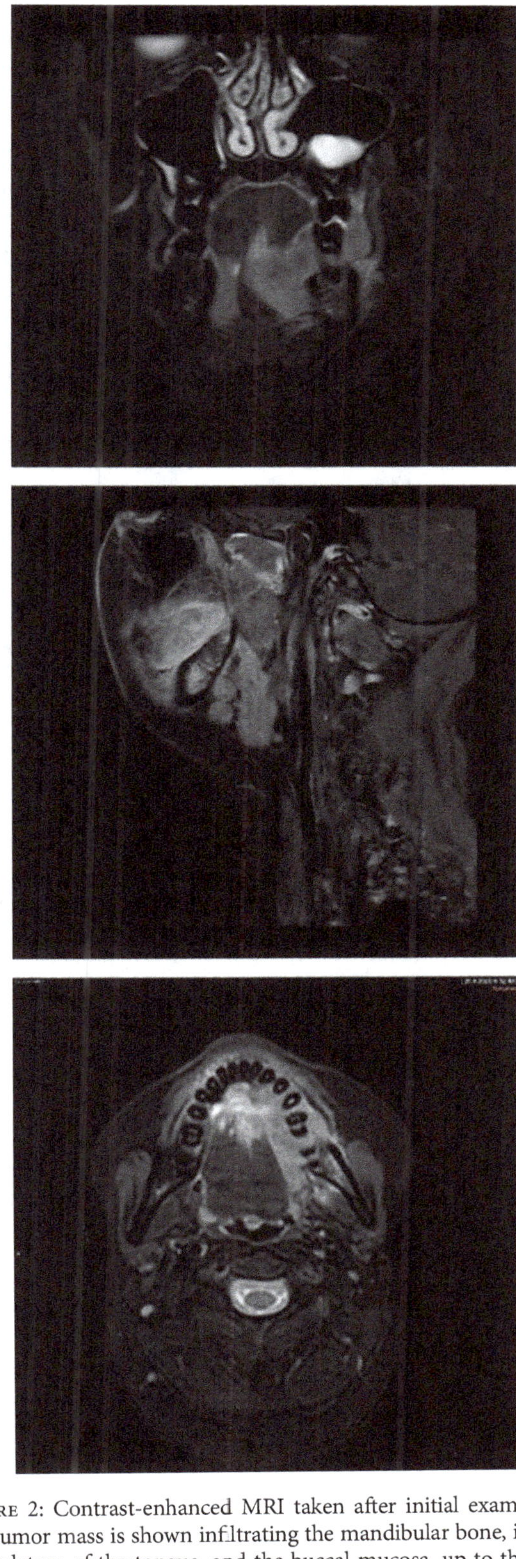

FIGURE 2: Contrast-enhanced MRI taken after initial examination. The tumor mass is shown infiltrating the mandibular bone, intrinsic musculature of the tongue, and the buccal mucosa, up to the depth of the mylohyoid muscle on the left side. Submandibular pathologic lymph node enlargement is also detected.

and 3). The disease was staged T4aN1M0, grade I. HPV testing with p16 and PCR was negative. The patient underwent mandibular resection with fibula osteocutaneous flap reconstruction with concomitant neck dissection, performed at levels Ia-IV. The patient was tracheostomized, and a PEG tube was inserted. A subsequent postoperative chemoradiotherapy to the tumor area to 65 Gy with a simultaneous 63 Gy to the neck metastases and up to 48 Gy to the uninvolved neck area in 2 Gy fractions was administered. Up to two weekly doses of concurrent chemotherapy with 50% reduced dose of cisplatin were administered. However, both doses inflicted major side effects with grade III mucositis, dysphagia, and hair loss, leading to chemotherapy discontinuation. Having completed the radiation treatment regime, the patient is now under follow-up.

3. Discussion

Fanconi anemia is a heterogeneous disease, characterized by hematological aberrations and congenital malformations. The patients are divided into different complementation groups in which the phenotype varies from mild to severe. A majority of FA patients develop bone marrow failure and subsequent pancytopenia within their first decade of life. However, an absence of hematological abnormalities, while rare, does not rule out FA [4, 5].

Generally, hematological abnormalities develop within the first decade of life. Currently, the treatment of choice for bone marrow failure is hematopoietic stem cell transplant (HSCT). The prognosis for HSCT has improved over the last decades, leading to increased numbers of patients surviving into adulthood. Thus, more FA patients also develop malignancies such as head and neck squamous cell carcinoma (HNSCC) [6].

It is estimated that patients affected by FA have a 500- to 1000-fold risk for HNSCC development, compared to the general population [4]. The risk for solid tumors in FA such as HNSCCs rises in early adulthood with a reported median between 20 and 32 years of age [5–7]. Chronic graft versus host disease arising in patients who have received HSCT is considered a major risk factor for HNSCC and is further

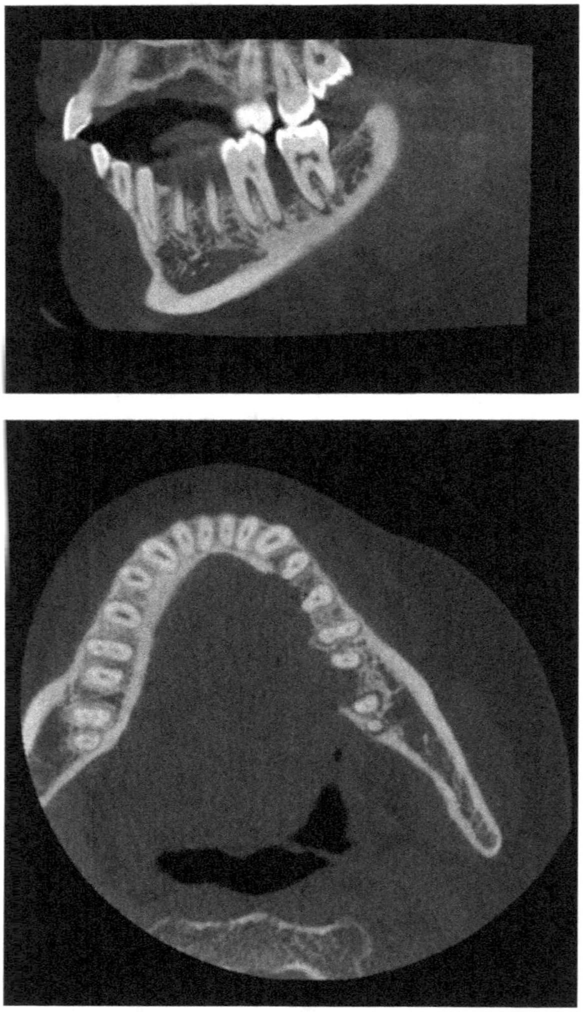

Figure 3: CBCT imaging of the lower jaw. Cortical bone destruction, affecting the lingual cortex that extends from the canine up to the second molar, is shown.

complicated by long-term immunosuppression [6]. Primarily, HNSCC develops in the oral cavity, most commonly the tongue and gingival areas [5, 8]. The diagnosis is typically made late with locoregional lymph node positivity, and HNSCC in FA patients is considered to be aggressive in nature. Additionally, an increased risk for multiple primary malignancies has also been reported [4, 5].

As our case demonstrates, standard treatment modalities for HNSCC are not a straightforward choice for patients with FA. Surgery is the primary therapeutic approach. Large reconstructions, free flaps, and lymph node evacuations are tolerated with comparable morbidity to non-FA patients, whereas chemotherapy (CTx) and radiation therapy (XRT) are complicated due to their high toxicity, driven by the defective DNA repair in FA [9]. FA patients typically develop complications such as severe mucositis, dysphagia, and hematological abnormalities despite experimentally attenuated XRT dosing [7], but small patient cohorts have also reported positive treatment tolerance [10]. Adjuvant therapies must therefore be carefully evaluated in order to avoid severe systemic complications. Therefore, early identification and aggressive surgical management are of the utmost importance in HNSCC treatment in FA, although adjuvant therapies are not categorically contraindicated owing to the poor prognosis of HNSCC in this cohort.

Some reports have shown increased prevalence of oral leukoplakia on FA patients who did not undergo a HSCT [11]. Nevertheless, the literature concerning the prevalence of erytroplakia, leukoplakia, or lichen planus lesions on FA patients is scanty at best, demonstrating an urgent need for further studies on early detection of oral premalignant lesions in these patients [12].

Human papillomavirus (HPV) is a known risk factor of HNSCC. In FA patients, the situation is less clear. Higher HPV prevalence with a broad spectrum of HPV types has been reported for FA patients, and experimental evidence further points toward a potential association between HPV and HNSCC in FA. However, the etiologic connection between HPV and HNSCC in FA remains to be determined [8, 13]. Regardless, HPV vaccination should be recommended for all FA patients.

Recently, Valleuer and coworkers reported the advantages of oral brush biopsy-based cytology to identify oral SCC or its precursor lesions at an early stage. This landmark study included 1233 brush biopsies from an unprecedentedly large cohort of 713 FA patients. They concluded that careful inspection of the oral cavity followed by brush biopsy of suspected lesions detects 63% of SCCs and its precursors at an early stage and negative cytology, especially when combined with DNA ploidy analysis, resulted in a benign course with a high specificity [14]. The benefits of brush biopsies in FA include low cost and minimal invasiveness in addition to potentially excellent sensitivity and specificity. However, the study employed the laboratory and pathologists of an expert cytopathology department, also with rigorously controlled ploidy analysis methodology. Therefore, should other hospitals consider routine oral screening of FA patients, employing adequately experienced cytopathologists and establishing well-controlled laboratory methods are also warranted.

Lastly, owing to the complexity of SCC treatment and the aggressive nature of the disease, we suggest that from early adulthood, patients with Fanconi anemia undergo a biannual screening of the oral cavity. We consider regular oral examinations, optimally performed by a specialist in oral diagnosis in an office properly equipped for oral examination, the only effective method of facilitating early detection of oral premalignancy and carcinoma. All the risk factors for HNSCC should also be addressed, a personalized plan for oral hygiene instructed with motivation for tobacco and alcohol abstinence. HPV vaccination should be recommended. Should a patient present with a leukoplakia or other premalignant mucosal lesions, follow-up examinations should be performed every 6-8 weeks, as stated by Kutler et al. [7] in order to increase survival and minimize morbidity caused by HNSCC for patients with this rare disease [10, 13].

References

[1] RESERVE IU-TDOrphanet: Fanconi anemia https://www.orpha.net/consor/cgi-bin/OC_Exp.php?Expert=84.

[2] A. D. Auerbach, "Fanconi anemia and its diagnosis," *Mutation Research/Fundamental and Molecular Mechanisms of Mutagenesis*, vol. 668, no. 1-2, pp. 4–10, 2009, Epub 2009 Feb 28.

[3] J. M. Amenábar, C. C. Torres-Pereira, K. D. Tang, and C. Punyadeera, "Two enemies, one fight: an update of oral cancer in patients with Fanconi anemia," *Cancer*, vol. 125, no. 22, pp. 3936–3946, 2019.

[4] D. I. Kutler, A. D. Auerbach, J. Satagopan et al., "High incidence of head and neck squamous cell carcinoma in patients with Fanconi anemia," *Archives of Otolaryngology – Head & Neck Surgery*, vol. 129, no. 1, pp. 106–112, 2003.

[5] C. P. Furquim, A. Pivovar, J. M. Amenábar, C. Bonfim, and C. C. Torres-Pereira, "Oral cancer in Fanconi anemia: review of 121 cases," *Critical Reviews in Oncology/Hematology*, vol. 125, pp. 35–40, 2018.

[6] C. Masserot, R. Peffault de Latour, V. Rocha et al., "Head and neck squamous cell carcinoma in 13 patients with Fanconi anemia after hematopoietic stem cell transplantation," *Cancer*, vol. 113, no. 12, pp. 3315–3322, 2008.

[7] D. I. Kutler, K. R. Patel, A. D. Auerbach et al., "Natural history and management of Fanconi anemia patients with head and neck cancer: a 10-year follow-up," *Laryngoscope*, vol. 126, no. 4, pp. 870–879, 2016, Epub 2015 Oct 20.

[8] R. Khoury, S. Sauter, M. Butsch Kovacic et al., "Risk of human papillomavirus infection in cancer-prone individuals: what we know," *Viruses*, vol. 10, no. 1, p. 47, 2018, Published 2018 Jan 20.

[9] A. Beddok, S. Krieger, L. Castera, D. Stoppa-Lyonnet, and J. Thariat, "Management of Fanconi Anemia patients with head and neck carcinoma: Diagnosis and treatment adaptation," *Oral Oncology*, vol. 108, p. 104816, 2020, Epub 2020 May 30.

[10] J. P. Lustig, G. Lugassy, A. Neder, and E. Sigler, "Head and neck carcinoma in Fanconi's anaemia–report of a case and review of the literature," *European Journal of Cancer. Part B, Oral Oncology*, vol. 31, no. 1, pp. 68–72, 1995.

[11] L. Grein Cavalcanti, K. F. Lyko, R. L. Araújo, J. M. Amenábar, C. Bonfim, and C. C. Torres-Pereira, "Oral leukoplakia in patients with Fanconi anaemia without hematopoietic stem cell transplantation," *Pediatric Blood & Cancer*, vol. 62, no. 6, pp. 1024–1026, 2015.

[12] E. Velleuer and R. Dietrich, "Fanconi anemia: young patients at high risk for squamous cell carcinoma," *Molecular and Cellular Pediatrics*, vol. 1, no. 1, p. 9, 2014.

[13] S. L. Sauter, S. I. Wells, X. Zhang et al., "Oral human papillomavirus is common in individuals with Fanconi anemia," *Cancer Epidemiology Biomarkers & Prevention*, vol. 24, no. 5, pp. 864–872, 2015, Epub 2015 Mar 25.

[14] E. Velleuer, R. Dietrich, N. Pomjanski et al., "Diagnostic accuracy of brush biopsy–based cytology for the early detection of oral cancer and precursors in Fanconi anemia," *Cancer Cytopathology*, vol. 128, no. 6, pp. 403–413, 2020, Epub 2020 Feb 5.

A Rare Case of Pyogenic Granuloma in the Tooth Extraction Socket

Yosuke Iijima,[1] Nami Nakayama,[1] Leona Kashimata,[1] Miki Yamada,[1] Ryutaro Kawano,[2] Shunsuke Hino,[1] Takahiro Kaneko,[1] and Norio Horie[1]

[1]*Department of Oral and Maxillofacial Surgery, Saitama Medical Center, Saitama Medical University, Saitama, Japan*
[2]*Department of Pathology, Saitama Medical Center, Saitama Medical University, Saitama, Japan*

Correspondence should be addressed to Yosuke Iijima; yoiijima@saitama-med.ac.jp

Academic Editor: Darko Macan

Pyogenic granuloma (PG) refers to a common, acquired, benign, and vascular tumor that arises in tissues such as the skin and mucous membranes. However, it is extremely rare for PG to arise from an empty socket after tooth extraction. Herein, we describe a rare case of PG that arose from the empty extraction socket of the second molar adjacent to a dentigerous cyst of the left mandibular wisdom tooth in a 57-year-old man. The patient's second molar was extracted during the same procedure in which the wisdom tooth and cyst were removed. Subsequently, at 42 days after surgery, an exophytic mass was found in the socket of the second molar. An excisional biopsy was performed, and the histopathological diagnosis was PG. Since the PG recurred 90 days after the surgery, a complete excision with bone curettage was performed. During the 12 months of follow-up, there has been no recurrence observed. In conclusion, as tooth extraction is a routine dental practice, clinicians should be aware that PGs can also develop from an extraction socket.

1. Introduction

Pyogenic granuloma (PG) refers to a common, acquired, benign, and vascular tumor that arises in tissues such as the skin and mucous membranes [1]. Although PGs were previously thought to be a reactive exaggerated granulomatous product, a recent classification by the International Society for the Study of Vascular Anomalies has classified PG, which is also known as lobular capillary hemangioma, as a benign vascular tumor [2]. In addition, epulis gravidarum, which appears in the gingiva of pregnant women and is well known to both dentists and oral surgeons, has also been included in this new classification of PG. With regard to the etiology of the development of PGs, it has been speculated that there is an association with female sex steroid hormones, in addition to certain kinds of drugs and viruses [3]. However, there are many cases where the etiology remains unclear.

The oral mucosa is a common site for PG, with the most frequent location found to be the gingiva followed by the lower lip and tongue [3]. Oral PG exhibits a solitary, red, sessile, or pedunculated papule that is very friable. The tumor easily bleeds and may be accompanied by surface ulceration [3]. Although PG is usually slow-growing, at times, it can show rapid growth, with large PG becoming lobulated [1, 4]. Histologically, PG consists of highly vascular granulation tissue with a variegated inflammatory infiltrate, but, with maturation, fibrosis is strongly observed [5].

Although the oral mucosa is a common site for PG, it is extremely rare for PG to arise from an extraction socket [6, 7]. In this case report, we present a rare case of PG that arose from a tooth extraction socket of the tooth that was adjacent to a dentigerous cyst, which was extracted at the same time as the removal of the cyst.

2. Case Report

A 57-year-old male was referred to our oral surgery clinic for the evaluation of a radiolucent image of his left mandible. Three weeks prior to being seen in our clinic, he visited a family dentist for the treatment of caries in his right maxillary tooth. At that time, a relatively large left mandibular radiolucent area, which was larger than that previously observed, was found. The patient's past history included hypertension, hemiplegia, dysarthria, and dysphagia. At the time of his initial examination, he was taking amlodipine besilate 2.5 mg/day. Radiographic examination showed impaction of the left mandibular wisdom tooth and a cystic radiolucent area spreading around the crown of the tooth (Figure 1). Oral examination demonstrated that there was no gingival swelling or tenderness in the area corresponding to the cyst and wisdom teeth. The patient's oral hygiene and periodontal status were fair. The clinical diagnosis was a dentigerous cyst of the left mandibular wisdom tooth. As results suggested that further expansion of the cyst was possible, after the consultation with the attending physician, the patient, and his family, a surgical treatment was planned. Under general anesthesia, the wisdom tooth and cyst were removed. The surgical procedure was performed using a triangular flap. This involved an incision from the distobuccal edge of the left first molar, dropping at a slightly oblique angle into the mandibular vestibule. The second incision made was a relieving incision that ran from the ramus to the distobuccal aspect of the first molar [8]. The left second molar was extracted at the same time, as the root apex was contained in the cyst. No abnormal findings were observed in the excision cavity of the cyst, the extracted mandibular second molar, or their extraction sockets. The surgical wound was sutured without complication. The histopathological diagnosis of the specimen was a dentigerous cyst (Figure 2). A follow-up was performed at approximately 1, 3, and 6 weeks after surgery. Around the time of his third follow-up, which was 42 days after his surgery, rapid proliferation of granulomatous tissue was found in the extraction socket of the second molar (Figure 3). However, the patient was not aware of when the mass first initially developed. The examination showed that the mass was slightly reddish, easily bled, was 13 × 8 mm in size, and was pedunculated from the mesial wall of the extraction socket of the second molar. There was no association found between the granulomatous tissue and the wound of the cyst. Due to a concern regarding the possibility of a malignant tumor, an excisional biopsy was performed. Figure 4 shows the excision site one week after the biopsy. A stump of the original mass was seen on the mesial wall of the extraction socket. Histopathologically, the specimen was partially covered by acanthotic squamous cell epithelium with ulceration and composed of granulation tissue with prominent capillary-sized vessels. In addition, there were large amounts of inflammatory infiltrate such as lymphocytes, plasma cells, and leukocytes present. The endothelial cells often had plump cytoplasm with a thick wall (Figure 5). Immunohistochemically, CD34, erythroblast transformation-specific-related gene (ERG), and WT-1 were positive for endothelial cells, with Ki-67 positivity found in approximately 5% of the epithelial cells (Figure 6). The histopathological diagnosis was PG. Although the growth of granulation tissue temporarily subsided, recurrence of the granulation tissue was found on the day of the follow-up, which corresponded to the 90th day after the surgery. As a result, we performed a complete removal with bone curettage, while the patient was under local anesthesia. Histopathological findings of the second specimen were similar to that for the first specimen, with the same diagnosis of PG. During the subsequent 12 months of follow-up, there has been no recurrence observed.

3. Discussion

Descriptions of PG in the extraction socket are extremely rare. Only 4 cases including our current case have been previously reported [6, 7]. Including our current case, all 4 of these cases exhibited a similar clinical presentation with an asymptomatic granulation tissue-like exophytic mass in the extraction socket. It has also been reported that this surface can be ulcerated due to the stimulation caused by occlusion and mastication. The period from tooth extraction to onset was reported to range from 1 to 2 months [6].

Histologically, PG consists of lobular aggregates of capillary-sized vessels, which are lined by plump endothelial cells, with scattered fibroblasts and various amounts of inflammatory infiltrate. Immunohistochemically, although these endothelial cells were positive for vascular markers such as CD31, CD34, factor VIII antigen, and WT-1, they were negative for glucose transporter protein isoform-1 (GLUT-1) [9, 10]. WT-1 is a tumor suppressor gene that plays an important role in regulating hematopoiesis and angiogenesis [9]. Ki-67, which is a proliferation marker, has been reported to exhibit a positive ratio for the Ki-67 labeling index of PG, ranging from 4 to 10% [9]. In the subjects with PG that arose from an empty socket, immunohistochemical staining was performed in one case, with results showing that CD31 was positive. Immunohistochemical staining in our current study also found that there was positive staining for CD34 and WT-1. In addition, ERG, which is essential in endothelial differentiation and angiogenesis, also showed positive staining [11]. The positivity of the Ki-67 labeling index in our current study was approximately 5%.

Etiologically, a history of trauma, hormonal factors, infection, and certain medications have all been suggested to be causes of PG [12–14]. Furthermore, BRAF mutations and potentially herpes virus type 1, Orf virus, and/or human papillomavirus type 2 have also been recently recognized to be an important part of the pathogenesis of PG [1, 15–19].

Although the oral mucosa can easily be affected by trauma, a history of trauma has only been reported in oral lesions in approximately 7% of all cases [9]. In our current case, the occurrence was thought to be related to a concomitant dentigerous cyst, as it occurred after the removal of this cyst. However, our findings strongly suggested that the PG was derived from the adjacent tooth extraction socket, as the base of the pedunculated PG was located on the mesial surface of the second molar extraction socket, which was a long distance from the cyst wound. Although this case occurred in the empty tooth extraction socket and it is known that the periodontal ligament disintegrates and disappears after tooth removal, our findings suggested that it was derived from the adjacent gingival cells rather than the periodontal ligament cells. Regardless, the findings for this case suggested an association with either tooth extraction or

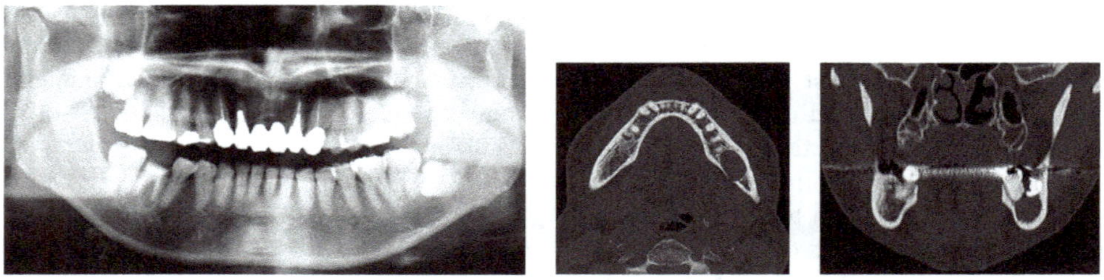

(a) (b) (c)

FIGURE 1: Photoradiograph of the impaction of the left mandibular wisdom tooth and surrounding cystic radiolucent image: (a) orthopantomogram; (b) computed tomography of axial image; (c) computed tomography of sagittal image.

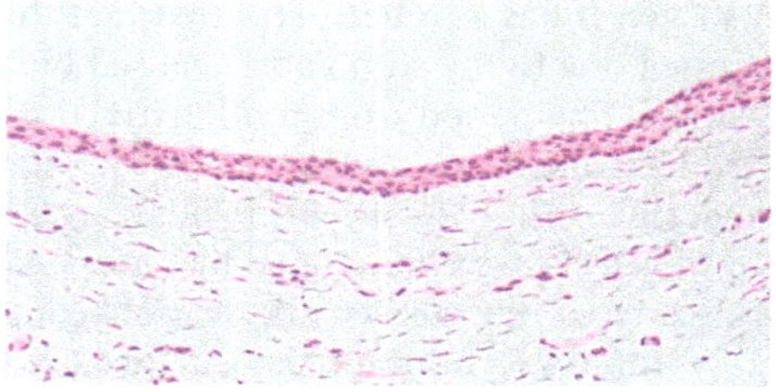

FIGURE 2: Photomicrograph of the dentigerous cyst. The cystic wall, which is covered by flat squamous cell epithelium, is composed of fibrous connective tissue with scarce inflammatory infiltrate (H-E staining, original magnification ×20).

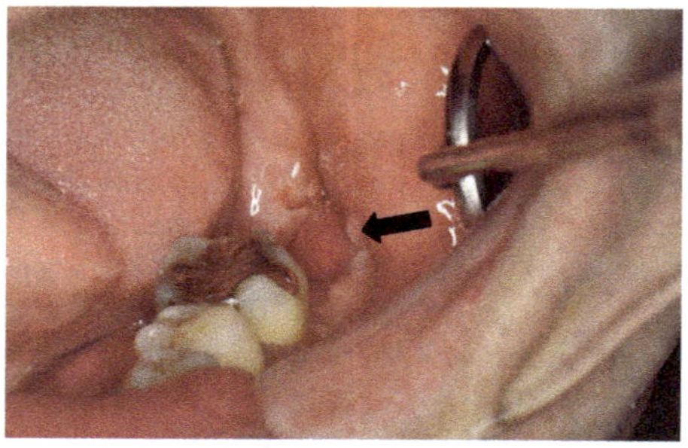

FIGURE 3: Reddish granular tissue that easily bleeds is observed protruding from the mesial wall of the extraction socket of the second mandible (arrow).

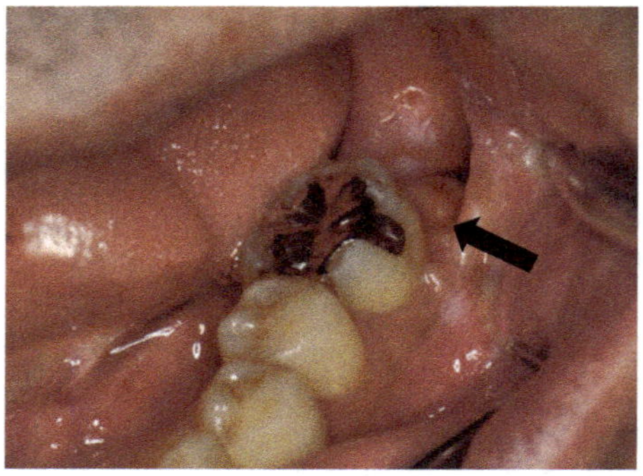

FIGURE 4: The excised site after one week. A stump of the mass can be seen on the mesial wall of the extraction socket (arrow).

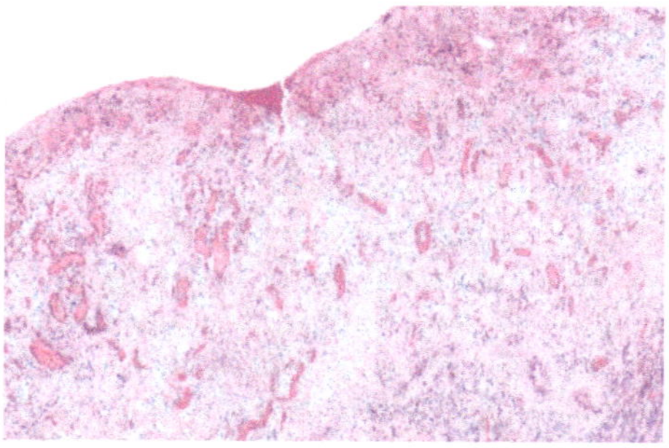

FIGURE 5: Photomicrograph of the mass in the tooth extraction socket. The specimen is partially covered with acanthotic squamous cell epithelium that is composed of granulation tissue with prominent small capillaries and large amounts of inflammatory infiltrate such as lymphocytes, plasma cells, and leukocytes. The endothelial cells often have plump cytoplasm (H-E staining, original magnification ×40).

trauma. Although tooth extraction is a clinically common practice, PGs originating from the extraction socket are very rarely observed during these procedures. The reason for this could possibly be that there are additional cofactors other than trauma. However, the precise reason remains unknown at the present time.

With regard to the effect of hormones on oral lesions, such as epulis gravidarum, it has been suggested that estrogens and other sex hormones can exaggerate the inflammatory responses in gingival tissue, particularly during pregnancy [20]. Medications that may cause PG include anticancer agents such as pyrimidine analogs, taxanes, epidermal growth factor receptor inhibitors, tyrosine kinase inhibitor and BRAF inhibitors, and immunosuppressants such as TNF-alpha antagonists and mTOR inhibitors [1, 21]. In these types of drug-associated cases, it has been reported that PG can occur in multiple sites. Therefore, care must be taken with regard to these drugs, as they have often been used for cancer chemotherapy in recent years.

Bacterial infection has additionally been considered to be a factor that can cause PG. Moreover, it has been suggested that periodontal disease was a factor associated with PG in one PG case that was related to an empty tooth extraction socket. Even so, it has been recently denied that the effects of a bacterial infection are associated with the pathology of PG, as there have yet to be any bacterial strains definitively identified [22]. However, it should be noted that the oral hygiene practice and periodontal status of our patient were fair and not exceedingly poor, respectively.

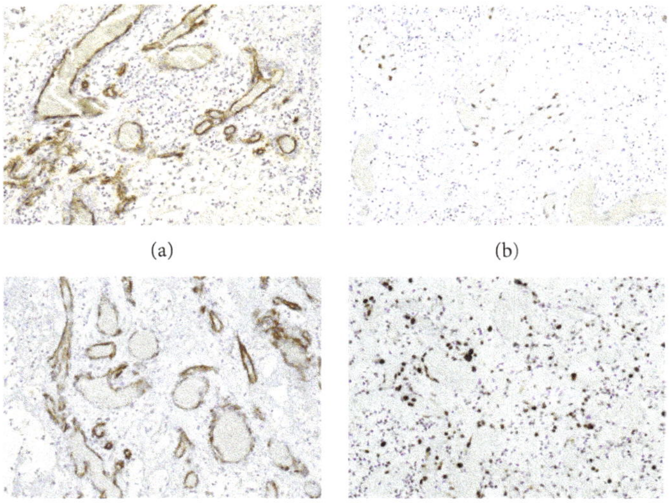

(a) (b) (c) (d)

FIGURE 6: Immunohistochemical staining. The endothelial cells are positive for CD34 (a), ERG (b), and WT-1 (c) (each original magnification ×100). Approximately 5% of the endothelial cells are positive for Ki-67 (d) (original magnification ×100).

Normally, it is uncommon for PGs to spontaneously regress. With regard to the treatment of oral PGs, surgical intervention is the preferred method. However, since PGs can sometimes reoccur, it has been reported that a complete excision of the entire lesion results in the lowest rate of recurrence. In addition, laser treatment may also be useful [6]. Even so, the effectiveness of using a conservative medication therapy has yet to be established. Furthermore, needless to say, there is a chance that epulis gravidarum may regress after the delivery [23].

The differential diagnosis of PG in the oral region includes the presence of a disease showing an exophytic mass-like growth. Thus, malignant tumors initially need to be considered. Moreover, malignant tumors include not only primary cancer but also hematological and metastatic cancers [24]. Benign tumors and inflammatory disease include findings such as peripheral fibroma and giant cell lesions [4]. In the case of maxillary tooth extraction, herniation of a sinonasal polyp is also possible [25]. Thus, a patient's medical history, radiographic examination, and blood tests can all be of assistance in the diagnosis. However, a histopathological search is essential for making a definitive diagnosis. In our current case, the histopathological search also proved to be very effective.

In conclusion, since tooth extractions are a routine dental practice, clinicians need to be aware that PGs can additionally develop from an extraction socket.

References

[1] U. Wollina, D. Langner, K. França, S. Gianfaldoni, T. Lotti, and G. Tchernev, "Pyogenic granuloma - a common benign vascular tumor with variable clinical presentation: new findings and treatment options," *Open access Macedonian journal of medical sciences*, vol. 5, no. 4, pp. 423–426, 2017.

[2] S. E. Mills, P. H. Cooper, and R. E. Fechner, "Lobular capillary hemangioma: the underlying lesion of pyogenic granuloma. A study of 73 cases from the oral and nasal mucous membranes," *The American Journal of Surgical Pathology*, vol. 4, no. 5, pp. 470–479, 1980.

[3] H. Jafarzadeh, M. Sanatkhani, and N. Mohtasham, "Oral pyogenic granuloma: a review," *Journal of Oral Science*, vol. 48, no. 4, pp. 167–175, 2006.

[4] B. D. Lakkam, M. Astekar, S. Alam, G. Sapra, A. Agarwal, and A. M. Agarwal, "Relative frequency of oral focal reactive overgrowths: an institutional retrospective study," *Journal of Oral and Maxillofacial Pathology: JOMFP*, vol. 24, no. 1, pp. 76–80, 2020.

[5] V. Marla, A. Shrestha, K. Goel, and S. Shrestha, "The histopathological spectrum of pyogenic granuloma: a case series," *Case reports in dentistry*, vol. 2016, Article ID 1323798, 2016.

[6] S. Ghadimi, N. Chiniforush, M. Najafi, and S. Amiri, "Excision of epulis granulomatosa with diode laser in 8 years old boy," *Journal of lasers in medical sciences*, vol. 6, no. 2, pp. 92–95, 2015.

[7] R. Leong and G. F. Seng, "Epulis granulomatosa: extraction sequellae," *General Dentistry*, vol. 46, no. 3, pp. 252–255, 1998.

[8] E. Bailey, W. Kashbour, N. Shah, H. V. Worthington, T. F. Renton, and P. Coulthard, "Surgical techniques for the removal of mandibular wisdom teeth," *Cochrane Database of Systematic Reviews*, vol. 7, no. 7, article Cd004345, 2020.

[9] K. Rastogi, L. Singh, N. A. Khan, S. Goyal, A. Khatri, and N. Gupta, "Benign vascular anomalies: a transition from morphological to etiological classification," *Annals of Diagnostic Pathology*, vol. 46, p. 151506, 2020.

[10] M. Seyedmajidi, S. Shafaee, G. Hashemipour, A. Bijani, and H. Ehsani, "Immunohistochemical evaluation of angiogenesis related markers in pyogenic granuloma of gingiva," *Asian Pacific Journal of Cancer Prevention*, vol. 16, no. 17, pp. 7513–7516, 2015.

[11] A. Moh-Moh-Aung, M. Fujisawa, S. Ito et al., "Decreased mi R-200b-3p in cancer cells leads to angiogenesis in HCC by enhancing endothelial ERG expression," *Scientific reports*, vol. 10, no. 1, article 10418, 2020.

[12] R. Krishnapillai, K. Punnoose, P. V. Angadi, and A. Koneru, "Oral pyogenic granuloma–a review of 215 cases in a South

Indian Teaching Hospital, Karnataka, over a period of 20 years," *Oral and Maxillofacial Surgery*, vol. 16, no. 3, pp. 305–309, 2012.

[13] B. M. Piraccini, S. Bellavista, C. Misciali, A. Tosti, D. de Berker, and B. Richert, "Periungual and subungual pyogenic granuloma," *The British Journal of Dermatology*, vol. 163, no. 5, pp. 941–953, 2010.

[14] A. A. Zarrinneshan, P. E. Zapanta, and S. J. Wall, "Nasal pyogenic granuloma," *Otolaryngology and Head and Neck Surgery*, vol. 136, no. 1, pp. 130-131, 2007.

[15] D. Biyik Ozkaya, B. Taskın, B. Tas et al., "Poxvirus-induced angiogenesis after a thermal burn," *The Journal of Dermatology*, vol. 41, no. 9, pp. 830–833, 2014.

[16] L. El Hayderi, A. Rübben, and A. F. Nikkels, "The alpha-herpesviridae in dermatology: herpes simplex virus types I and II. German version," *Hautarzt*, vol. 68, no. 3, pp. 181–186, 2017.

[17] L. Groesser, E. Peterhof, M. Evert, M. Landthaler, M. Berneburg, and C. Hafner, "_BRAF_ and _RAS_ mutations in sporadic and secondary pyogenic granuloma," *The Journal of Investigative Dermatology*, vol. 136, no. 2, pp. 481–486, 2016.

[18] M. Ran, M. Lee, J. Gong, Z. Lin, and R. Li, "Oral acyclovir and intralesional interferon injections for treatment of giant pyogenic granuloma-like lesions in an immunocompromised patient with human Orf," *JAMA Dermatology*, vol. 151, no. 9, pp. 1032–1034, 2015.

[19] O. T. Vázquez-Martínez, A. González-Betancourt, M. C. Barboza-Cerda et al., "Human papillomavirus type 2 associated with pyogenic granuloma in patients without clinical evidence of warts," *International Journal of Dermatology*, vol. 55, no. 7, pp. 745–750, 2016.

[20] A. Hugoson, "Gingival inflammation and female sex hormones. A clinical investigation of pregnant women and experimental studies in dogs," *Journal of Periodontal Research. Supplement*, vol. 5, pp. 1–18, 1970.

[21] X. Roussel, R. Charollais, E. Deconinck, E. Daguindau, and A. Brion, "Pyogenic granuloma during ibrutinib therapy for B-cell neoplasia," *JCO Oncology Practice*, vol. 16, no. 12, pp. 834–836, 2020.

[22] A. Mariotti and M. Mawhinney, "Endocrinology of sex steroid hormones and cell dynamics in the periodontium," *Periodontology 2000*, vol. 61, no. 1, pp. 69–88, 2013.

[23] S. Løes and K. Tornes, "Misinterpretation of histopathological results as an important risk factor for unneeded surgery - case report of a "near miss" event in a pregnant woman," *Patient Safety in Surgery*, vol. 2, no. 1, p. 14, 2008.

[24] A. Fasanmade, M. Pring, J. Pawade, P. Guest, and C. Bell, "Rapidly progressing mass of anterior mandible following a dental extraction," *Oral Surgery, Oral Medicine, Oral Pathology, Oral Radiology, and Endodontics*, vol. 109, no. 3, pp. 330–334, 2010.

[25] J. L. Prasad, T. J. Robbins, R. J. Vargo, M. Sosovicka, and K. F. Summersgill, "Intraoral herniation of a sinonasal polyp: an underreported complication of maxillary extraction?," *Journal of Oral and Maxillofacial Surgery*, vol. 78, no. 11, pp. 1909–1918, 2020.

27

Minimally Invasive Resin-Bonded Inlay-Retained Cantilever Fixed Dental Prosthesis: A Clinical Report

Albandari Bin-Rubayan[1], **Abdulaziz Samran**[2,3] **and Ali Alqerban**[4,5]

[1]*Ministry of Health (SCFHS), Prosthodontics Program (Training Center: Department of Restorative and Prosthetic Dental Sciences, College of Dentistry, Dar Al Uloom University), Riyadh, Saudi Arabia*
[2]*Department of Restorative and Prosthetic Dental Sciences, School of Dentistry, Dar Al-Uloom University, Riyadh, Saudi Arabia*
[3]*Department of Prosthodontics, School of Dentistry, Ibb University, Yemen*
[4]*Department of Preventive Dental Sciences, College of Dentistry, Prince Sattam Bin Abdulaziz University, Alkharj, Saudi Arabia*
[5]*Department of Preventive Dental Science, Dar Al Uloom University, Riyadh, Saudi Arabia*

Correspondence should be addressed to Abdulaziz Samran; asamran@dau.edu.sa

Academic Editor: Asja Celebic

This clinical report demonstrates the treatment of a healthy adult patient referred for prosthodontic treatment after orthodontic treatment with a resin-bonded inlay-retained cantilever fixed dental prosthesis (IRCFDP). The purpose of this report was to demonstrate the esthetic, functional, and conservative properties of a resin-bonded IRCFDP fabricated from monolithic zirconia which can be placed in posterior area in certain situations. Acceptable esthetics with a conservative and functional result were achieved by using a resin-bonded inlay-retained cantilever fixed dental prosthesis (IRCFDP). All laboratory and clinical procedures of this case report are described.

1. Introduction

Replacement of missing teeth area can be accomplished with resin-bonded fixed dental prostheses (FDPs), conventional fixed dental prostheses (FDPs), implant-supported FDPs, or removable dentures. Conventional FDPs typically require the removal of 50% to 70% of sound dental tissue [1, 2] which has been reported to lead to damage tooth vitality in 10% of the FDPs [3, 4]. For that reason, these options are indicated when the adjacent teeth are extensively restored or damaged. Tooth structure can be preserved with adhesively placed resin-bonded FDPs.

Metal resin-bonded fixed dental prostheses (RBFDPs) have been recommended as a conservative option to conventional FDPs [5–8]. However, when a 2-retainer design is used, debonding of one abutment often results in caries that is not perceived by the patient. Ceramic anterior RBFDPs were first described in the 1990s and have been used to replace posterior teeth in certain situations [9]. Ceramic cantilever RBFDPs were suggested by Kern et al. [10] since their clinical study of ceramic RBFDPs with two retainers exhibited high fracture rates within the first year after insertion. The cantilever design leads to reduced shear and tensile forces compared with splinting two abutments teeth with differential movement [11]. In addition, when cantilever RBFDPs debond, the patient will immediately notice [12]. In a report of 10-year follow-up study, the survival rate of cantilever ceramic RBFDPs was 98.2% [13], which was better than that of two-retainer RBFDPs [14]. A zirconia inlay-retained fixed dental prosthesis (IRFDP) design was suggested by Wolfart and Kern [15], and Bishtia et al. [16] tested a new design for inlay-retained cantilever fixed dental prostheses (IRCFDPs) in an in vitro study. This design represents a conservative solution which can be applied in some patients, such as those with existing restorations or caries and when an implant-supported prosthesis is contraindicated. The aim of this clinical report was to describe the replacement of a missing mandibular right first molar with a computer-aided design and computer-aided manufacture (CAD-CAM) resin-bonded IRCFDP made of zirconia ceramic.

2. Case Report

A healthy 42-year-old man visited the Department of Prosthodontics of Dar Aluloom University seeking a replacement for his missing mandibular right first molar which had been extracted several years ago after unsuccessful endodontic treatment (Figure 1). His dental history also included orthodontic treatment for about two years to correct malocclusion (crowding in some areas and spacing in other areas because of his missing four first molars). The orthodontist referred him to the prosthodontic clinic to restore the narrow space in the mandibular right first molar area, which had not been closed by the orthodontic treatment. The clinical investigation revealed a narrow mandibular first molar space that contraindicated for implant placement (Figure 2). In addition, the mandibular right second molar had an occlusal amalgam restoration with occlusal recurrent caries (Figure 3). The majority of teeth were vital, and the oral hygiene was good. A periapical radiograph revealed a deep existing amalgam restoration in the mandibular right second molar, with no periapical abscesses or other significant findings. After making primary impressions for diagnostic casts and consultation with other specialists, a treatment plan was formulated to replace the missing tooth with a minimally invasive resin-bonded IRCFDP [17]. The patient was informed about the risk of the proposed treatment and its alternatives, including a conventional cantilever FDP and IRFDP. After rubber dam placement, the existing amalgam restoration on the second right molar and the caries were removed, providing a cavity for the inlay retainer, which followed the preparation principles for ceramic inlay restorations [18]. The inlay cavity was prepared without bevels with fine-grit diamond rotary instruments by removing sharp margins, smoothing the pulpal floor, and preparing two retainer-wings buccally and lingually. The enamel surface was reduced by approximately 0.5 mm to provide a 3 × 4 mm enamel area for bonding (Figure 4). The reduction was parallel to the path of insertion of the inlay retainer. After abutment preparation, polyvinyl siloxane impression material was used for the final impression (Take 1 Advanced; Kerr Corp) in a stock tray and poured with Type IV dental stone (Fujirock; GC Corp). The stone cast was scanned with a laboratory scanner. The resin-bonded IRCFDP was designed as an inlay retainer with buccal and lingual retainer wings and a second premolar pontic and milled from an A2 zirconia shade block (Cercon HT Full Contour Zirconia; Dentsply Sirona) (Figures 5 and 6).

After sintering, the framework was seated on the cast after minor corrections, and then, the marginal fit and internal fit were checked intraorally using an explorer and a silicone indicator paste (Fit Checker, GC Corp). The silicone indicator paste exhibited a homogeneous and thin thickness which was accepted. For the inlay retainer, the minimum thickness was 3 mm, and for the buccal and lingual retainer wings, it was 0.7 mm. The dimensions for the proximal connector were approximately 4 mm in height and 4 mm in width. After try-in stage (Figure 7) and to remove the residues of the saliva and blood, the bonding surface of resin-bonded IRCFDP was cleaned using hot water steamer. Then, the bonding surface of the inlay retainer and the buccal and lingual retainer wings were airborne-particle abraded with 50 μm Al_2O_3 for 10 seconds with 0.1 MPa pressure [19]. After that, the prosthesis was ultrasonically cleaned for

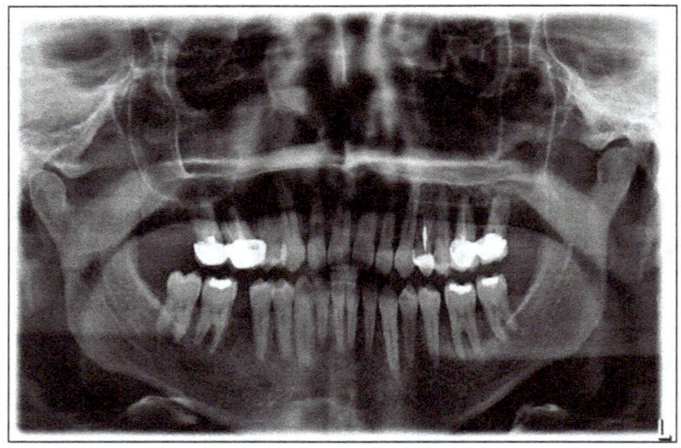

FIGURE 1: Pretreatment panoramic radiograph of initial patient presentation.

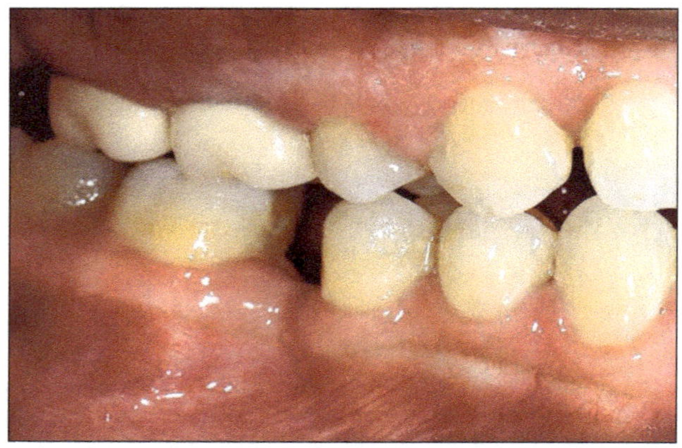

FIGURE 2: Pretreatment lateral view of mandibular arch.

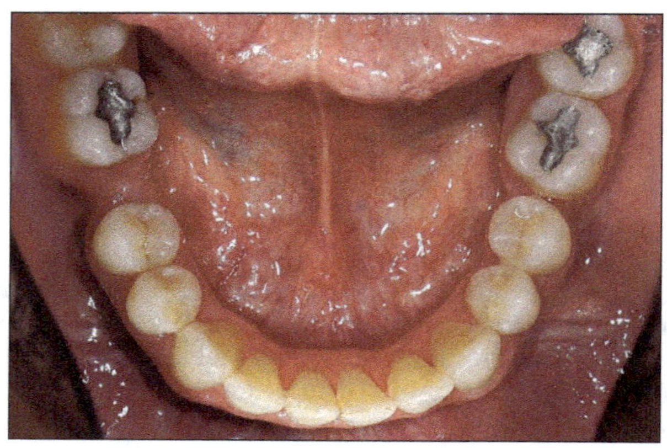

FIGURE 3: Pretreatment occlusal view of mandibular arch.

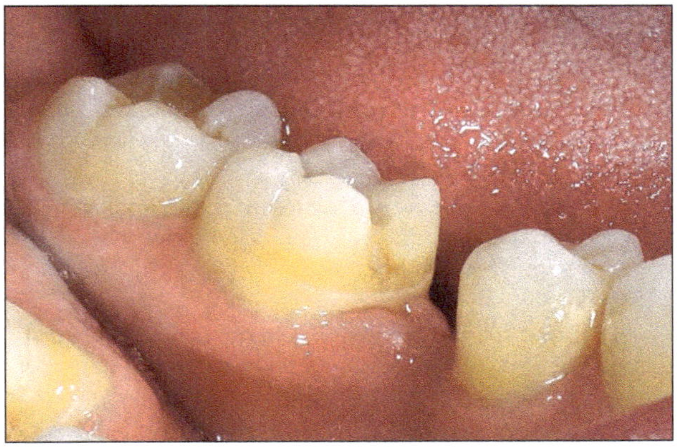

FIGURE 4: The mandibular right second molar after preparation.

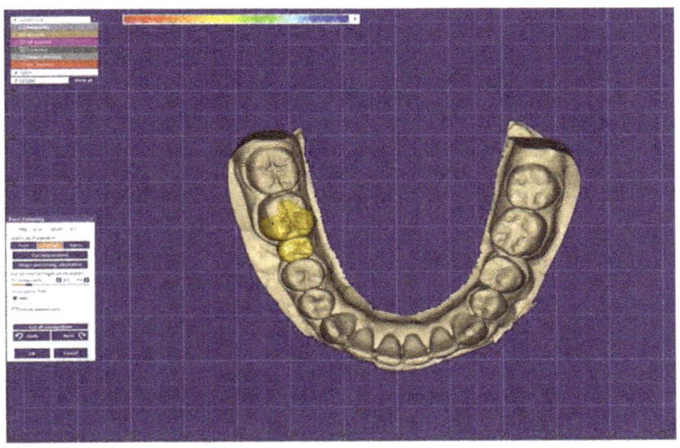

FIGURE 5: Computer-aided designed framework (occlusal view).

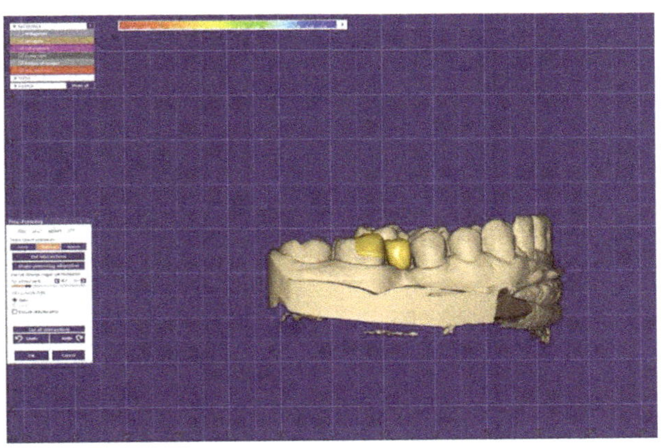

FIGURE 6: Computer-aided designed framework (buccal view).

3 minutes in alcohol path to remove the abrasive residues. Consequently, the resin-bonded IRCFDP was stored in a special container while the preparation surfaces of the abutment tooth are cleaned and treated for the next cementation process.

A rubber dam was applied during adhesive cementation, and the abutment tooth was cleaned with pumice. Then, the preparation surfaces of the abutment tooth were etched with a 37% phosphoric acid gel (Cica; Promedica) for 15-30 sec (according to the tooth structure; dentin or enamel). Then, the acid etch gel was sprayed off with water for 15 sec, and

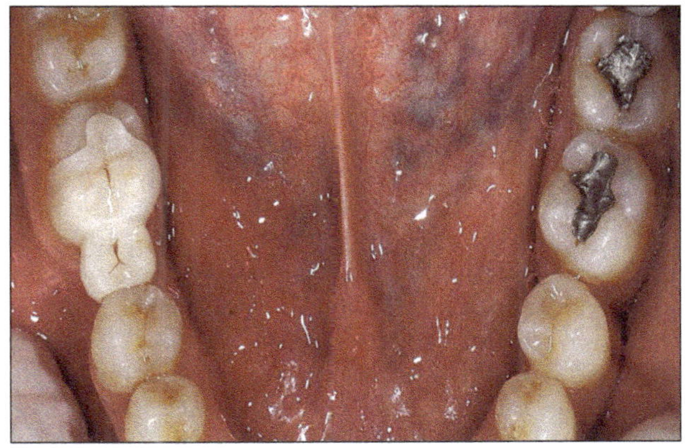

FIGURE 7: Evaluation of resin-bonded inlay-retained cantilever fixed dental prosthesis before cementation.

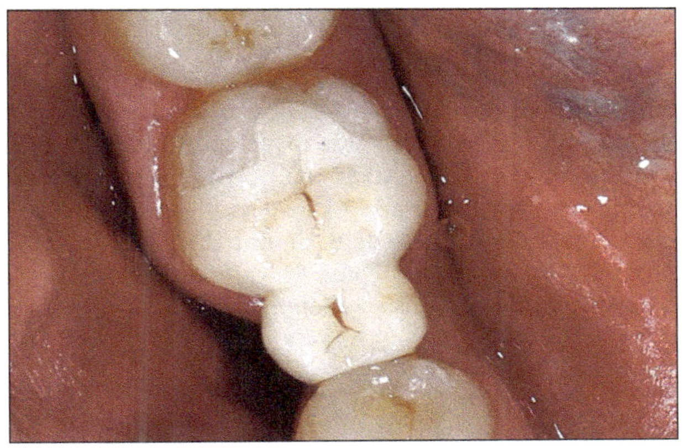

FIGURE 8: Occlusal view of resin-bonded inlay-retained cantilever fixed dental prosthesis immediately after insertion.

the tooth was thoroughly dried with air stream. After that, the enamel and dentin walls were conditioned with corresponding primer (Compobond LCM Primer; Promedica) which was mixed according to manufacturer's instructions and applied for 30 seconds before dispersing the excess using gentle oil-free air stream. Then, the adhesive material (Compobond LCM Adhesive; Promedica) was mixed according to manufacturer's instructions and applied for 15 seconds before removing the excess using gentle oil-free air stream and light cured for 15 sec. Finally, bonding surfaces of the prosthesis were primed with a ceramic primer (Aureocem DC Ceramic Primer; Promedica) using a microbrush. The primer was left for 60 s, and the excesses were removed with an oil-free air stream. After that, the cement (Aureocem DC Automix, Promedica) was distributed over the resin-bonded IRCFDP bonding surfaces, and the prosthesis was seated in place (Figure 8). Steady finger pressure was applied during the setting time. After cementation, the function and occlusion were checked using articulator papers.

3. Discussion

This clinical report describes replacing the narrow space of a missing mandibular right molar with an esthetic and conservative resin-bonded IRCFDP fabricated from monolithic zirconia. The esthetics of this zirconia resin-bonded IRCFDP were excellent, better than the metal-ceramic FDP. Although this technique has been recommended only as an interim technique of replacing of missing teeth, however, its conservative preparation, esthetic, and reported survival rate suggest that it may be considered as a definitive treatment choice in certain situations [6, 13, 20–22]. The framework of the current resin-bonded IRCFDP was made of monolithic zirconia material based on laboratory studies that reported higher fracture load for zirconia-based IRFDPs than those made from lithium disilicate ceramic [23–25]. This resin-bonded IRCFDP design was developed to overcome the high failure rate of previous IRFDP designs which might not be recommended for clinical indications [26–28]. The presence of wings in this design reduced stress on the inlay retainer caused by torsion forces applied nonaxially and to increase the enamel surface area for bonding. Similar retainer wings have been used in previous studies with cantilevered ceramic resin-bonded FDPs [20, 29].

Disadvantages of this design included the poor color match of the resin-bonded IRCFDP to the adjacent natural teeth because the prosthesis was made completely of monolithic zirconia (Figure 6). Additionally, the wings were somewhat bulky which added approximately 0.1 to 0.2 mm to the tooth contour. A suggested minimum thickness of 0.6 to 0.7 mm was used for the zirconia wings, and the tooth preparation was minimal in this area (approximately 0.5 mm) [17].

4. Conclusion

An esthetic and conservative approach to replacing the narrow space of a missing posterior molar with a resin-bonded IRCFDP fabricated from monolithic zirconia was described. After a conservative tooth preparation, a resin-bonded IRCFDP with buccal and lingual wings was fabricated from monolithic zirconia. The patient was so satisfied and pleased with the aesthetics and functional results. This treatment option helped maintain the abutment and the adjacent teeth. Clinical follow-up is important to determine the success rate of this type of prosthesis.

Acknowledgments

The authors would like to thank the Deanship of Graduate Studies and Research in Dar Aluloom University for its support.

References

[1] D. Edelhoff and J. A. Sorensen, "Tooth structure removal associated with various preparation designs for posterior teeth," *The International Journal of Periodontics & Restorative Dentistry*, vol. 22, no. 3, pp. 241–249, 2002.

[2] D. Edelhoff and J. A. Sorensen, "Tooth structure removal associated with various preparation designs for anterior teeth," *The Journal of Prosthetic Dentistry*, vol. 87, no. 5, pp. 503–509, 2002.

[3] K. Langeland, "Dentin and pulp reactions to cavity and crown preparation. Survey of literature," *Annual Meeting - American Institute of Oral Biology*, vol. 23, pp. 73–88, 1966.

[4] K. Langeland and L. K. Langeland, "Pulp reactions to cavity and crown preparation," *Australian Dental Journal*, vol. 15, no. 4, pp. 261–276, 1970.

[5] A. L. Rochette, "Attachment of a splint to enamel of lower anterior teeth," *The Journal of Prosthetic Dentistry*, vol. 30, no. 4, pp. 418–423, 1973.

[6] M. Wood, M. Kern, V. P. Thompson, and E. Romberg, "Ten-year clinical and microscopic evaluation of resin-bonded restorations," *Quintessence International*, vol. 27, no. 12, pp. 803–807, 1996.

[7] D. F. Howe and G. E. Denehy, "Anterior fixed partial dentures utilizing the acid-etch technique and a cast metal framework," *The Journal of Prosthetic Dentistry*, vol. 37, no. 1, pp. 28–31, 1977.

[8] G. J. Livaditis and V. P. Thompson, "Etched castings: an improved retentive mechanism for resin-bonded retainers," *The Journal of Prosthetic Dentistry*, vol. 47, no. 1, pp. 52–58, 1982.

[9] M. Kern, H. Knode, and J. R. Strubb, "The all-porcelain, resin-bonded bridge," *Quintessence International*, vol. 22, no. 4, pp. 257–262, 1991.

[10] M. Kern and J. R. Strub, "Bonding to alumina ceramic in restorative dentistry: clinical results over up to 5 years," *Journal of Dentistry*, vol. 26, no. 3, pp. 245–249, 1998.

[11] B. Mourshed, A. Samran, A. Alfagih, A. Samran, S. Abdulrab, and M. Kern, "Anterior cantilever resin-bonded fixed dental prostheses: a review of the literature," *Journal of Prosthodontics*, vol. 27, no. 3, pp. 266–275, 2018.

[12] M. Kern and R. Glaser, "Cantilevered all-ceramic, resin-bonded fixed partial dentures: a new treatment modality," *Journal of Esthetic Dentistry*, vol. 9, no. 5, pp. 255–264, 1997.

[13] M. Kern, N. Passia, M. Sasse, and C. Yazigi, "Ten-year outcome of zirconia ceramic cantilever resin-bonded fixed dental prostheses and the influence of the reasons for missing incisors," *Journal of Dentistry*, vol. 65, pp. 51–55, 2017.

[14] A. van Dalen, A. J. Feilzer, and C. J. Kleverlaan, "A literature review of two-unit cantilevered FPDs," *The International Journal of Prosthodontics*, vol. 17, no. 3, pp. 281–284, 2004.

[15] S. Wolfart and M. Kern, "A new design for all-ceramic inlay-retained fixed partial dentures: a report of 2 cases," *Quintessence International*, vol. 37, no. 1, pp. 27–33, 2006.

[16] S. Bishti, C. Jakel, M. Kern, and S. Wolfart, "Influence of different preparation forms on the loading-bearing capacity of zirconia cantilever FDPs. A laboratory study," *Journal of Prosthodontic Research*, vol. 63, no. 3, pp. 347–353, 2019.

[17] M. Kern, *Resin-Bonded Fixed Dental Prostheses: Minimally Invasive–Esthetic–Reliable*, Quintessence Publishing, 2019.

[18] J. B. Summitt, J. W. Robbins, T. J. Hilton, R. S. Schwartz, and J. Dos Santos Jr., "Esthetic Inlays and Onlays," in *Fundamentals of operative dentistry A contemporary approach*, pp. 514–528, Quintessence Publishing Co, 2006.

[19] S. M. Wegner, W. Gerdes, and M. Kern, "Effect of different artificial aging conditions on ceramic-composite bond strength," *The International Journal of Prosthodontics*, vol. 15, no. 3, pp. 267–272, 2002.

[20] M. Kern, "Single-retainer resin-bonded fixed dental prostheses as an alternative to orthodontic space closure (and to single-tooth implants)," *Quintessence International*, vol. 49, no. 10, pp. 789–798, 2018.

[21] M. Kern, "Fifteen-year survival of anterior all-ceramic cantilever resin-bonded fixed dental prostheses," *Journal of Dentistry*, vol. 56, pp. 133–135, 2017.

[22] M. Kern and M. Sasse, "Ten-year survival of anterior all-ceramic resin-bonded fixed dental prostheses," *The Journal of Adhesive Dentistry*, vol. 13, no. 5, pp. 407–410, 2011.

[23] M. A. Kilicarslan, P. S. Kedici, H. C. Kucukesmen, and B. C. Uludag, "In vitro fracture resistance of posterior metal-ceramic and all-ceramic inlay- retained resin-bonded fixed partial dentures," *The Journal of Prosthetic Dentistry*, vol. 92, no. 4, pp. 365–370, 2004.

[24] C. A. Mohsen, "Fracture resistance of three ceramic inlay-retained fixed partial denture designs. An in vitro comparative study," *Journal of Prosthodontics*, vol. 19, no. 7, pp. 531–535, 2010.

[25] S. Wolfart, K. Ludwig, A. Uphaus, and M. Kern, "Fracture strength of all-ceramic posterior inlay-retained fixed partial dentures," *Dental Materials*, vol. 23, no. 12, pp. 1513–1520, 2007.

[26] D. Edelhoff, H. Spiekermann, and M. Yildirim, "Metal-free inlay-retained fixed partial dentures," *Quintessence International*, vol. 32, no. 4, pp. 269–281, 2001.

[27] S. Harder, S. Wolfart, S. Eschbach, and M. Kern, "Eight-year outcome of posterior inlay-retained all-ceramic fixed dental prostheses," *Journal of Dentistry*, vol. 38, no. 11, pp. 875–881, 2010.

[28] S. Wolfart, F. Bohlsen, S. M. Wegner, and M. Kern, "A preliminary prospective evaluation of all-ceramic crown-retained and inlay-retained fixed partial dentures," *The International Journal of Prosthodontics*, vol. 18, no. 6, pp. 497–505, 2005.

[29] M. Kern, "Clinical long-term survival of two-retainer and single-retainer all-ceramic resin-bonded fixed partial dentures," *Quintessence International*, vol. 36, no. 2, pp. 141–147, 2005.

28

Delayed Diagnosis of Unilateral Mandibular Condylar Fracture in a Posterior Edentulous Patient

Sahani Anupama and Pilana Vithanage Kalani Shihanika Hettiarachchi

Department of Oral Medicine and Periodontology, Faculty of Dental Sciences, University of Peradeniya, Sri Lanka

Correspondence should be addressed to Pilana Vithanage Kalani Shihanika Hettiarachchi; kalaniz2004@yahoo.com

Academic Editor: Giuseppe Alessandro Scardina

Background. Fractures of the mandible are common in elderly patients, and among them, condylar fractures are the most frequent type. A change in occlusion is the most common physical finding in patients with fractures of the mandible. Therefore, it is challenging to identify mandibular fractures in posterior edentulous patients due to the lack of posterior occlusal contacts. It is crucial to do radiological investigations in such patients to exclude fractures. *Case Presentation.* This article describes a case of delayed diagnosis of a unilateral mandibular condylar fracture for a week's duration and treating the condition as temporomandibular pathology in a posterior edentulous, 52-year-old patient. *Conclusion.* This clinical case highlights the importance of radiological investigations and occlusal analysis for early diagnosis of condylar fractures, particularly in posterior edentulous patients, lacking posterior occlusal contacts.

1. Introduction

Among facial bone fractures, mandible fracture has the highest incidence next to nasal bone fractures [1]. Out of mandibular fractures, condylar fractures are the most frequent accounting for between 29% and 52% of all mandibular fractures [2]. Binding of the mandibular ramus with high stiffness and mandibular condyle head with low stiffness can be considered the reason for the high incidence of mandibular condylar fractures [1].

The main causative factor for maxillofacial fractures including condylar fractures is road traffic accidents, violence, industrial hazards, falls, and sports accidents. Falls are the main etiology for maxillofacial trauma in children and geriatric patients, and falls are mostly responsible for mandible fractures in the latter group [3, 4].

Condylar fractures are most commonly missed on clinical examination. Therefore, condyle fractures are diagnosed with the help of both clinical and radiological assessment [5]. Clinical signs such as jaw deviation, mouth opening limitation, malocclusion, and edema of the preauricular region can be indicative of fractures of the condylar process [6]. A change in occlusion is the most common physical finding in patients with fractures of the mandible including condylar fractures [5]. But it is difficult to rely on this feature in patients who lack posterior occlusal contacts due to posterior edentulousness. Therefore, in these kinds of patients, we need to rely on radiographic evaluation to exclude condylar fractures.

Nogami et al. found that the incidence of fracture in the condylar region was significantly lower in patients with contacted molars in the maxilla and mandible as compared to affected patients with noncontact molars and suggested that contacted molars in the maxilla and mandible have an influence on condyle fractures in elderly individuals [4].

A mandibular condyle fracture may cause long-term complications such as mandibular growth and functional disorders and chronic temporomandibular joint (TMJ) complications such as TMJ ankylosis especially in children [1]. Therefore, to prevent these complications, early recognition and management of condylar fracture are paramount. This report describes the case of delayed diagnosis of a unilateral condylar fracture in a posterior edentulous 52-year-old

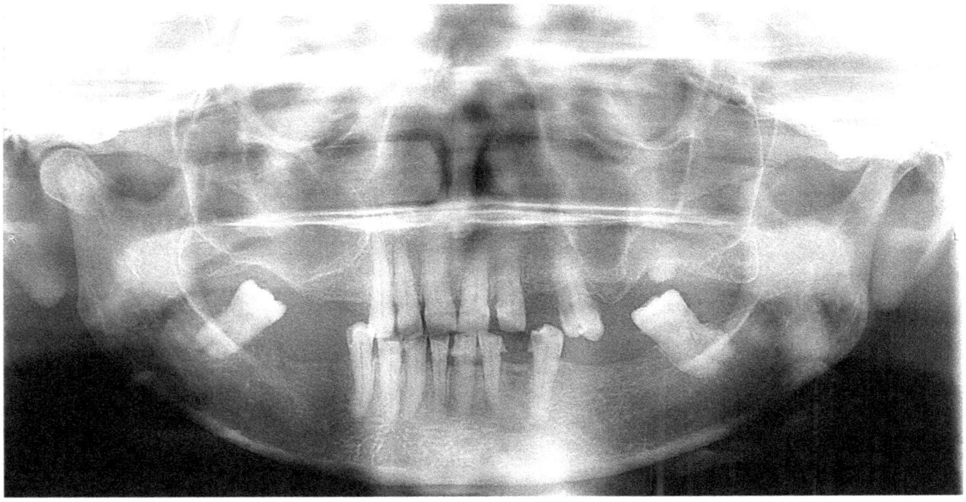

FIGURE 1: Panoramic radiograph demonstrating the condylar fracture on the right side.

patient, highlighting the importance of initial radiological examination in such cases.

2. Case History

A 52-year-old female patient was presented to the Oral Medicine Clinic of Dental Teaching Hospital, Peradeniya, with chief complaint of pain on the right-side TMJ region for 1-week duration. Patient had a history of fall a month ago due to an epileptic attack and hitting an object in the right-side TMJ region during the fall. The patient had presented to a local hospital initially and was treated with a course of analgesics which had been ineffectual; therefore, the patient sought medical advice from a specialist centre. Past medical history revealed that the patient was under antiepileptic medication for epilepsy for 30 years. She had no known allergies.

Examination revealed tenderness of the right-side TMJ region and slight restriction of mouth opening. No deviation of the mandible was observed. Intraoral examination showed that the patient was partially edentulous and had no posterior occlusal contacts. Out of the molar teeth, only 37 and 47 were present. Laceration or hematoma was not observed on the mucosa. No other significant findings were observed in the oral cavity.

Based on the clinical picture, TMJ disorder was suspected at the outpatient department. Therefore, the patient was initially treated with analgesics, muscle relaxants, and heat fermentation of the said region. Also, advice was given on self-care and to take a soft diet, and a review appointment was scheduled after a week. However, as the patient was symptomatic and there was no improvement of the condition, she has sought treatment from our clinic, where she was investigated with a panoramic radiographic examination. This revealed a fracture of the right-side condylar neck (Figure 1). The patient was referred immediately to the oral and maxillofacial unit for further management.

3. Discussion

Fractures of the mandible occur with a greater frequency in the elderly, and fractures of the condylar process of mandible are common injuries that account for 20-62% of all mandibular fractures [6]. The incidence of mandibular condylar fractures is higher in males compared to females [2, 4]. On the contrary, in the present case, the patient was a female.

The etiology for the condylar fracture documented in this case mirrors the existing literature in which accidental falls were the commonest cause [3, 4]. Also, the etiology of mandibular fractures is different between males and females; females had a higher incidence of mandibular fractures due to falls while males had a higher incidence due to road traffic accidents [7]. This fact was evident in the present case where the patient was female and had an accidental fall due to an epileptic attack.

Studies suggest that patients with epilepsy treated with antiepileptic drugs may be at an increased risk for bone disease including changes in bone turnover, osteoporosis, alterations in bone quality, and most importantly fractures [8]. However, mandible fracture cases have rarely been reported [9]. This case report belongs to that category. It is a widely known fact that epileptic seizures may be associated with fractures and dislocations either owing to the falls associated with the seizure or, indeed, owing to the mechanism of the seizure itself. In this case, it was due to the fall associated with the seizure. In addition, it is well established that antiepileptic drugs increase fracture risk by an average of twofold to sixfold [9]. In the present case, as the patient was on antiepileptic drugs for a long period of time, it can be speculated that this may have been one of the reasons for the fracture to have occurred.

There are many reasons which can contribute to condylar fractures in the elderly. Werning et al. showed that osteoporosis is an independent risk factor for the development of maxillofacial fractures in the elderly [10]. Osteoporosis can be defined as a common metabolic bone disease characterized by low bone mass, microarchitectural weakening leading to bone fragility, and increased fracture risk. Osteoporosis predominantly affects elderly women as the rate of bone loss increases after menopause in women. Women show an estrogen-related bone loss commencing at menopause, mainly in trabecular bone, followed by a slower loss of both trabecular and cortical bones 4–8 years later [11]. It is a known fact that osteoporosis results in reduced jaw bone mass as well as alterations of the mandibular structure, especially of the inferior border [12]. Also, antiepileptic drugs have also been shown to cause osteoporosis and bone fractures in the absence of vitamin D deficiency [9]. Hence, in the present case, the patient may have had osteoporosis as the patient was a postmenopausal women and was using antiepileptic drugs. This may have contributed to the condylar fracture.

Bisphosphonates are the most widely used class of antiresorptive drugs. Bisphosphonate use plays a primary role in the management of metastatic bone diseases as well as osteoporosis. In patients suffering from metastatic bone diseases, bisphosphonates provide significant protection against skeletal complications, in particular against fractures. But one of the serious side effects of bisphosphonates can be considered the bisphosphonate-related osteonecrosis of the jaws (BRONJ). This condition can even lead to pathological fractures of the mandible [13]. But the above factors may not have contributed to the condylar fracture in the current case as the patient was not on bisphosphonates.

Nogami et al. found that incidence of fracture in the condylar region was significantly lower in patients with contacted molars in the maxilla and mandible as compared to affected patients with noncontacted molars and advanced the hypothesis that the presence of contacted molars may work as "a vertical stop" and be a protective element for the condyle [4]. Hasegawa et al. showed that the risk of condylar fractures was significantly higher in patients without occlusal support or mandibular third molars [14]. This was highlighted in this case where the patient had no posterior occlusal contacts as out of all the molars only 37 and 47 were present.

Zhou et al. examined the influence of unerupted mandibular third molars on the incidence of condyle fractures and found a significantly higher incidence of fractures in the condylar region in patients without than in those with unerupted third molars [2]. This case agrees with this finding as the mandibular third molars were absent in this patient.

The patient's history and the clinical examination are helpful in the diagnosis of condylar fractures but radiographs are probably the most important aid as condylar fractures are most commonly missed on clinical examination [5]. This was evident in this case as the diagnosis of condylar fracture was missed at the initial presentation due to the lack of clinical signs, and also, initially, a TMJ disorder was suspected. This was mainly due to the posterior edentulousness of the patient, and as a result, alterations in the occlusion were not evident. Therefore, the authors would like to emphasize the importance of radiological evaluation in such patients at the initial presentation to exclude condylar and/or mandibular fractures.

Routine plain radiological investigations that aid in the diagnosis of condylar fracture include oblique views, posteroanterior view, and Towne's view [5]. Computed tomography (CT) is considered a gold standard for the radiographic evaluation of fractures of the mandibular condyle process. It can be used to evaluate both bony and soft tissue changes, and multiplanar evaluation is an added advantage. However, the routine use of CT for mandibular fractures is not justified due to the high cost and increased radiation exposure [6]. Panoramic radiograph is the most comprehensive view possible with a single film and provides good visualization of the entire mandible including the condylar region; therefore, it is commonly used by many clinicians as an ideal screening view for mandibular fractures [5, 6]. In the present case as well, panoramic radiograph was used as the radiological diagnostic aid in which the condylar fracture was identified.

Complications of mandibular condylar fractures includes nonunion, malunion, malocclusion, TMJ derangement, traumatic arteritis, ankylosis of TMJ, condyle resorption, growth disorders mainly in young patients, and facial asymmetry [1]. To prevent these, it is important that the condylar fractures are diagnosed and managed early.

4. Conclusion

Although condylar fractures are common in elderly patients, they are frequently overlooked by the clinicians. In the geriatric population, the dental elements tend to decrease in number, and posterior edentulousness is a common presentation among them. In such patients presenting with pain in the TMJ region, it is eminent to not only rely on clinical features but also carry out radiological evaluation to exclude condylar fractures and/or mandibular fractures at the initial presentation itself. This will aid in early identification and management of condylar fractures, preventing the possible complications.

Consent

Written informed consent was obtained from the patient for publication of this case report and any accompanying images.

Authors' Contributions

PVKSH conceptualized the work, organized the order of events in the patient's management, and interpreted the results. SA helped with the writing of the article. PVKSH and SA performed the review of the literature. All authors agree to be accountable for all aspects of the work. All authors read and approved the final manuscript.

References

[1] K. Y. Choi, J. D. Yang, H. Y. Chung, and B. C. Cho, "Current concepts in the mandibular condyle fracture management part I: overview of condylar fracture," *Archives of Plastic Surgery*, vol. 39, no. 4, pp. 291–300, 2012.

[2] H. H. Zhou, Q. Liu, G. Cheng, and Z. B. Li, "Aetiology, pattern and treatment of mandibular condylar fractures in 549 patients: a 22-year retrospective study," *Journal of Cranio-Maxillo-Facial Surgery*, vol. 41, no. 1, pp. 34–41, 2013.

[3] S. Nogami, K. Yamauchi, G. B. Bottini et al., "Fall-related mandible fractures in a Japanese population: a retrospective study," *Dental Traumatology*, vol. 35, no. 3, pp. 194–198, 2019.

[4] S. Nogami, K. Yamauchi, T. Yamashita et al., "Elderly patients with maxillofacial trauma: study of mandibular condyle fractures," *Dental Traumatology*, vol. 31, no. 1, pp. 73–76, 2015.

[5] K. G. Sriraam and K. R. A. Vignesh, "Diagnosis and management of mandibular condyle fractures," in *Oral and Maxillofacial Surgery*, pp. 119–137, Intech Open, 2021.

[6] T. Sidal and D. A. Curtis, "Fractures of the mandible in the aging population," *Special Care in Dentistry*, vol. 26, no. 4, pp. 145–149, 2006.

[7] R. Sawazaki, S. M. Júnior, L. Asprino, R. W. Moreira, and M. De Moraes, "Incidence and patterns of mandibular condyle fractures," *Journal of Oral and Maxillofacial Surgery*, vol. 68, no. 6, pp. 1252–1259, 2010.

[8] J. F. Annegers, L. J. Melton III, C. Sun, and W. A. Hauser, "Risk of age-related fractures in patients with unprovoked seizures," *Epilepsia*, vol. 30, no. 3, pp. 348–355, 1989.

[9] K. Yalcin, S. Celalettin, U. Fatih, M. G. Şenol, and C. Tuncer, "Mandible fractures during epileptic seizure: two case reports," *European Journal of Plastic Surgery*, vol. 32, pp. 253–255, 2009.

[10] J. W. Werning, N. M. Downey, R. A. Brinker et al., "The impact of osteoporosis on patients with maxillofacial trauma," *Archives of Otolaryngology – Head & Neck Surgery*, vol. 130, no. 3, pp. 353–356, 2004.

[11] A. Gulsahi, "Osteoporosis and jawbones in women," *Journal of International Society of Preventive and Community Dentistry*, vol. 5, no. 4, pp. 263–267, 2015.

[12] B. D. Lee and S. C. White, "Age and trabecular features of alveolar bone associated with osteoporosis," *Oral Surgery, Oral Medicine, Oral Pathology, Oral Radiology, and Endodontics*, vol. 100, no. 1, pp. 92–98, 2005.

[13] S. Otto, C. Pautke, S. Hafner et al., "Pathologic fractures in bisphosphonate-related osteonecrosis of the jaw-review of the literature and review of our own cases," *Craniomaxillofacial Trauma & Reconstruction*, vol. 6, no. 3, pp. 147–154, 2013.

[14] T. Hasegawa, H. Sadakane, M. Kobayashi et al., "A multicentre retrospective study of mandibular fractures: do occlusal support and the mandibular third molar affect mandibular angle and condylar fractures?," *International Journal of Oral and Maxillofacial Surgery*, vol. 45, no. 9, pp. 1095–y1099, 2016.

The First Clinical use of Augmented Reality to Treat Salivary Stones

Anna Lysenko,[1] Alexandra Razumova,[2] Andrey Yaremenko,[2] Rustam Mirzakhmedov,[3] Anna Zubareva,[4] and Marina Chibisova[5]

[1]*Department of Maxillofacial Surgery, Research Institute of Dentistry and Maxillofacial Surgery, Russia*
[2]*Department of Dental Surgery and Maxillofacial Surgery, First Pavlov State Medical University, Russia*
[3]*Create Unique 3D Filters, Russia*
[4]*Department First Pavlov State Medical University, Russia*
[5]*Department of Radiology in Dentistry, Private Educational Institution SPb INSTOM, Private Educational Institution St. Petersburg Institute of Post-Graduate Dentistry, Russia*

Correspondence should be addressed to Alexandra Razumova; alserova@yandex.ru

Academic Editor: Giuseppe Alessandro Scardina

In this study, we report our first experience of applying the concretion visualization method using augmented reality technology. A clinical case of a new surgical intervention on the parotid salivary gland with the localization of salivary stone in its parenchyma is considered. During additional diagnostics, it was found that the size of the concretion exceeds 5 mm which did not allow us to use the endoscopic technologies. That was the reason for the choice of surgical intervention external access using salivary stone visualization with the help of augmented reality. The preoperative procedures included making the upper jaw cast model, fitting the model and individual mouthguard with an X-ray contrast marker and marker slot. In addition to this, computed tomography of the head and neck using a mouthguard was made. During surgery under general anesthesia with nasal intubation, the mouthguard together with the marker is installed in the patient's mouth and the surgeon puts on the glasses to visualize the stone image in place of its localization. This method enables to visualize the salivary stone on all surgery stages no matter what type of approach is used or performing hydropreparation. That is why using the augmented reality appears promising and is to be studied further.

1. Introduction

Salivary stone condition is a polyetiological pathology of the salivary glands. The primary factor of stone formation is still not discovered. That is why the main method to treat salivary stones is to remove the salivary stones or the gland extirpation [1].

Most often a stone is localized in the submandibular salivary glands, rarer in the parotid salivary glands with the incidence reported up to 20% [2]. Surgical intervention in this area can lead to both operative and postoperative complications such as the facial nerve branch damage or formation of fistulous tract. That is why development of new organ preserving methods of salivary stone treatment is an important issue of the contemporary maxillofacial surgery. Using modern methods such as sialoendoscopy is not always available due to the very expensive equipment needed and a specialized training to be performed [3]. Today, the augmented reality technique is steadily implemented in our everyday life and is integrated with the picture of reality not distorting it [4]. In February 2018 in the Almazov National Medical Research Center, a memorandum about establishing a national project called "Digital Healthcare" was signed. It is aimed at implementing and developing digital technologies in the Russian Federation healthcare [5]. That is why it enables us to implement its potential in medicine as well, particularly, in the maxillofacial surgery. The ability to combine the reality and virtual reality with the first one prevailing as well as the total

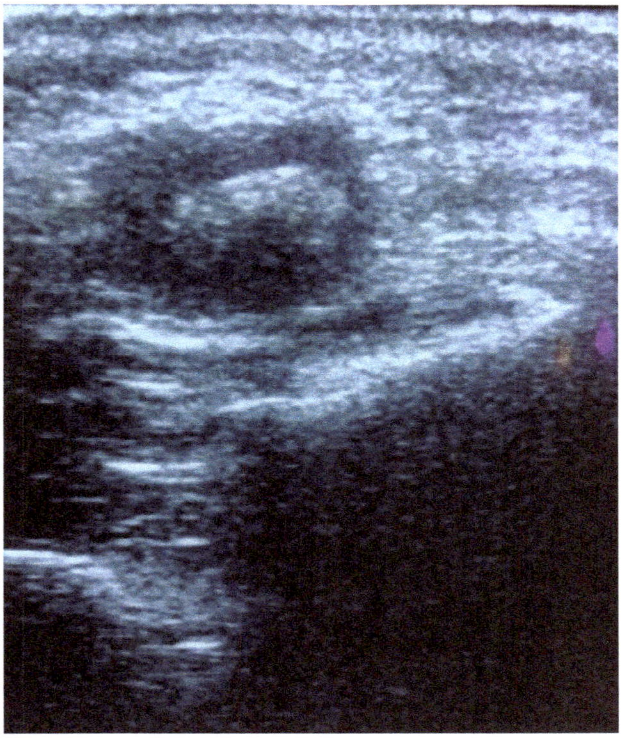

FIGURE 1: Echography of the patient M. left parotid gland showing the hyperechogenic mass with 3×5 mm acoustic shadow.

interactivity of all "artificial" objects and their 3D presentation, the ability to evaluate it from all aspects, and their interaction with the real world allow us to work out the newest surgical method in case of stone removal from the parotid salivary gland parenchyma.

2. Materials and Methods

A female patient M. 33 years old presented on the Oncology Department #8 (Maxillofacial Surgery Department), I.P. Pavlov SPbSMU, with pain and swelling in the preauricular area from the left side, becoming enlarged while eating.

2.1. Past Medical History. The first time the patient noted the pain syndrome and the parotid gland enlargement from the left side was 10 years ago during the meals. During this time, the symptoms resolved spontaneously. A year before the admission to the Oncology Department #8 (Maxillofacial Surgery Department), I.P. Pavlov SPbSMU, the patient had undergone in some other hospital an in-patient ultrasound examination of the salivary glands showing the stone. They performed only intraoral drainage in the Stenonov duct projection with its dissection. Though, after the inflammatory process subsided, the pain and enlargement of the parotid salivary gland did not resolve. The patient presented to the Oncology Department #8 (Maxillofacial Surgery Department), I.P. Pavlov SPbSMU, for surgery arrangement.

2.2. Status Localis. Examination showed hyperplasia of the parotid salivary gland from the left side. The skin of the pre-

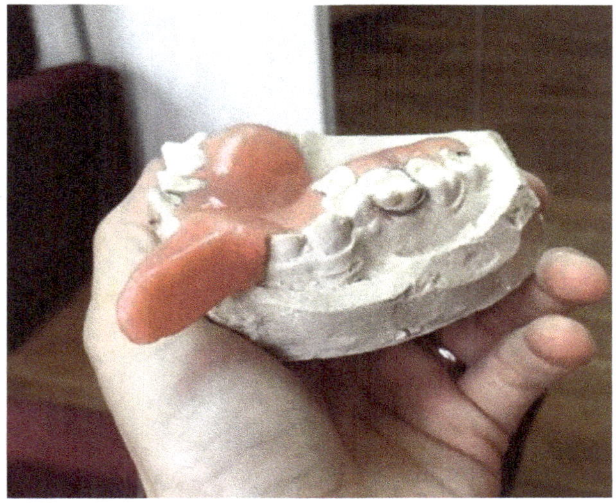

FIGURE 2: Individual occlusal splint with a radiopaque marker.

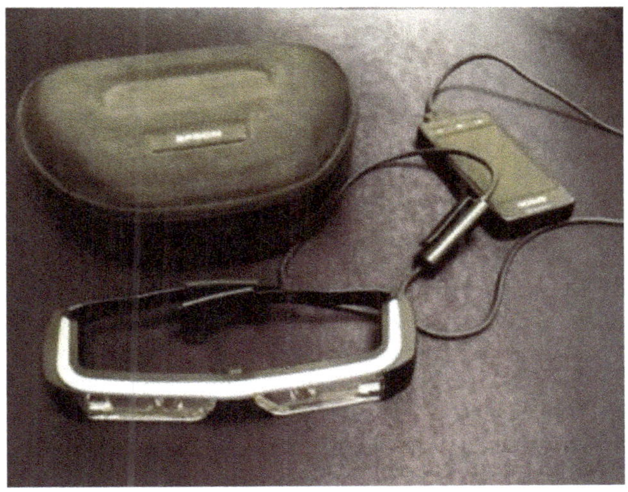

FIGURE 3: Augmented reality glasses (company: Epson Moverio BT-200, eyepieces resolution 960×540 px, weight: 88 g).

auricular masticatory area from the left side is not changed in color. The parotid salivary gland is dense but painless on palpation. While massaging the parotid salivary gland, there is a little amount of pure saliva secreted. The oral cavity is sanitized. The oral mucous membrane is pink, smooth, and shiny. The Stenonov duct opening is slightly deformed; there is a scar changed mucous membrane of the cheek.

After the basic examinations, additional diagnostics were prescribed.

The echography picture during the large salivary gland ultrasound examination showed dilatation of the outflow duct; there, a hyperechogenic mass with 3×5 mm acoustic shadow was visualized (Figure 1).

There were no signs of purulent liquefaction of the parotid salivary gland found. Considering the stone size and scar deformation of the duct as well as its localization, we decided to refuse from removing the stone using a wire basket and sialoendoscope and to apply the method of augmented reality to visualize the salivary stone.

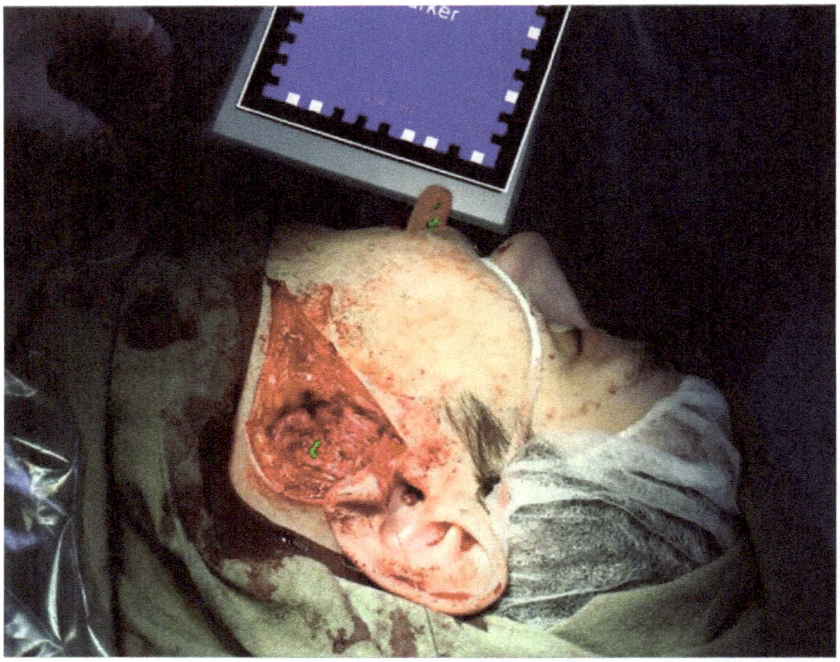

FIGURE 4: Salivary stone removal surgery using augmented reality techniques (the concretion is located in the surface layer of the parotid gland parenchyma).

Preoperatively, the cast model was made, and the individual mouthguard was produced having an X-ray contrast marker with the marker slot (Figure 2).

A spiral computed tomography with the individual mouthguard was performed to transmit the image to the augmentation reality glasses.

The surgery is performed under endotracheal anesthesia with nasal intubation. The patient had her individual mouthguard on the lower jaw. After that, the surgeon put on the AR glasses (Figure 3).

In the real-time regimen, the surgeon was able to see the virtual picture of the stone localization in the parotid salivary gland (Figure 4).

After that, an S-shaped incision [6] in the preauricular region of the skin and subcutaneous hypoderm was made; the flap was made and the capsule incised. The part of the duct where the stone was visualized was bluntly selected and incised and the stone was removed. Then, a stent was installed and fixed in the oral cavity to prevent stricture formation of the duct. The wound was sutured layer by layer.

3. Discussion

In this clinical case, the technique of using augmented reality to visualize the concrement during the surgical intervention of salivary stone removal using external access is shown. At present, minimally invasive methods for removing parotid gland salivary stones exist and these methods are performed using sialoendoscopy with the wire basket or laser, chemical and shock wave lithotripsy. However, if there is a narrowing, stricture, or cicatricial deformity of the salivary gland duct, using of these methods is not possible. The technique we are developing allows to change the view on surgical treatment of patients with salivary stone disease. It is based on thorough preoperative preparation and an individual approach to each patient so an individual mouthguard with a tap is made and computed tomography is also performed. Augmented reality technology allows to visualize the concrement in the operating field and shows an accurate localization of it in the salivary gland duct. Thus, augmented reality technology can reduce the time of surgery and force the postoperative recovery period. However, it is not possible to calculate the depth of the concretion and it is also necessary to reduce the localization errors of the salivary stone virtual image. If these disadvantages are eliminated, it is possible to reduce the length of the incision and the volume of surgery to the minimum possible.

4. Conclusion

The use of the augmented reality technique for concretion visualization during the surgical intervention of salivary stone removal by external access was effective, and there was no any postoperative complications. However, randomized controlled clinical trials with longer follow-up periods should be conducted in order to compare the effectiveness of this technique, its injury rate, and the possibility of using it in the daily practice of a maxillofacial surgeon.

Consent

Patient consent was obtained from the patients.

Authors' Contributions

Yaremenko A.I. is the head of the Department of Dental Surgery and Maxillofacial Surgery who coordinated our work. Lysenko A.V. and Razumova A.Y. performed the operation on the patient, as well as observed after it. Mirzakhmedov R.R. made the individual splint with a radiopaque marker. Chibisova M. A. and Zubareva A.A. performed radiological examination before and after the operation.

References

[1] P. J. Bradley, *Salivary Gland Disorders and Diseases: Diagnosis and Management*, P. J. Bradley and O. Guntnas-Lichus, Eds., Georg Thieme Verlag, 2011.

[2] L. T. Roland, S. A. Skillington, and M. A. Ogden, "Sialendoscopy-assisted transfacial removal of parotid sialoliths: a systematic review and meta-analysis," *Laryngoscope*, vol. 127, no. 11, pp. 2510–2516, 2017.

[3] D. S. Deenadayal and V. Bommakanti, "Sialendoscopy: a review of 133 cases," *International Journal of Otolaryngology and Head & Neck Surgery*, vol. 5, no. 1, pp. 28–33, 2016.

[4] A. C. Profeta, C. Schilling, and M. McGurk, "Augmented reality visualization in head and neck surgery: an overview of recent findings in sentinel node biopsy and future perspectives," *British Journal of Oral and Maxillofacial Surgery*, vol. 54, no. 6, pp. 694–696, 2016.

[5] O. V. Chernenko, "Tekhnologii dopolnennoy i virtualnoy realnosti s meditsine: analiz konkurentnogo landshafta," *Ekonomika nauki*, vol. 4, no. 1, pp. 69–80, 2018.

[6] T. Kopeć, W. Szyfter, and M. Wierzbicka, "Sialoendoscopy and combined approach for the management of salivary gland stones," *European Archives of Oto-Rhino-Laryngology*, vol. 270, no. 1, pp. 219–223, 2013.

30

Third Molar Displacement into Submandibular Space

Mirlany Mendes Maciel Oliveira,[1] Rodrigo da Franca Acioly,[2] Dennis Dinelly de Souza,[2] Bruno Araújo da Silva,[2] and Daniel Do Carmo Carvalho[2]

[1]*Bucomaxilofacial Surgery and Traumatology Clinical Hospital of the Federal University of Uberlândia (HC-UFU), Uberlândia, Minas Gerais, Brazil*
[2]*Buccomaxillofacial Surgery, Department of Buccomaxillofacial Surgery and Traumatology, Hospital Geral de Roraima, Boa Vista, RR, Brazil*

Correspondence should be addressed to Mirlany Mendes Maciel Oliveira; mirlany.mendess@gmail.com

Academic Editor: Daniel Torres-Lagares

There are various accidents and complications that may occur during extraction of dental elements. The displacement of dental elements to other facial spaces is one kind of the possible complications, and there may be significant physical and psychological results for the patient. The treatment for this kind of occurrence may vary from a conservative technique to surgical procedure, what will depend on clinical characteristics, symptoms, the location of the dental element, and its relation to adjacent structures. The objective of this article is to report a clinical case of the displacement of a lower third molar tooth into the submandibular space during its extraction, followed by surgical removal through extraoral approach, with proservation for the next two years when patient evolved to paresthesia of the inferior alveolar nerve.

1. Introduction

The extraction of dental elements is one of the most common procedures in the dental surgeons' routine, either for a general dentist or an oral and maxillofacial surgeon. However, as all other procedures in the dental field, the simplest oral surgeries can also present occurrence of accidents and complications [1].

Several accidents during dental extractions can occur, which include fractured mandible, damage to nervous structures, and displacement of the element into facial spaces [2].

The displacement of teeth to neighboring spaces is a rare intraoperative accident in dental surgery and it can cause physical and psychological damage to the patient [1]. The possible causes of teeth displacement may be associated with excessive pressure, lack of experience of the professional, inadequate use of the surgical equipment, and anatomic characteristics of the patient [2, 3].

Lingually located teeth or deeply impacted molars present a higher risk of displacement to other facial spaces [4]. According to Aznar-Arasa et al. [3], the most common location of displacement is into the maxillary sinus. Other places include submandibular space, lingual space, infratemporal fossa, oral space, pterygomandibular space, and lateral pharyngeal space [2, 5].

The symptoms after teeth displacement into facial spaces may vary from asymptomatic cases to pain report, edema, and mandible trismus, and based on these findings, it is indicated a choice between the removal of the dental element and a conservative treatment [3].

The open surgical technique, together with appropriate use of pressure and placement of retractors of the tongue region, can help minimize the occurrence of this kind of complication [4, 6, 7].

The present article is aimed at reporting a clinical case of the transoperative displacement of a lower third molar tooth into the submandibular space.

2. Case Report

Male patient, 21 years old, with leucoderma, denied underlying diseases or allergies, attended to the Oral and Maxillofacial

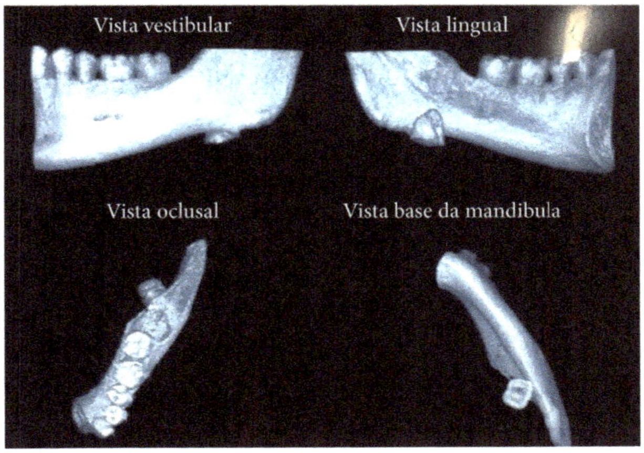

Figure 1: Computed tomography 3D reconstruction.

Surgical and Trauma Service of the General Hospital of Roraima-HGRR, with the main symptomatology of pain and edema after an attempt of extraction of the left lower third molar which evolved with complication transoperative of displacement to adjacent spaces. The patient reported that during the attempt to extract the dental element, he felt symptoms of intense pain and he was communicated of the transoperative accident. After the displacement of the dental element, the surgeon dentist attempted the removal of the tooth by using specially one of the fingers, but without success. After image examination of a cone beam computed tomography, the diagnosis of displacement of the third molar into submandibular space was confirmed. The management adopted was the procedure to remove the dental element under general anesthesia, and through an extraoral access on the left submandibular region, an incision in layers was made and the dental element was completely removed. The surgical procedure was performed without further complications, and there was a review of hemostasis, suture of layers using thread vicryl 3-0, external suture using nylon thread 5-0, and review of the systems (Figures 1–3).

After 2 years of proservation, the patient presents preserved masticatory functions, satisfactory mouth opening, and the occurrence of alveolar inferior nerve paresthesia.

3. Discussion

Nowadays, the extraction of dental elements is a routine procedure in dental offices. However, individual analysis of each case is needed to perform this procedure.

The surgeon should not underestimate the procedure by considering it easy at first; there should be an efficient preoperative analysis, and after the extraction, a clinical and radiographic analysis of the place the tooth element has been removed from [6, 8].

Surgeon dentists who perform third molar extractions should consider the local characteristics of the dental element in order to evaluate the level of difficulty the surgical procedure might present. These characteristics include level of impactation, root format, dental inclination, and bone density [4, 9].

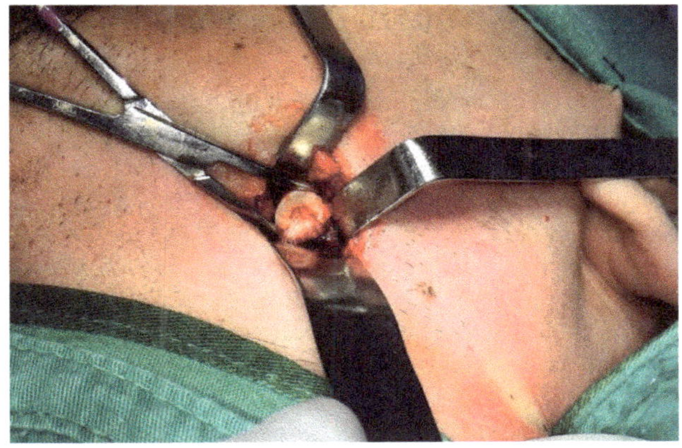

Figure 2: Removal of dental element by extraoral access.

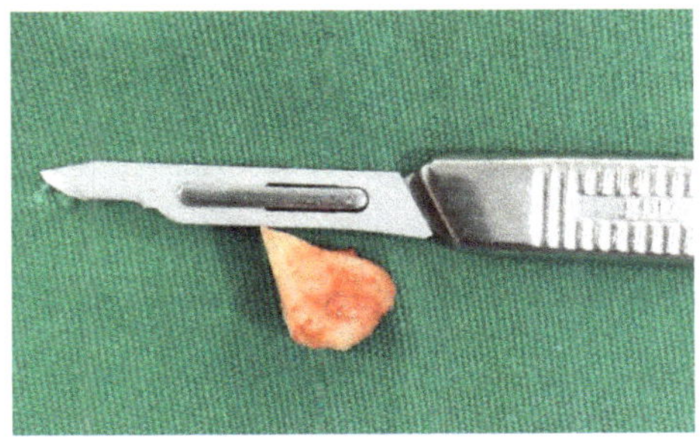

Figure 3: Third molar removed.

Bimanual examination can help finding the fragment location, associated to radiograph and tomography images, seeking for the exact local, especially in cases of lower tooth displacement. The advantages of external pressure include avoiding displacement of the fragment, elevation of the mouth floor, and palpation of the area. However, this approach is not recommended if patients present edema or obesity [1]. In case displacement of a dental element into facial spaces occurs, careful thinking should indicate the management procedures to be adopted. Attempts of immediate removal with lack of skills or lack of anatomic and surgical knowledge may worsen the condition by deepening the fragment or moving it into adjacent spaces [5].

If fragments are bigger than 5 mm, there should be a surgical procedure, but if fragment is smaller than 5 mm and it is not palpable, the conservative treatment can be an option. However, if dental element is left for a long period of time, it is possible that there will be reaction to a foreign body as well as the possibility of infection in the neck spaces [4].

The surgeon experience is an important aspect to be considered, but it is not determinant for the occurrence of teeth displacement into facial spaces, because both general surgeon dentists and specialists in Oral and Maxillofacial Surgery may face the occurrence of this kind of accident.

In the international literature, it is possible to find other accidents related to dental removal which include the displacement of a dental high-speed piece bur into submandibular space and a broken needle dislodged into the prevertebral space [5, 10, 11].

4. Conclusion

The displacement of dental elements is a rare accident, but potentially serious. Although third molars are the dental elements mostly involved in displacement into facial spaces, the other teeth can also be responsible for these accidents. Thus, the case should be sent to an Oral and Maxillofacial surgeon to provide adequate diagnosis, verify the exact location of the dental fragment through imaging exams, and plan the removal or not of the element, based on clinical characteristics, location, noble adjacent structures, and size of the element located in the neighboring facial spaces.

References

[1] S. Zhao, Z. Huang, T. Geng, and L. Huang, "Intraoral management of iatrogenically displaced lower third molar roots in the sublingual space: a report of 2 cases," *International Journal of Clinical and Experimental Medicine*, vol. 8, no. 10, pp. 19591-19595, 2015.

[2] W. Chang, T. Chang, K. Chiu, C. Wu, and Y. Chen, "Accidental iatrogenic displacement of the mandibular third molar into the lateral pharyngeal space-a case report," *Tawian J Oral Maxillofac Surg*, vol. 25, pp. 119–126, 2014.

[3] L. Aznar-Arasa, R. Figueiredo, and C. Gay-Escoda, "Iatrogenic displacement of lower third molar roots into the sublingual space: report of 6 cases," *Journal of Oral and Maxillofacial Surgery*, vol. 70, no. 2, pp. e107–e115, 2012.

[4] M. A. Nusrath and R. J. Banks, "Unrecognised displacement of mandibular molar root into the submandibular space," *British Dental Journal*, vol. 209, no. 6, pp. 279-280, 2010.

[5] S. Yalcin, I. Aktas, Y. Emes, and B. Atalay, "Accidental displacement of a high-speed handpiece bur during mandibular third molar surgery: a case report," *Oral Surgery, Oral Medicine, Oral Pathology, Oral Radiology, and Endodontics*, vol. 105, no. 3, pp. e29–e31, 2008.

[6] P. Bozkurt and E. Erdem, "Management of upper and lower molars that are displaced into the neighbouring spaces," *British Journal of Oral and Maxillofacial Surgery*, vol. 55, pp. 49–52, 2017.

[7] A. Campbell and B. J. Costello, "Retrieval of a displaced third molar using navigation and active image guidance," *Journal of Oral and Maxillofacial Surgery*, vol. 68, no. 2, pp. 480–485, 2010.

[8] N. Medeiros and G. Gaffrée, "Accidental displacement of inferior third molar into the lateral pharyngeal space: case report," *Journal of Oral and Maxillofacial Surgery*, vol. 66, no. 3, pp. 578–580, 2008.

[9] C. E. Sverzut, A. E. Trivellato, A. T. Sverzut, F. P. Matos, and R. B. Kato, "Removal of a maxillary third molar accidentally displaced into the infratemporal fossa via intraoral approach under local anesthesia: report of a case," *Journal of Oral and Maxillofacial Surgery*, vol. 67, no. 6, pp. 1316–1320, 2009.

[10] K. Kamburoglu, S. Kursun, and B. Oztas, "Submandibular displacement of a mandibular third molar root during extraction: a case report," *Cases Journal*, vol. 3, no. 1, article 8, 2010.

[11] B. Sahin, S. Yildirimturk, Y. Sirin, and B. Basaran, "Displacement of a broken dental injection needle into the perivertebral space," *Journal of Craniofacial Surgery*, vol. 28, no. 5, pp. e474–e477, 2017.

31

Definitive Obturator Fabrication for Partial Maxillectomy Patient

M. Singh, I. K. Limbu, P. K. Parajuli, and R. K. Singh

Department of Prosthodontics and Crown-Bridge, B P Koirala Institute of Health Sciences, Dharan, Nepal

Correspondence should be addressed to M. Singh; drmiramiracle@gmail.com

Academic Editor: Gilberto Sammartino

Maxillectomy defects can result in oroantral communication that causes difficulty in mastication and deglutition, impaired speech, and facial disfigurement. The prosthodontist plays an important role in the rehabilitation of such defects with obturators. This paper describes a clinical report of fabricating a definitive obturator with a cast metal framework using a single flask and one-time processing method for an acquired maxillary defect. A tripodal design was selected for this case. Rest was placed on the premolars and molars of both quadrants of the maxilla. Complete palate as the major connector was designed to ensure maximum distribution of the functional load to the tissue. Indirect retainer was planned on the right first premolar. Direct retention was provided by the I-bar clasp placed on the left first premolar, circumferential clasp on the right first premolar, and embrasure clasp between the right first and second molars. Thus, this definitive prosthesis rehabilitated the patient by providing better masticatory efficiency, improving the clarity of speech and quality of life of the patient.

1. Introduction

Palatal defects may result from congenital malformations, trauma, disease, pathologic changes, radiation burns, or surgical intervention [1]. These defects predispose the patient to hypernasal speech, leakage of fluid into a nasal cavity, and impaired masticatory function. Such defects need special prosthesis to establish oronasal seal which can be provided by obturator prosthesis [2]. The Glossary of Prosthodontic Terms defines an obturator as "a maxillofacial prosthesis used to close a congenital or acquired tissue opening, primarily of the hard palate and/or contiguous alveolar or soft tissue structures" [3]. The degree of obturator extension into the defect varies according to the configuration of the defect, character of its lining tissue, and functional requirements for stabilization, support, and retention of the prosthesis [4]. The open hollow obturator has disadvantages such as accumulation of food, debris, and mucus inside the hollow part leading to malodor and an increase in weight. The closed hollow obturator prevents water and food retention, enables cleaning, and has a reduced weight and maximum extension [5]. The size of the defect, number of remaining teeth, amount of remaining bony structures, and ability of the patient to adapt to the prosthesis are few factors that affect the prognosis of the treatment.

2. Case Report

A 38-year-old female presented to the Department of Prosthodontics and Crown-Bridge for the prosthetic rehabilitation of postmaxillectomy defect resulting from squamous cell carcinoma of the left maxilla 12 months back. The patient complained of difficulty in mastication, nasal regurgitation of fluids, and nasal tone in her voice. She had worn surgical and interim obturator. Intraoral examination revealed well-healed surgical defect in the maxilla involving part of the hard palate, alveolar ridge, and maxillary tuberosity creating an oroantral communication. All teeth posterior to the first premolar were missing on the left quadrant of the maxilla (Figure 1). Masticatory and phonetic functions of the patient were affected. After a thorough examination, the defect was classified as Aramany's Class II maxillary defect. The treatment plan was made to rehabilitate this patient with a definitive obturator with a cast metal framework.

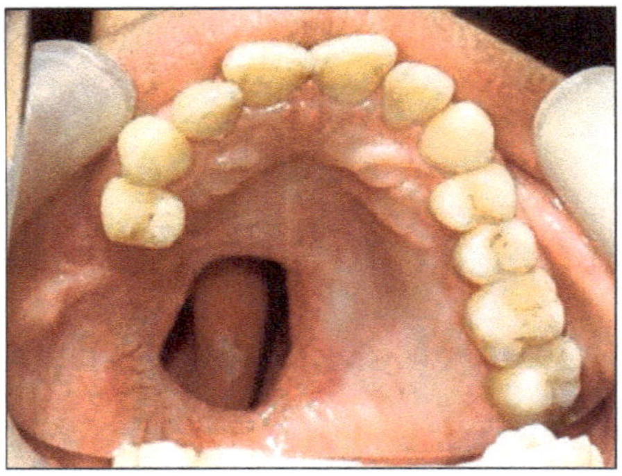

FIGURE 1: Intraoral defect of the palate.

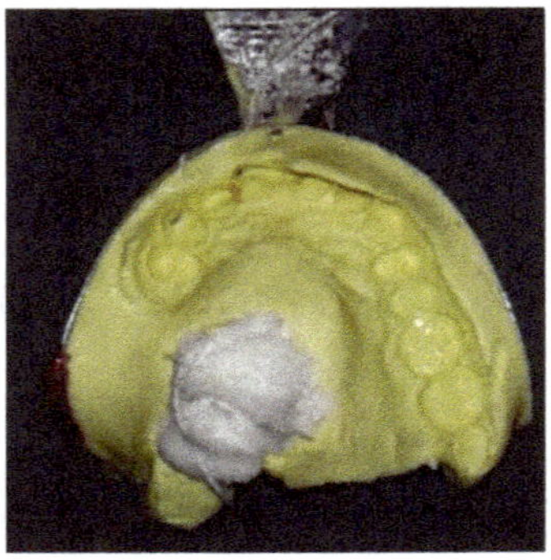

FIGURE 2: Primary impression.

3. Procedure

The primary impression was made using irreversible hydrocolloid (Zelgan 2002, DENTSPLY) (Figure 2) and was poured with dental stone (Kalstone, Kalabhai) to obtain a primary cast (Figure 3). The defect was blocked with a gauze piece lubricated with petroleum jelly prior to impression making. The primary cast was then surveyed on a surveyor (MARATHON-Surveyor 103 Complete Milling Units # 100769), and the framework was designed. The design included a tripodal obturator design with complete palate as the major connector. Indirect retainer was planned on the right first premolar, and direct retention was provided by the I-bar clasp placed on the left first premolar, circumferential clasp on the right first premolar, and embrasure circumferential clasp on the right first and second molars. Rest seat preparations on 14, 16, 17, and 24 were carried out to receive rest of the cast metal framework following the principles of Aramany's Class II obturator design. Impression of preprosthetic mouth preparation was made with medium body elastomer (Reprosil, DENTSPLY), and the cast was poured with type IV dental stone (Kalstone, Kalabhai Karson).

A tripodal configuration for the cast metal framework was designed. Designs of the cast metal framework were transferred on the cast, and a cast metal framework was fabricated and checked intraorally for fit and retention (Figure 4). Border molding was done using green stick impression compound (DPI pinnacle tracing sticks), and final impression of defect was made with light viscosity addition silicone impression material (Reprosil, DENTSPLY Caulk, USA). Pick-up impression was made over it with irreversible hydrocolloid (Zelgan 2002, DENTSPLY) and perforated stock tray (Figure 5). Master cast was poured and jaw relation was recorded and transferred to a semiadjustable articulator (Hanau Wide Vue Articulator) (Figure 6). Teeth were arranged on the metal framework, and wax try-in was carried out.

After try-in, waxed up obturator was processed conventionally with flasking, dewaxing, and packing using heat-polymerizing acrylic resin (Trevalon Denture Material, DENTSPLY India Pvt. Ltd., India) (Figure 7). Finishing and polishing of the obturator prosthesis were done (Figures 8 and 9). It was then inserted into the patient's mouth after

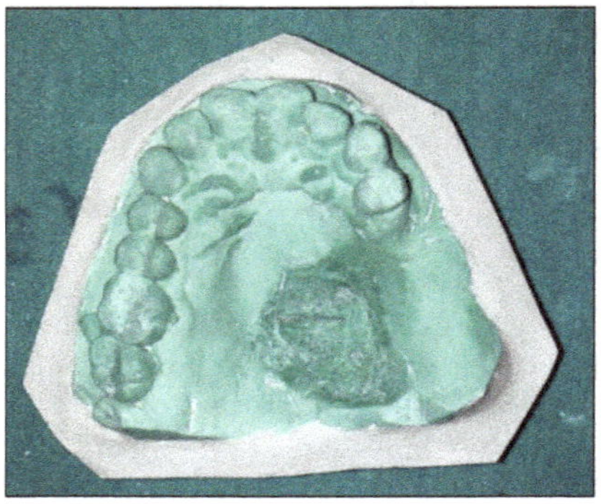

FIGURE 3: Primary cast.

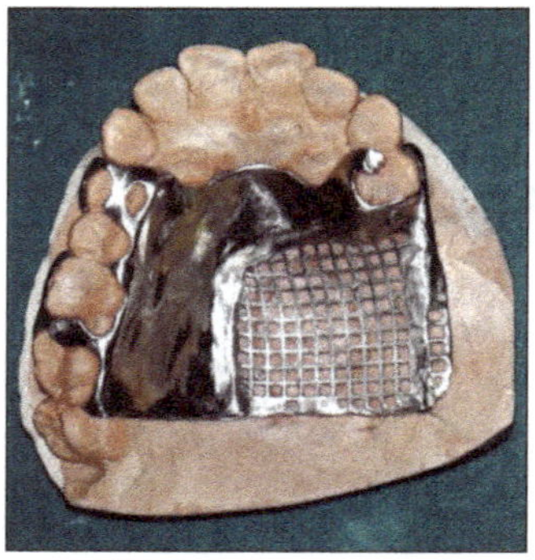

FIGURE 4: Metal framework of the obturator.

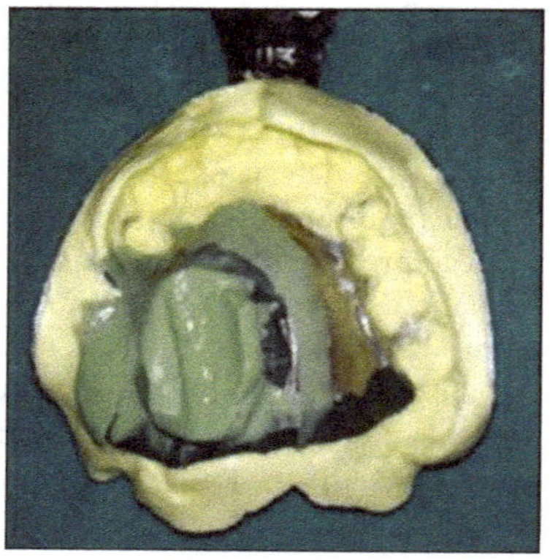

FIGURE 5: Pick-up impression.

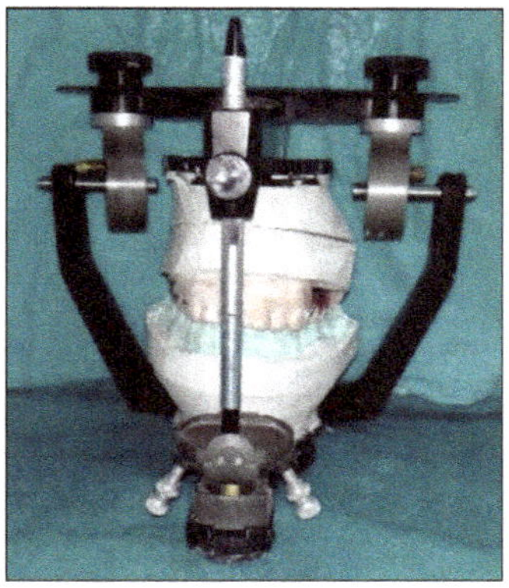

Figure 6: Teeth arrangement.

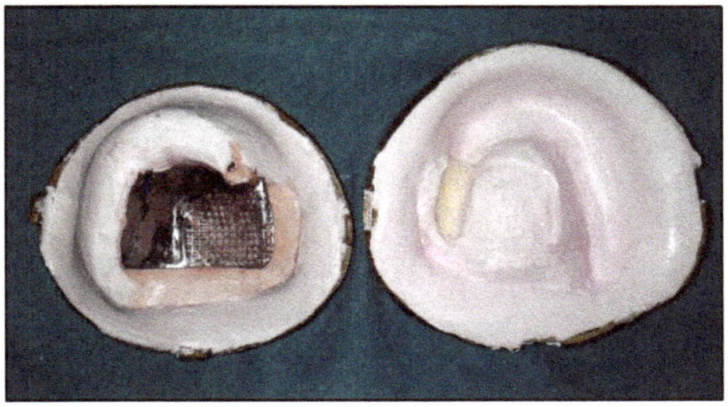

Figure 7: After dewaxing.

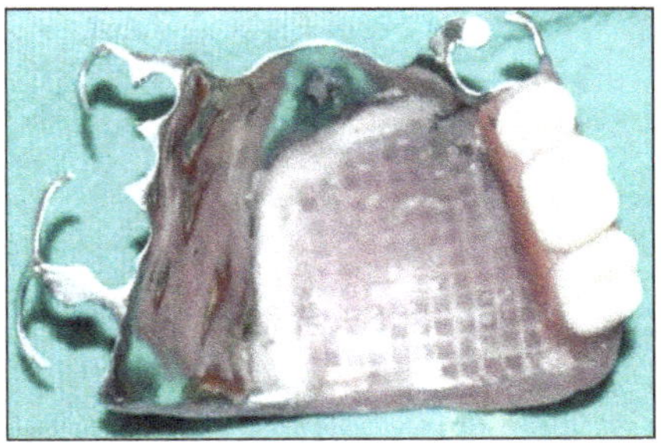

Figure 8: Occlusal view of prosthesis.

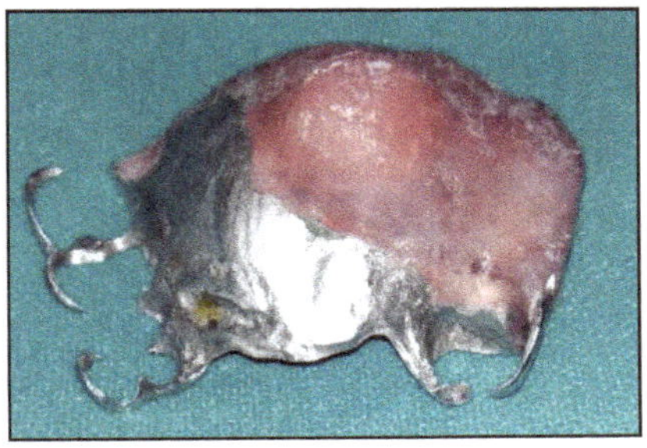

Figure 9: Impression view of prosthesis.

intraoral adjustments (Figures 10 and 11). The patient was happy and satisfied with her improved function, speech, and esthetics. The patient was instructed about the maintenance of the prosthesis and periodic recall check-up.

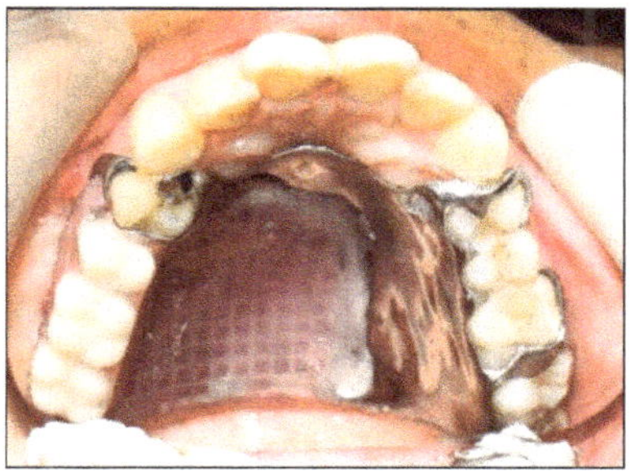

Figure 10: Prosthesis in situ.

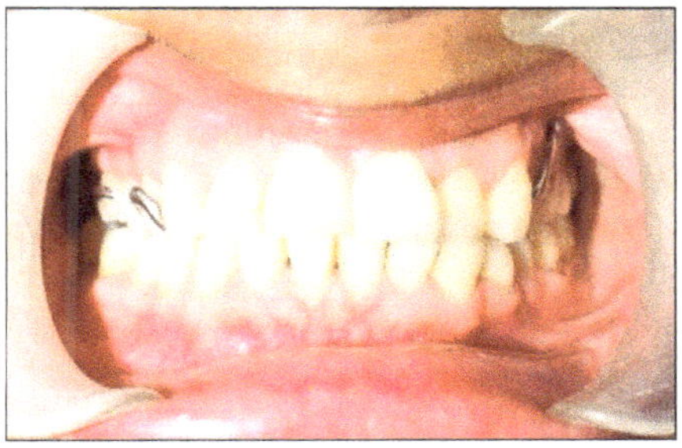

Figure 11: After prosthesis insertion.

4. Discussion

Obturator prosthesis plays a crucial role in the recovery of oral function in postsurgical maxillectomy patients [1]. Framework designs for obturators may vary based on the classification system of the defect. All removable obturator prosthesis should be dictated by basic prosthodontic principles which include broad stress distribution, cross arch stabilization with the use of a rigid major connector, and stabilizing and retaining components at locations within the arch to best minimize dislodging functional forces [4].

A tripodal design was selected for this case. Support of the prosthesis was provided by the remaining teeth, palate, and rest. Rest was prepared on the right and left first premolars and first and second molars of the right quadrant of the maxilla. Complete palate was designed to ensure maximum distribution of the functional load to the tissue. Indirect retainer was planned on the right first premolar. Direct retention was provided by the I-bar clasp placed on the left first premolar, circumferential clasp on the right first premolar, and embrasure circumferential clasp between the right first and second molars [6–8].

In dentate patients, the remaining teeth play an important role in providing retention, support, and stability to the obturator. Retention can be achieved from the remaining teeth or ridge, lateral part of the defect, soft tissue undercut, and scar band. Stabilization and indirect retention components must be positioned effectively to retard the movement of the defect extension portion away from its terminal position [9].

Different types of retentive aids such as magnets, snap-on (friction-type) attachments, acrylic buttons, retentive clips, and implants are used for the conventional obturator prosthesis. The use of implant is a new advancement in maxillofacial prosthodontics. They effectively improve the retention of prosthesis without the help of other appliance. However, cost, health of the patient, and bone qualities are some of the factors which limit the use of implants [10].

The advantages of metal framework obturator prosthesis are the longevity of the prosthesis and thermal conductivity of metal which made it sensitive to temperature change [4, 5].

5. Conclusion

The great challenge in rehabilitating a hemimaxillectomy patient is to obtain adequate retention, stability, and support. Thorough knowledge and skills coupled with a better understanding of the needs of the patients enable the successful rehabilitation of such patients. Definitive obturator prosthesis fabricated with maximum extension and proper design rehabilitates the patient by improving masticatory efficiency, increasing the clarity of speech and quality of life.

References

[1] F. Keyf, "Obturator prostheses for hemimaxillectomy patients," *Journal of Oral Rehabilitation*, vol. 28, no. 9, pp. 821–829, 2001.

[2] J. Rieger, J. Wolfaardt, H. Seikaly, and N. Jha, "Speech outcomes in patients rehabilitated with maxillary obturator prostheses after maxillectomy: a prospective study," *International Journal of Prosthodontics*, vol. 15, no. 2, pp. 139–144, 2002.

[3] K. J. Ferro, S. M. Morgano, C. F. Driscoll et al., "The glossary of prosthodontic terms," *Journal of Prosthetic Dentistry*, vol. 94, no. 1, pp. 10–92, 2005.

[4] I. Kumar, M. B. Kandarphale, V. Aanand, J. Mohan, and P. Kalaignan, "Definitive obturator for a maxillary defect," *Journal of Integrated Dentistry*, vol. 2, no. 3, pp. 1–4, 2017.

[5] K. Hori, T. Miyamoto, T. Ono et al., "One step polymerizing technique for fabricating a hollow obturator," *Journal of Prosthodontic Research*, vol. 57, no. 4, pp. 294–297, 2013.

[6] M. A. Aramany, "Basic principles of obturator design for partially edentulous patients. Part I: classification," *Journal of Prosthetic Dentistry*, vol. 40, no. 5, pp. 554–557, 1978.

[7] M. A. Aramany, "Basic principles of obturator design for partially edentulous patients. Part II: design principles. 1978 [classical article]," *Journal of Prosthetic Dentistry*, vol. 86, no. 6, pp. 562–568, 2001.

[8] G. R. Parr, G. E. Tharp, and A. O. Rahn, "Prosthodontic principles in the framework design of maxillary obturator prostheses," *Journal of Prosthetic Dentistry*, vol. 93, no. 5, pp. 405–411, 2005.

[9] M. E. Gowda, M. S. Mohan, K. Verma, and I. D. Roy, "Implant rehabilitation of partial maxillectomy edentulous patient," *Contemporary Clinical Dentistry*, vol. 4, no. 3, pp. 393–396, 2013.

[10] R. Gurjar, S. Kumar, H. Rao, A. Sharma, and S. Bhansali, "Retentive aids in maxillofacial prosthodontics—a review," *International Journal of Contemporary Dentistry*, vol. 2, no. 3, pp. 84–88, 2011.

Glass Ionomer Subgingival Matrix Technique to Restore a Tooth with Severe Root Resorption for Implant Site Development

Ahmad Y. Imam[1] **and Raghad A. Al-Dabbagh**[2]

[1]*Oral and Maxillofacial Prosthodontics Department, Faculty of Dentistry, King Abdulaziz University, Jeddah, Saudi Arabia*
[2]*Oral and Maxillofacial Rehabilitation Department, Faculty of Dentistry, King Abdulaziz University, Jeddah, Saudi Arabia*

Correspondence should be addressed to Ahmad Y. Imam; amahmowd@kau.edu.sa

Academic Editor: Sukumaran Anil

Here, we present the multidisciplinary, patient-specific management of a patient with severe external root resorption and bone loss in a maxillary anterior tooth. The tooth was provisionally noninvasively restored with glass ionomer subgingival matrix in preparation for forced orthodontic extrusion, papillary preservation, and implant placement. This approach enables clinicians to control infection within and around the resorbed tooth and then to use it as an anchor for slow forced tooth eruption to correct bone and mucogingival deformities. Aesthetic and functional outcomes were clinically and radiographically satisfactory. The advantages and disadvantages of this technique are discussed.

1. Introduction

Trauma to the face and dentition is common and can often have significant repercussions for the individual [1]. The consequences of such trauma can include immediate or delayed aesthetic problems, with or without underlying infections [2]. To achieve predictable outcomes, the management should be timely, patient-specific, and multidisciplinary [3, 4]. Additionally, such patients will need life-long regular follow-up to prevent or manage complications for optimal aesthetics and function [4].

One complication of traumatic dental injury is external root resorption. Injury to the tooth may lead to displacement or removal of the protective precementum layer followed by colonization with multinucleated cells along the root surface. These cells then initiate the resorptive process and may continue to do so depending on the presence of inflammation or pressure [5]. Early diagnosis is sometimes difficult, because this type of resorption progresses slowly and can initially be asymptomatic. However, clinical presentations such as pink tooth discoloration, localised irregularities in gingival contour, and oedematous gingival tissue, with or without gingival bleeding on probing, could be indicative of external root resorption [6]. Management of such lesions depends on the etiological factor or the source of continuous infection. For example, if the source of infection was the pulp, then the recommendation is intracanal medication with calcium hydroxide for 6-12 months [7]. However, delayed or incorrect treatment may lead to severe root resorption that would deem the tooth nonrestorable.

Another complication of dental trauma and associated infection is loss of the supporting tooth structure (bone and soft tissue), which may compromise aesthetic and functional outcomes of treatment. Augmenting horizontal bony defects may be more predictable than the less predictable management of vertical bone loss [8]. Nonsurgical enhancement of bone and soft tissue with forced slow orthodontic extrusion of hopeless teeth may predictably improve bone and soft tissue volume, thus enhancing final restoration aesthetics [9]. Furthermore, this increased vertical bone height and width may further improve the positioning and stability of immediately placed implants and the subsequent outcome [10].

Here, we describe a case of reestablished aesthetics and function in a patient with long-standing severe root resorption due to trauma to a maxillary central incisor. The tooth was provisionally nonsurgically restored with a glass ionomer

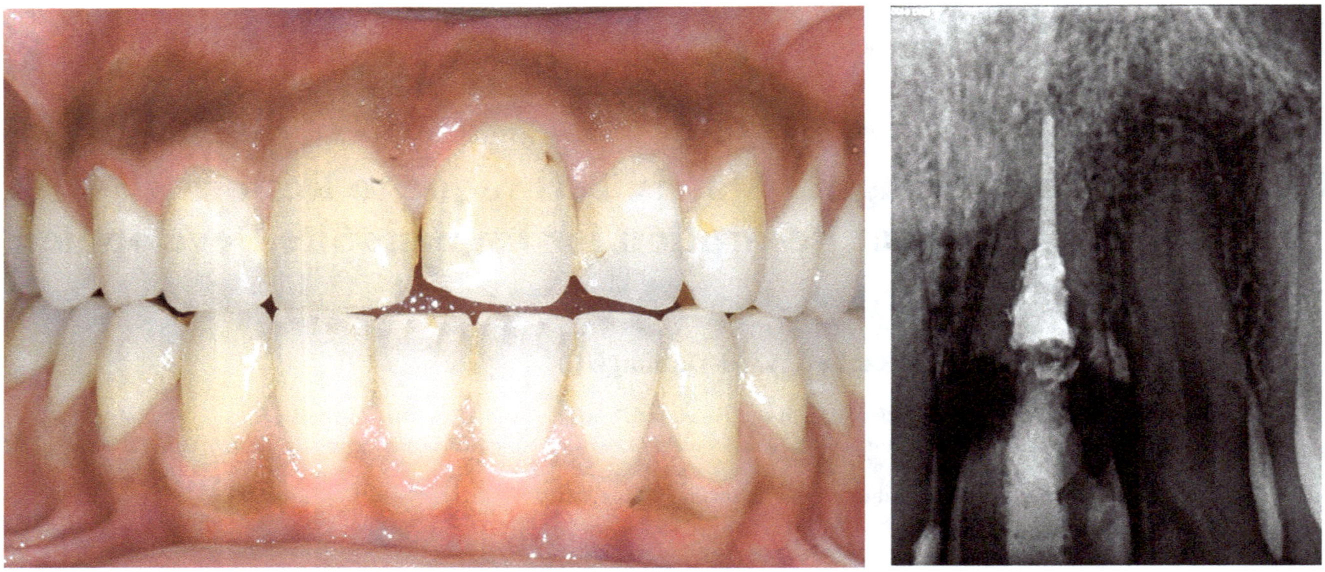

(a) (b)

FIGURE 1: Preoperative clinical and radiographic presentation of tooth #21. (a) Intraoral frontal view shows associated gingival recession and an uneven incisal plane. (b) Periapical radiograph shows extensive root resorption affecting the coronal third of the root.

(GI) subgingival matrix (which we term the "Imam matrix") in preparation for forced orthodontic extrusion, papillary preservation, and implant placement.

2. Case Description

A 45-year-old man was referred by a periodontist colleague at a private practice (UniDents, Jeddah, Saudi Arabia). The patient reported severe mobility, bleeding, and pain related to the maxillary left front tooth and a history of trauma ten years ago. There had been several attempts at root canal treatment by general dentists and endodontists. Clinically, tooth #21 had grade III mobility, recession, a 7 mm pocket, and soft tissue inflammation. He had a high smile line, uneven anterior incisal plane, and a class I incisal relationship (Figure 1(a)). Radiographically, tooth #21 was root canal treated, had communicating root resorption affecting the coronal third of the root, and interproximal, labial, and palatal bone resorption (Figure 1(b)).

After obtaining patient consent, a multidisciplinary treatment plan was commenced. The plan for tooth #21 included (1) nonsurgical removal of all pathologic tooth structure; (2) nonsurgical provisional restoration of the tooth by creating a subgingival glass ionomer (GI) matrix ("Imam matrix"), cemented fiber post, and composite core; (3) fabrication of a provisional crown and definitive cementation; (4) forced orthodontic tooth extrusion; (5) extraction of the tooth; (6) immediate implant placement; and (7) prosthetic restoration.

A putty index (Virtual, Ivoclar Vivadent) was taken prior to tooth preparation, and local anesthesia (lidocaine 2%, Lignospan® standard) was administered. Next, all pathological tooth structures were removed with a diamond bur (gold bur, KOMET) including the existing defective restoration. Gutta percha was removed with a fiber post drill (medium size, 3M, Saint Paul, MN) to leave 3-4 mm at the apical area of the root canal. Bleeding was minimized with a saline-soaked cotton pellet placed on the palatal aspect of the tooth and left for a couple of minutes. Then, paper points were placed into the canal to dry the canal initially and then to maintain canal patency. Next, GI restoration (Fuji IX, GC America Inc., Alsip, IL) was placed palatally, packed with an alcohol swab, and shaped with a plastic filling instrument (HF-PFIDD56, Henry Schein Australia) to build the missing proximal and palatal walls of the root and crown. To ensure bonding of the GI restoration to the deep cervical root margins, it was properly packed with an alcohol swab. Once the GI had set, the paper points were removed from the canal and an access cavity was prepared to leave a 1 mm subgingival band of GI isolating the canal space from the surrounding tissue (fiber post drill; 3M) (Figure 2).

The canal was then acid etched with phosphoric acid following the manufacturer's instructions (Scotchbond™ Universal Etchant, 3M ESPE), rinsed, and dried in preparation for fiber post placement. Dual-cure, self-adhesive resin cement was injected into the canal (RelyX™ Unicem, 3M), and the fiber post (3M) was placed in position. Excess was removed, and the cement was light cured following the manufacturer's instructions. The tooth was then prepared (S6882, KOMET), ensuring all margins were placed at sound tooth structure. Then, the putty index was used to prepare the provisional crown (Protemp, 3M). Video 1 shows step-by-step the process of fabricating the GI matrix. The provisional crown was finished, polished (Enhance Finishing discs, Dentsply Sirona), and cemented with polycarboxylate cement (Poly-F Plus cement BONDEXE, Dentsply). Excess cement was removed, and occlusion was checked.

The patient was then referred to an orthodontist to perform slow orthodontic extrusion. Extrusion of tooth #21 took seven months, including two months for retention. Clinical

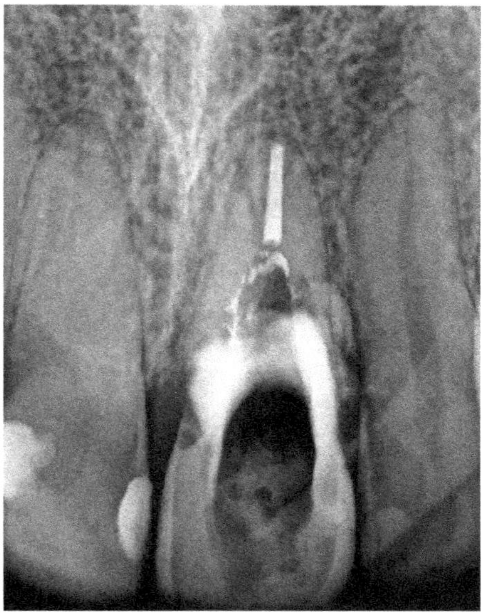

FIGURE 2: GI subgingival "Imam matrix" that sealed the resorptive root defect.

and radiographic images suggested sufficient formation of bone and soft tissue (Figures 3(a) and 3(b)). The labial gingival recession at tooth 21 was reduced to a level that was satisfactory to the patient.

After achieving satisfactory nonsurgical bone and soft tissue augmentation around tooth #21, the patient was referred back to his periodontist for atraumatic extraction of the tooth (Figure 4) and immediate implant placement (Keystone, Lifecore) and loading with a provisional crown (Figures 5(a) and 5(b)). Six months later, a definitive screw-retained zirconia crown was fabricated (dynamic abutment solution) (Figure 6). The patient maintenance protocol included biannual appointments for clinical and radiographic assessment.

3. Discussion

Here, we restored the aesthetics and function of a traumatized tooth by provisionally repairing a nonrestorable maxillary central incisor with severe root resorption for implant site development. In this patient, the central maxillary incisor had recession, mobility, and severe communicating root resorption affecting the coronal third of the root. The treatment plan involved provisionally restoring the tooth, correcting supporting hard and soft tissue volume through slow forced orthodontic extrusion, extraction of the tooth, and finally implant placement. This approach was chosen for interdental papillae preservation, predictable vertical bone augmentation, and achieving a fixed, aesthetically and functionally pleasing restoration throughout treatment.

Restoring a central maxillary incisor with a single implant is aesthetically challenging [11], even more so when there is significant horizontal and vertical bone loss. The main objective is to achieve an osseointegrated dental implant surrounded by healthy soft and hard tissue and placed in a position that enables the dentist to mimic contralateral tooth gingiva position and contour, interdental papillae, and crown shape and shade [11]. Preprosthetic improvement of implant site topography can be achieved either surgically or nonsurgically. Surgical augmentation could include guided tissue regeneration [12], bone and soft tissue graft procedures [13], ridge splitting [14], and distraction osteogenesis [15]. However, surgical augmentation procedures are invasive and painful, can be associated with bleeding and infections, and produce uncertain outcomes when restoring vertical bony defects [13].

In contrast, nonsurgical augmentation involves slow forced orthodontic eruption of nonrestorable teeth, which is predictable and noninvasive, needs patient compliance, and is time consuming [9, 16]; in this case, the patient's exacting personality helped ensure compliance. During orthodontic extrusion, bone and gingival volume increase as a result of stretching of periodontal fibers. These fibers elongate, and osteoblastic cells lay down bone. When this force is slow, gingival tissue follows the newly deposited bone [17].

To use nonrestorable teeth to prepare implant sites, the aim is to eliminate infection prior to noninvasive orthodontic bone and soft tissue augmentation. This patient's central maxillary incisor had severe communicating root resorption affecting the entire coronal third of the root, and there was a proximal and palatal bone loss. Access to the infected part of the root was achieved nonsurgically to remove all infected tooth structure. Then, the resorbed part of the root was sealed with a GI restoration to create the Imam matrix. GI restorations are commonly used to repair external root resorption [18, 19]. The tooth was then reenforced with a fiber post, composite core, and a provisional crown that was definitively cemented. Accessibility and hemorrhage control were challenging but manageable with the aim of controlling infection and enabling the use of this nonrestorable tooth as an anchor for forced extrusion.

The central incisor was previously root canal treated, and the apical root canal treatment was satisfactory with no associated apical radiolucency. Accordingly, after sealing the root defect with the GI restoration, the canal was accessed coronally and the remaining gutta percha was removed to retain the apical 3-5 mm intact. The canal was shaped and irrigated before placement of the fiber post and composite core. Seven months later (orthodontic extrusion), all the surrounding bone tissue looked radiographically normal with no signs or symptoms of infection. Thus, retaining the existing apical seal in this case was sufficient to prevent bacterial percolation into the apical area.

One main advantage of this approach is that it achieves a fixed, aesthetically and functionally pleasing restoration throughout treatment. In this patient, the central incisor suffered from severe mobility and bleeding due to the extensive root resorption that led to the separation of the crown from the root. The provisional restoration of such a tooth was achievable after fabricating the Imam matrix and strengthening it with a fiber post and provisional crown. The tooth was retained until the site was ready for immediate implant placement with an interim crown.

However, this technique might be challenging to achieve. Visual accessibility and hemorrhage control might hinder the

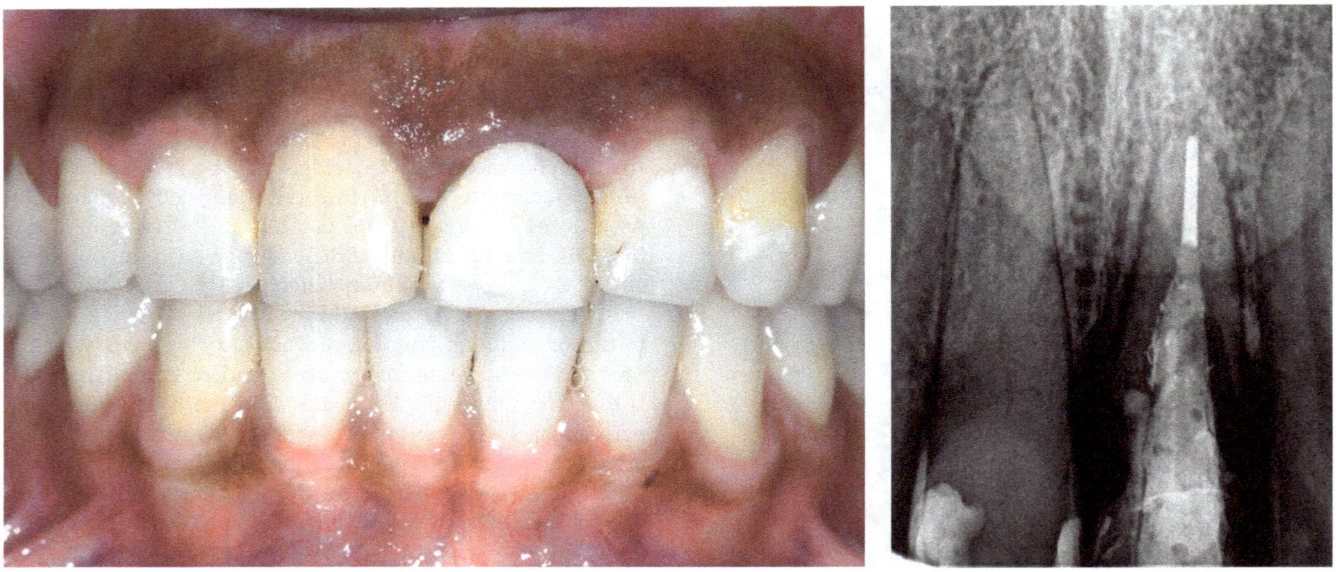

(a) (b)

Figure 3: Clinical and radiographic presentation after orthodontic extrusion of tooth 21. (a) Intraoral frontal view showing the coronal relocation of the gingival margin and preservation of interdental papillae. (b) Periapical radiograph showing the coronal repositioning of the apex of the tooth and bone fill proximally.

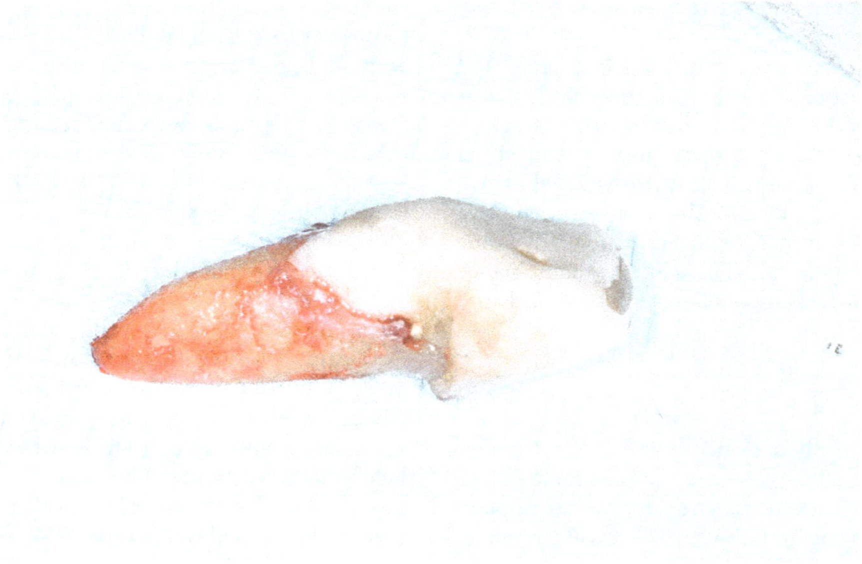

Figure 4: Extracted tooth 21 with well-adapted deep margins of the provisional restoration.

bonding of the GI restoration to deep sound tooth margin. If a proper seal and bonding had not been achieved, then extraction with surgical socket preservation methods and bone and soft tissue augmentation techniques would have been alternative options. Indeed, the surgical approach has been used with a predictable outcome when bone surrounding the tooth was preserved post extraction [20]. However, in this patient, there was a significant vertical bone loss from the onset, reaching the middle third of the root, and using surgical bone and soft tissue augmentation techniques would have a compromised aesthetic outcome [13].

Although this approach was time consuming, expensive, multidisciplinary, and highly dependent on patient compliance, it produced a predictable and satisfying aesthetic and functional long-term outcome. Yet, the surgical approach would as well be time consuming and expensive when staged. To our best knowledge, this is the first report to show that provisionally and nonsurgically restoring teeth with extensive root resorption can be achieved by fabricating a GI subgingival "Imam matrix," fiber post, composite core, and provisional crown. This provisional restorative technique created an infection-free environment and a sufficiently

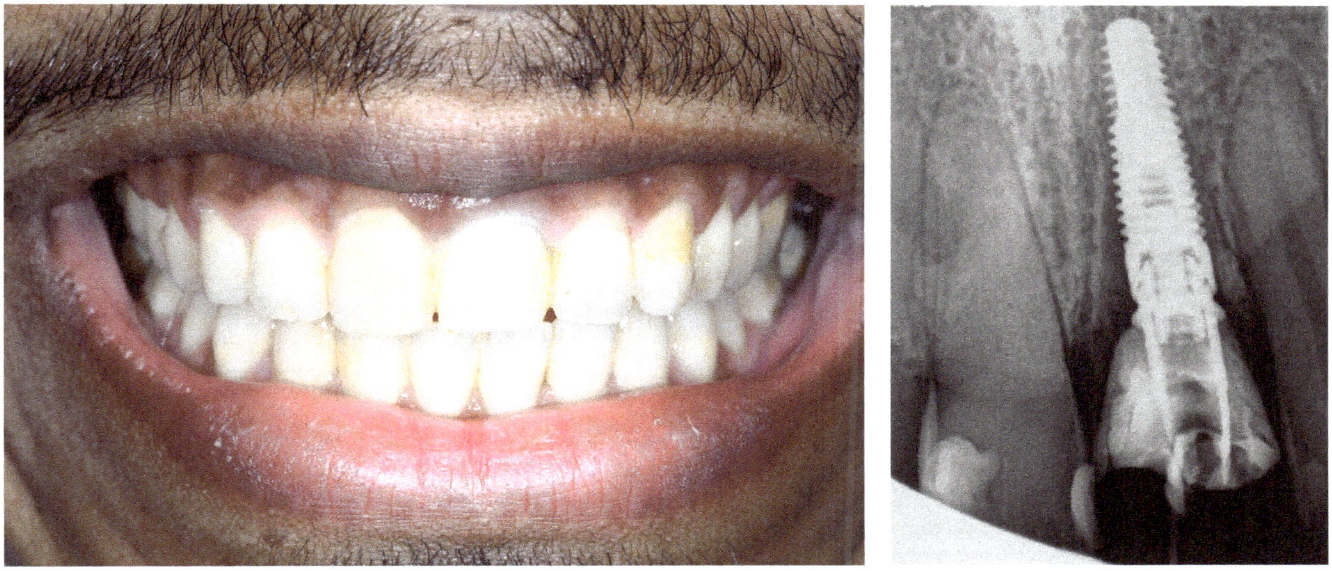

(a) (b)

FIGURE 5: Clinical and radiographic presentation of the immediately placed implant with provisional restoration for tooth #21. (a) Intraoral frontal view. (b) Periapical radiograph.

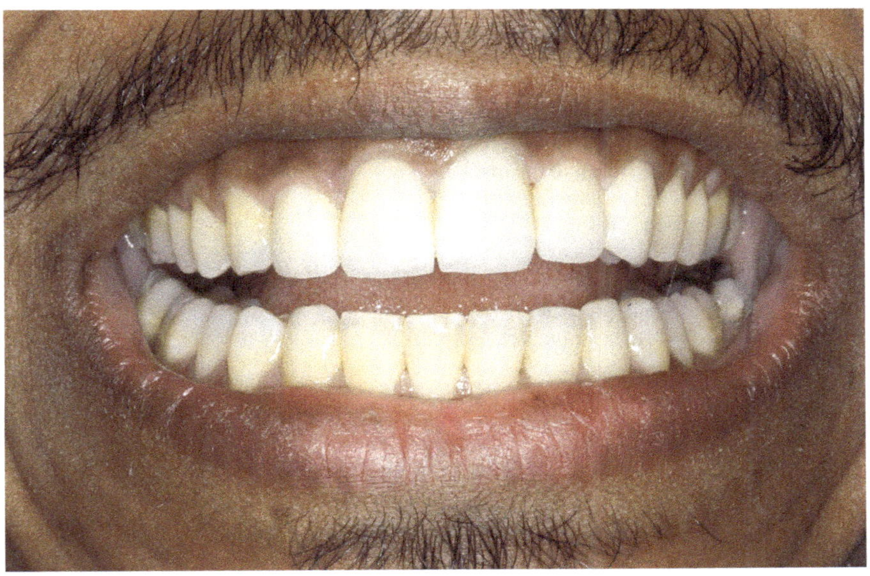

FIGURE 6: Postoperative clinical presentation of the definitive implant-supported crown of tooth 21.

strong tooth to withstand forced eruption for implant site development.

4. Summary

This case illustrates the importance of a timely, patient-specific, and multidisciplinary treatment plan. Our management allowed the patient to transition from tooth to implant-supported crown without the use of a removable partial denture. Additionally, a satisfactory aesthetic and functional outcome, with minimal surgical intervention, was achieved.

Abbreviations

GI: Glass ionomer.

Acknowledgments

The authors would like to thank Prof. Ali Al-Ghamdi (periodontist) and Dr. Wael Elias (orthodontist) for their contribution in the multidisciplinary treatment provided to the presented case. We would like to thank as well Dr. Noha Alkordy for her efforts in developing the presented video.

References

[1] E. E. Petersson, L. Andersson, and S. Sorensen, "Traumatic oral vs non-oral injuries," *Swedish Dental Journal*, vol. 21, no. 1-2, pp. 55–68, 1997.

[2] J. O. A. F. Andreason and L. Andersson, *Text Book and Colour Atlas of Traumatic Injuries to the Teeth*, Copenhagen, Denmark, Blackwell Munksgaard, 4th edition, 2007.

[3] Y.-H. Chou, J. K. du, S. T. Chou et al., "An interdisciplinary treatment approach combining orthodontic forced eruption with immediate implant placement to achieve a satisfactory treatment outcome: a case report," *Clinical Implant Dentistry and Related Research*, vol. 15, no. 1, pp. 113–120, 2013.

[4] D. Schwartz-Arad, L. Levin, and M. Ashkenazi, "Treatment options of untreatable traumatized anterior maxillary teeth for future use of dental implantation," *Implant Dentistry*, vol. 13, no. 2, pp. 120–128, 2004.

[5] Z. Fuss, I. Tsesis, and S. Lin, "Root resorption - diagnosis, classification and treatment choices based on stimulation factors," *Dental Traumatology*, vol. 19, no. 4, pp. 175–182, 2003.

[6] G. S. Heithersay, "Clinical, radiologic, and histopathologic features of invasive cervical resorption," *Quintessence International*, vol. 30, no. 1, pp. 27–37, 1999.

[7] L. Andersson, "New guidelines for treatment of avulsed permanent teeth," *Dental Traumatology*, vol. 28, no. 2, p. 87, 2012.

[8] A. R. Rokn, A. Saffarpour, R. Sadrimanesh et al., "Implant site development by orthodontic forced eruption of nontreatable teeth: a case report," *The Open Dentistry Journal*, vol. 6, no. 1, pp. 99–104, 2012.

[9] H. Salama and M. Salama, "The role of orthodontic extrusive remodeling in the enhancement of soft and hard tissue profiles prior to implant placement: a systematic approach to the management of extraction site defects," *The International Journal of Periodontics & Restorative Dentistry*, vol. 13, no. 4, pp. 312–333, 1993.

[10] L. Chambrone and L. A. Chambrone, "Forced orthodontic eruption of fractured teeth before implant placement: case report," *Journal of the Canadian Dental Association*, vol. 71, no. 4, pp. 257–261, 2005.

[11] R. S. de Molon, E. D. de Avila, J. A. de Souza et al., "Forced orthodontic eruption for augmentation of soft and hard tissue prior to implant placement," *Contemporary Clinical Dentistry*, vol. 4, no. 2, pp. 243–247, 2013.

[12] N. U. Zitzmann, P. Scharer, and C. P. Marinello, "Long-term results of implants treated with guided bone regeneration: a 5-year prospective study," *The International Journal of Oral & Maxillofacial Implants*, vol. 16, no. 3, pp. 355–366, 2001.

[13] S. Winkler, "Implant site development and alveolar bone resorption patterns," *The Journal of Oral Implantology*, vol. 28, no. 5, pp. 226–229, 2002.

[14] T. Shimoyama, T. Kaneko, S. Shimizu, D. Kasai, T. Tojo, and N. Horie, "Ridge widening and immediate implant placement: a case report," *Implant Dentistry*, vol. 10, no. 2, pp. 108–112, 2001.

[15] C. Aparicio and O. T. Jensen, "Alveolar ridge widening by distraction osteogenesis: a case report," *Practical Procedures & Aesthetic Dentistry*, vol. 13, pp. 663–668, 2001.

[16] S. L. Rasner, "Orthodontic extrusion: an adjunct to implant treatment," *Dentistry Today*, vol. 30, pp. 104–106, 2011.

[17] T. Mantzikos and I. Shamus, "Forced eruption and implant site development: an osteophysiologic response," *American Journal of Orthodontics and Dentofacial Orthopedics*, vol. 115, no. 5, pp. 583–591, 1999.

[18] S. Y. Kim and S. E. Yang, "Surgical repair of external inflammatory root resorption with resin-modified glass ionomer cement," *Oral Surgery, Oral Medicine, Oral Pathology, Oral Radiology, and Endodontics*, vol. 111, no. 4, pp. e33–e36, 2011.

[19] L. F. Silveira, C. F. Silveira, J. Martos, E. M. Piovesan, and J. B. Cesar Neto, "Clinical technique for invasive cervical root resorption," *Journal of Conservative Dentistry*, vol. 14, no. 4, pp. 440–444, 2011.

[20] G. Kotsakis, V. Chrepa, N. Marcou, H. Prasad, and J. Hinrichs, "Flapless alveolar ridge preservation utilizing the "socket-plug" technique: clinical technique and review of the literature," *The Journal of Oral Implantology*, vol. 40, no. 6, pp. 690–698, 2014.

33

A Clinicopathological Report of Four Cases of Squamous Odontogenic Tumor-Like Proliferations in Odontogenic Cysts: Suggested Opinions regarding this Unusual Nature

Massoumeh Zargaran[1] and **Setareh Shojaei**[2]

[1]*Department of Oral and Maxillofacial Pathology, Faculty of Dentistry, Kurdistan University of Medical Sciences, Sanandaj, Iran*
[2]*Department of Oral& Maxillofacial Pathology, School of Dentistry, Hamadan University of Medical Sciences, Hamadan, Iran*

Correspondence should be addressed to Massoumeh Zargaran; massoumehzargaran@gmail.com

Academic Editor: Vlaho Brailo

Distinguishing squamous odontogenic tumor-like proliferations (SOTLPs) is important in odontogenic cysts to avoid misinterpretation such as a squamous odontogenic tumor, well-differentiated squamous cell carcinoma, and acanthomatous type of ameloblastoma. This study is aimed at reporting 4 cases of these clinicopathological proliferations in order to shed more light on the importance of distinguishing them from other similar types. 150 odontogenic cysts were studied in which four cases (2.66%) with SOTLPs were identified including 2 radicular cysts, 1 dentigerous cyst, and 1 odontogenic keratocyst. These proliferations were observed in the cysts' wall particularly adjacent to the epithelial lining. All cysts had inflammation while 3 cases showed budding from the epithelial cyst lining. The findings suggested that lining of odontogenic cysts could be a source of SOTLPs, and inflammation probably played an effective role in their development. Its incidence was 2.66% in the present study. Although SOTLPs are not frequent in odontogenic cysts, their identification is important to prevent wrong histopathologic interpretation and treatment.

1. Introduction

Squamous odontogenic tumor (SOT) is a rare benign neoplasm with odontogenic epithelium origin. SOT growth is slow/gradual, but it might invade the trabecular bone and infiltrate into its adjacent tissues. This tumor histopathologically is described as the proliferation of well-differentiated squamous epithelial cells that create islands and nests located in a fibrous stroma [1]. SOT should be differentiated histopathologically from a similar feature called a squamous odontogenic tumor-like proliferation (SOTLP) [1–3].

SOTLPs are a rare phenomenon [2, 4]. These proliferations occur in the walls of odontogenic cysts [1, 3, 5, 6] while they are morphologically similar to epithelial islands that form SOT [1–3]. In spite of this similarity, there is no evidence of neoplastic transformation [1–3]; in fact, its biological behavior and prognosis is different from SOT [2, 3, 7]. Histopathological appearance of SOTLPs overlaps with that of some other neoplasms like the acanthomatous type of ameloblastoma and the well-differentiated squamous cell carcinoma (SCC) [1–3]. Due to this similarity in microscopic appearance, SOTLPs can be misinterpreted by a pathologist who is not aware of the subtle differences between this phenomenon and other stated lesions [2–4]. The present study is aimed at reporting 4 cases of odontogenic cysts with SOTLPs and comparing them with other reports in this regard.

2. Case Report

150 odontogenic cysts (inflammatory or developmental) belonging to the archive of the Department of Oral Pathology, Faculty of Dentistry, Hamadan University of Medical Sciences, were studied using an optical microscope. All hematoxylin and eosin (H&E) slides were carefully inspected for presence of SOTLPs. Presence of several squamous

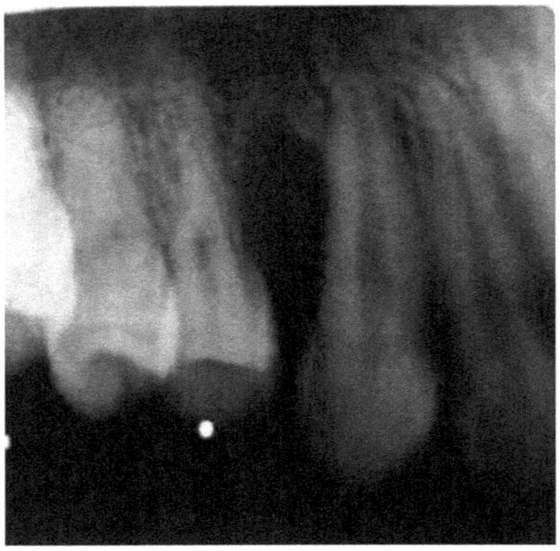

FIGURE 1: Radiography image of a unilocular, cystic radiolucent lesion between the maxillary first premolar and canine.

epithelial islands that were morphologically similar to SOT was considered as a histopathological criterion for diagnosing SOTLPs [3].

Clinical information was obtained from the patients' records. Four cases including 2 radicular cysts, 1 dentigerous cyst, and 1 odontogenic keratocyst (OKC) were detected with SOTLPs; three cases were in men (75%) and one in a woman (25%). All patients were white, between 18 and 28 years old, and 2 cysts were in the maxilla and 2 in the mandible. Radiographical appearances of the lesions in the records of the patients were described as unilocular, cystic, or well-circumscribed radiolucency (Figure 1). These radiographical appearances and the records of intraoperative findings for all samples were interpreted as cystic lesions, and gross descriptions of them were matched to a cystic nature.

Histopathologically, SOTLPs were observed as islands in various sizes consisting of well-differentiated squamous cells with bland appearance within the connective tissue wall of the cyst especially adjacent to the cyst lining (Figures 2(a) and 2(b)). The peripheral cells of these islands were flat, and some were cubic basaloid cells. Dyskeratotic cells, keratin pearl formation, microcyst formation, and mitosis were not observed in any of the islands. All detected cysts had inflammatory components as primary or secondary in nature. Changes such as hyperplasia, desquamation, and/or lining replacement with granulation tissue were observed in the epithelial lining of lesions. The inflammation type of the cysts was chronic, and it mainly consisted of lymphocytes and/or plasma cells. Degree and intensity of the inflammations were mild to moderate and were dispersed. Budding from the epithelial lining was observed in 3 cases (Figures 3 and 4), and 1 case represented nests and epithelial cords consistent with rests of Malassez.

3. Discussion

Almost 60 odontogenic cysts with STOLPs were reported in English language articles searched in PubMed and MEDLINE particularly by Sala-Pérez et al. [1–3, 5–9]. These four cases found in the present study should be added to previously reported cases. In fact, there are only a few case series reporting STOLPs, most of which reported only one case, and their clinicopathological information did not seem to be adequate when compared with the present study [1, 7–9] except for Parmar et al. [2] and Wright [3].

Out of 150 odontogenic cysts investigated in the present study, 4 cases were found with SOTLPs (2.66%). The number of cases reported by Parmar et al. was more than that in this study; their percentage of SOTLPs cases was 3.4%. The range of patients' age in the Parmar et al. and Wright studies [2, 3] was 28-80 and 31-65 years old, respectively, whereas it was 18-28 for the current study. Histopathologically, no pearl keratin, dyskeratotic cells, and microcyst formation were observed in epithelial islands in this study unlike Parmar et al. [2]. However, absence of mitosis and presence of chronic inflammation mostly formed of lymphocytes and/or plasma cells were similar to Parmar et al. [2]. Degree of inflammation was mostly moderate to severe for Parmar et al. [2], but it was mild to moderate for this study although inflammation distribution was diffused for both. Budlike extensions and presence of rest of Malassez were observed in some samples of both studies too.

SOTLPs are rare histopathological findings [2, 4] with unknown etiology [1, 4]. However, there are different opinions on epithelial origin of SOTLPs including the following:

(I) The odontogenic epithelial remnants particularly the rest of Malassez could be proposed as an important source of such epithelial proliferations [3, 4] because of (a) the proliferative ability of these remnants which apparently had an important role in the pathogenesis of odontogenic cysts, (b) their squamous differentiation in some of the cases [4], and (c) the closeness of the cysts with SOTLPs to the root of the teeth [3]. Islands and epithelial cords with inactive appearance consistent with the rest of Malassez were observed in 1 case of this study and 4 cases reported by Parmar et al. [2] with no evidence of hyperplasia or squamous differentiation

(II) Inflammatory reactive hyperplasia of cyst lining was also mentioned as STOLPs' origin [10]. In this study, STOLPs were adjacent to the epithelial lining of cysts which became hyperplastic or desquamated and was replaced with granulation tissue. They were observed in the cases of the dentigerous cyst and OKC in the regions whose epithelial lining had neither typical morphology nor diagnostic criteria. In Wright's study, 3 of 4 dentigerous cysts had inflammation and the histopathological appearance of the epithelial lining was not typical [3]

(III) Another suggestion was hyperplasia with the form of budding in the epithelial lining of radicular cysts in response to a subsided inflammation, because these budlike extensions usually occurred in areas without inflammation and they were histopathologically similar to the squamous epithelial islands in the cyst wall [2]. However, the buddings were found in radicular cysts and OKC with/without subsided

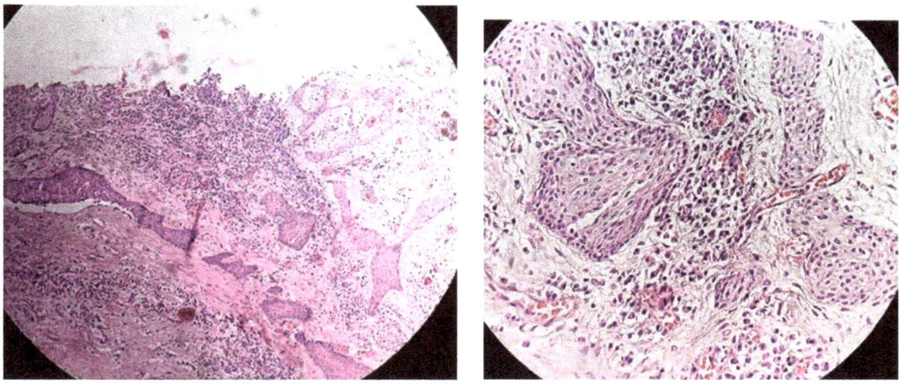

(a) (b)

Figure 2: (a) Islands of various sizes consisting of well-differentiated squamous cells with bland appearance within the connective tissue wall of the cyst; H&E, ×10. (b) Islands of various sizes consisting of well-differentiated squamous cells with bland appearance within the connective tissue wall of the cyst; H&E, ×40.

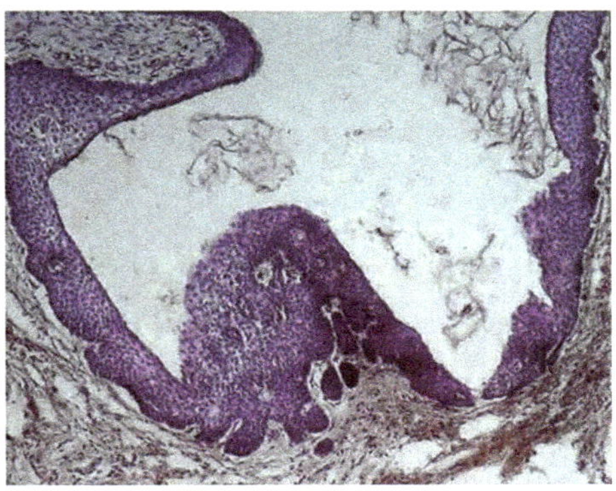

Figure 3: Budding from the epithelial lining of OKC; H&E, ×10.

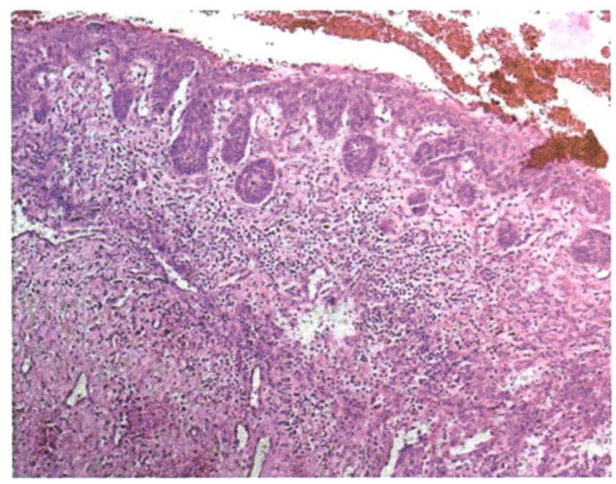

Figure 4: Budding from the epithelial lining of the radicular cyst; H&E, ×10.

inflammation in the present study. Hence, it seemed that the buddings in the epithelial lining necessarily were not a consequence of subsided inflammation

Moreover, this study found that hyperplasia and budding in the epithelial lining of the cyst might be the direct origin of SOTLPs. Even in cases where the epithelium lining was desquamated or replaced with granulation tissue, these changes seemed to have occurred in the lining after budding and separation of squamous odontogenic tumor like islands. Consequently, the source of epithelial lining of odontogenic cysts could be considered as the indirect origin of SOTLPs.

In addition to that, the role of inflammation in SOTLPs seemed to be unknown [2]. Parmar et al. [2] suggested that, due to finding SOT-like islands in inflammation-free areas, inflammation might not be the initial stimulus for SOTLPs in radicular cysts. The results also revealed the role of inflammation as the stimuli of SOTLPs although it was not considered as the only definitive cause of these proliferations since few samples were found with SOTLPs. Considering that SOTLPs were present in only four cases of primary/secondary inflammatory odontogenic cysts in this study, there might be other unknown factors influencing this phenomenon.

In fact, SOTLPs were morphologically similar to SOT although they did not seem to have any tendency to develop a solid tumor [1–3]. Like Wright's study [3], all samples of the current study had radiographically a provisional diagnosis of a cyst, and they were all cystic in terms of gross description.

Care must be taken that the overlapping histopathological features of SOTLPs, ameloblastoma (especially the acanthomatous type), and well-differentiated SCC do not lead to misdiagnosis. Ameloblastoma typically has islands with peripheral columnar ameloblast-like cells which have a clear cytoplasm and nucleus reverse polarity [2]. In this study, the peripheral cells of all islands were flat with eosinophilic cytoplasm to cuboidal basaloid with little cytoplasm. Budlike extensions off the epithelial lining of the cyst and the presence of islands of squamous cells adjacent to the lining made the lesions so similar to islands of SCC. Therefore, they could be mistaken for a primary intraosseous SCC arising in an odontogenic cyst. The SCC islands have cytologic atypia including altered nuclear cytoplasmic ratios, nuclear hyperchromatism, and mitotic activity [2]. In present study, the islands were free of any malignant features such as cellular atypia seen in SCC.

4. Conclusion

The findings of this study suggested that SOTLPs likely originated from the odontogenic cyst lining and inflammation might play a role for their development. STOLPs were considered as a rare histopathological finding, and their incidence was 2.66% in the present study. Although SOTLPs were not frequent in odontogenic cysts, their diagnosis was very important. The pathologists' lack of knowledge and their neglecting the specific features of SOTLP may lead to histopathological misinterpretation and consequently an improper treatment. As a result, the sophisticated and subtle differences of SOTLPs must be carefully understood to distinguish them from other lesions with similar appearance in order to avoid radical and unnecessary surgeries.

References

[1] S. Sala-Pérez, V. Marco-Molina, and C. Gay-Escoda, "Squamous odontogenic tumor-like proliferation in a radicular cyst: a case report," *Journal of Clinical and Experimental Dentistry*, vol. 5, no. 5, pp. e298–e301, 2013.

[2] R. M. Parmar, R. B. Brannon, and C. B. Fowler, "Squamous odontogenic tumor-like proliferations in radicular cysts: a clinicopathologic study of forty-two cases," *Journal of Endodontia*, vol. 37, no. 5, pp. 623–626, 2011.

[3] J. M. Wright Jr., "Squamous odontogenic tumorlike proliferations in odontogenic cysts," *Oral Surgery, Oral Medicine, and Oral Pathology*, vol. 47, no. 4, article 0030422079902597, pp. 354–358, 1979.

[4] J. A. G. P. Oliveira, I. M. Costa, and A. M. Loyola, "Squamous odontogenic tumor-like proliferations (SOT-LP) versus intraosseous squamous cell carcinoma in residual cyst," *Journal of Oral and Maxillofacial Surgery*, vol. 64, no. 8, p. 1325, 2006.

[5] G. Anneroth and L. S. Hansen, "Variations in keratinizing odontogenic cysts and tumors," *Oral Surgery, Oral Medicine, and Oral Pathology*, vol. 54, no. 5, pp. 530–546, 1982.

[6] D. J. Hodgkinson, J. E. Woods, D. C. Dahlin, and D. E. Tolman, "Keratocysts of the jaw. Clinicopathologic study of 79 patients," *Cancer*, vol. 41, no. 3, pp. 803–813, 1978.

[7] J. H. S. Simon and J. L. Jensen, "Proliferaciones con apariencia de tumor odontogenico escamoso en quistes periapicales," *Journal of Endodontia*, vol. 11, no. 10, pp. 446–448, 1985.

[8] T Unal, M. Gomel, and O. Gunel, "Squamous odontogenic tumor-like islands in a radicular cyst: report of a case," *Journal of Oral and Maxillofacial Surgery*, vol. 45, no. 4, pp. 346–349, 1987.

[9] G. S. Leventon, R. P. Happonen, and J. R. Newland, "Squamous odontogenic tumor," *The American Journal of Surgical Pathology*, vol. 5, no. 7, pp. 671–677, 1981.

[10] H. P. Philipsen and P. A. Reichart, "Squamous odontogenic tumor (SOT): a benign neoplasm of the periodontium. A review of 36 reported cases," *Journal of Clinical Periodontology*, vol. 23, no. 10, pp. 922–926, 1996.

34

Minimally Invasive Surgery for Clinical Crown Lengthening using Piezoelectric Ultrasound

Ana Carolina Monachini Marcantonio,[1] Guilherme José Pimentel Lopes de Oliveira,[2] Cássio Rocha Scardueli,[1] Camila Chiérici Marcantonio,[1] Rosemary Adriana Chiérici Marcantonio,[1] and Elcio Marcantonio Jr.[1]

[1]*Department of Diagnosis and Surgery, Univ. Est. Paul. - UNESP, Araraquara 14801-903, Brazil*
[2]*Department of Periodontology/Implantology, Dental School, Federal University of Uberlândia-UFU, Uberlândia 38405-266, Brazil*

Correspondence should be addressed to Elcio Marcantonio Jr.; elciojr@foar.unesp.br

Academic Editor: Kevin Seymour

This case report is aimed at describing a flapless, minimally invasive clinical crown lengthening with an osteotomy performed using a piezoelectric ultrasound. A female patient complained about the amount of gum that was exposed when she smiled, which caused aesthetic discomfort. After a clinical examination, it was confirmed that the patient had excessive gum exposure in the upper arch of the dental region for teeth 14 to 24 when she smiled. The tomographic exam showed that bone tissue was at the level of the enamel-cementum junction, and gingival tissue covered a part of the anatomic crown. Virtual analysis using digital smile design (DSD) demonstrated that enlarging the clinical crowns would provide better aesthetics. The excess gingival tissue was removed from the gingival margin region with the aid of a mockup without interference to the interdental papillae. Then, osteotomy was performed using piezoelectric ultrasound until there was a 2.5 mm distance from the top of the bone crest to the new gingival margin. In the postoperative period, good repositioning of the gingival margin, absence of postoperative complications, and rapid healing of the gingival tissue were verified. After 6 months, a good aesthetic outcome was observed with stability in the level of the periodontal tissues obtained via the crown-lengthening technique. It can be concluded that the minimally invasive clinical crown-lengthening technique was effective in repositioning the gingival margin with no postoperative complications.

1. Introduction

The use of minimally invasive surgical techniques has been a trend in medicine and dentistry because they result in good clinical outcomes with minimal complications during the postoperative phase [1, 2]. Using minimally invasive surgical techniques has been related to reduced postoperative discomfort [3], reduced consumption of analgesic and anti-inflammatory drugs [4], reduced length of hospitalization, and, consequently, reduced time required to return to normal activities [4]. Thus, although the use of the new technologies may increase the cost of the surgical procedure, the patient's earlier return to normal life may generate benefits that makes the procedure more cost effective than if conventional surgical techniques are applied [5].

Specifically, in the dentistry field, efforts have been made to develop minimally invasive surgical techniques, such as the use of a surgical microscope [6], computed tomographic-guided surgeries [7], and the use of planning software, such as digital smile design (DSD), that assist in predicting the tissue to be excised for patient's oral rehabilitation [8]. The use of these technologies has promoted advances in minimally invasive techniques, such as the development of ultraconservative flaps with minimal detachment [9]. Minimally invasive surgical techniques have been indicated for the harvest of intraoral bone grafts [10], coverage of gingival recessions with subepithelial connective tissue grafts [6], treatment of periodontal bone defects [2], and immediate implant placement [11] with high levels of success and reduced patient morbidity.

One of the possible indications for the use of minimally invasive surgery is anterior crown lengthening indicated due to passive eruption disturbances. In this condition, the top of the bony crest is close to the cementum-enamel junction, and simply removing the gingival tissue is not sufficient to predictably expose the clinical crown over long follow-up periods [12, 13]. Indeed, a previous study described a minimally invasive technique for clinical crown lengthening with or without the aid of a microscope, showing that the flapless technique and osteotomy with a microchisel was as effective as the use of the open-flap technique promoting less side effects [12]. The osteotomy procedure can alternatively be performed with a piezoelectric ultrasound [14, 15]. This type of tool has the potential to remove the bone tissue without causing damage to the root surface and soft tissue and may be the most suitable for crown-lengthening surgical procedures that use a flapless technique during osteotomy.

Thus, the objective of this case report was to present a minimally invasive crown-lengthening technique with papilla preservation and an osteotomy performed by piezoelectric ultrasound.

2. Case Presentation

A 22-year-old female patient complained about the amount of gingiva that was exposed when she smiled, which caused aesthetic discomfort for the patient. In the anamnesis, the patient reported not having any systemic problems, not continuously using any medication, and not being a smoker. A clinical examination confirmed the presence of an excessive exposure of the gingiva in the upper arch of teeth 14 to 24 (Figure 1(a)). The periodontal examination, which consisted of an analysis of gingival marginal bleeding, bleeding on probing, periodontal probing depth, and gingival margin position using a millimeter probe, confirmed that the periodontal tissues were in a healthy condition. In addition, conical beam tomography with an oral retractor was ordered to evaluate the bone and gingival tissue associated with the upper anterior teeth, and molding and photographs were also ordered.

The tomography showed that the bone tissue was at the level of the enamel-cementum junction and that the gingival tissue covered part of the anatomic crown (Figure 1(b)). Virtual planning was also performed using DSD, which showed the need to increase the size of the clinical crowns for better aesthetics (Figure 1(c)). With these data, it was shown that the patient suffered from altered passive eruption and, therefore, would need an osteotomy to enlarge the clinical crown. After this diagnosis, a flapless, minimally invasive surgical technique with piezoelectric ultrasound to perform the osteotomy and a mockup to guide the removal of soft tissue was proposed for the patient.

Surgical planning was performed by DSD with the patient's smile photos and crown measurements using an 80% width to length ratio. After design of the optimal teeth, the distance from the cementum-enamel junction to the top of the bone crest and the position of the gingival margin in relation to the enamel-cementum junction was measured by tomographic analysis (Figure 2(a)). These measures were used as a reference for the wax model and mockup (Figure 2(b)). In addition, these measurements were used with tomography to plan the amount of osteotomy needed to maintain the biological space without recurrence of coronary covering by the gingival tissue.

With the mockup in position, the projection of what the gingival condition would look like after the surgical procedure was shown to the patient. After patient approval, the clinical crown-lengthening procedure was performed; this procedure consisted of marking the soft tissue height to be removed (Figure 3(a)) and a sulcular incision to allow the removal of a gingival collar at the buccal face around all anterior and upper teeth without interfering with the interproximal region.

After removing the gingival collar, the need for bone tissue removal due to the proximity of the new gingival margin was detected, since the bone tissue was practically at the level of the enamel-cementum junction (Figure 3(b)). A flapless osteotomy procedure was performed at the buccal bone with the aid of a piezoelectric ultrasound that induces bone tissue wear by ultrasonic vibrations (Figure 3(c)). According to the treatment plan, approximately 2.5 mm of bone was removed around all of the upper anterior teeth. Osteotomy was performed with minimal invasiveness, cutting only the bone tissue without causing damage to the root surface (Figure 3(d)).

Then, the osteotomy height was confirmed by probing (Figure 3(d)), with the immediate results demonstrating an increase in the clinical crown length with minimal soft tissue trauma (Figure 3(e)). After 6 months, a good aesthetic result was observed with stability in the results obtained in the clinical crown-lengthening technique (Figure 3(f)). Figure 4 shows the initial condition (Figure 4(a)) and final clinical condition 14 days after the surgical procedure (Figure 4(b)).

3. Discussion

This case report shows a flapless, minimally invasive clinical crown-lengthening technique and osteotomy performed with piezoelectric ultrasound with a good clinical outcome; it was possible to correct the altered passive eruption with no complications in the postoperative period.

Altered passive eruptions are one of the main indications for clinical crown-lengthening procedures [12]. In these cases, the margin of the bone tissue does not normally migrate apically after the establishment of dental occlusion, which results in an excessive covering of the clinical crown [13] and causes discomfort to the patients regarding the aesthetics of the upper teeth. Usually, the treatment of this type of condition is indicated in cases where there is presence of thick gingival phenotypes associated with a keratinized gingival width higher than 2 mm [12]; however, the occurrence of root exposure or return of the gingival margin in an excessive coronal position after the treatment are possible findings that should be carefully evaluated during the follow-up visits.

The conventional surgical procedure in these cases would be to remove excess gingival margin tissue with a flap detachment and osteotomy until the establishment of biological distances; however, because it is sometimes necessary to open the flaps and because the osteotomy is a more intense dental

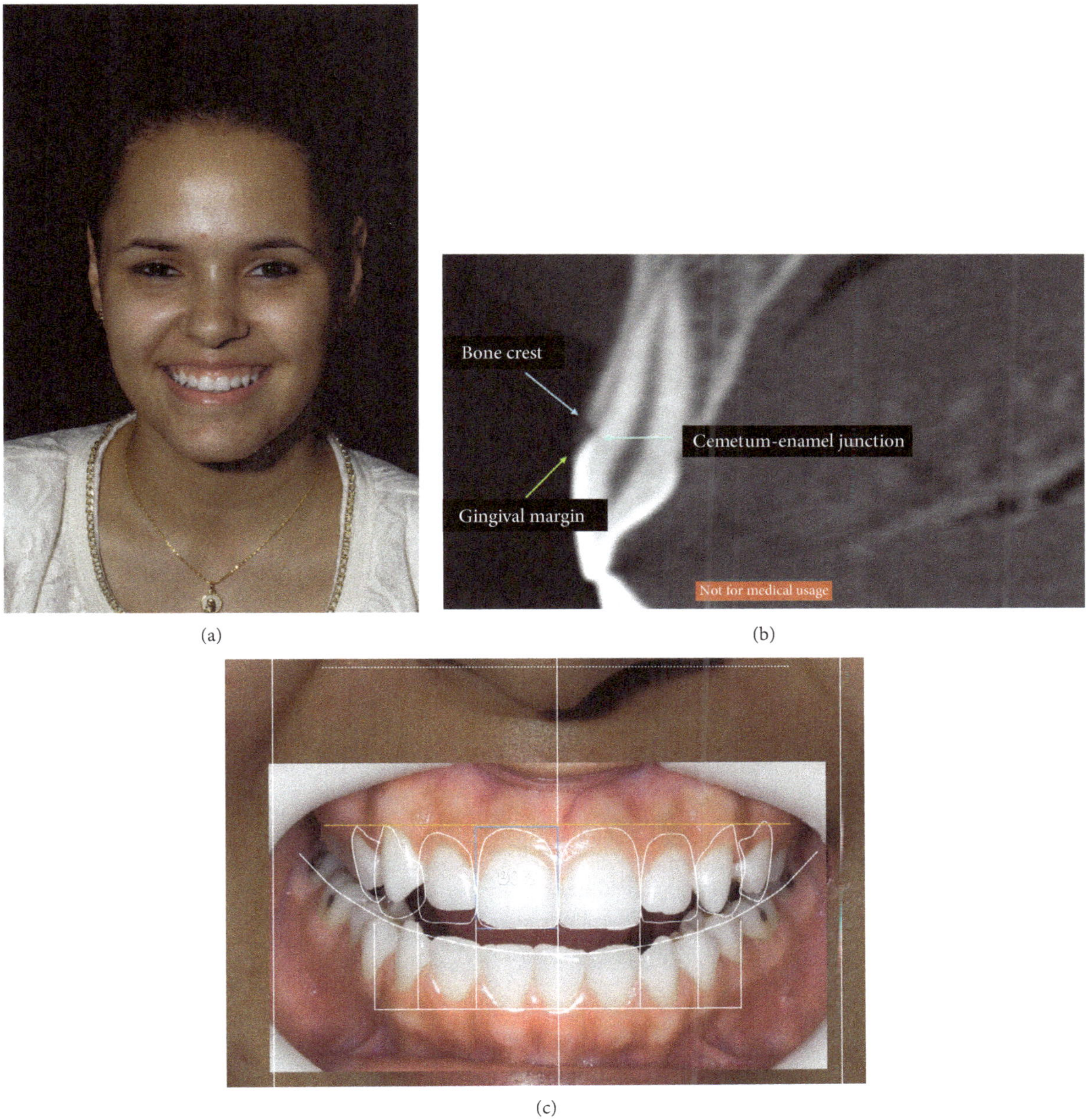

FIGURE 1: Initial diagnosis. (a) Initial condition of the patient where it is possible to observe a large gingival exposure when smiling. (b) Tomographic analysis showing that the top of the bone crest was practically at the level of the enamel-cementum junction. (c) DSD planning that showed the need to increase the length of the clinical crowns for better aesthetics.

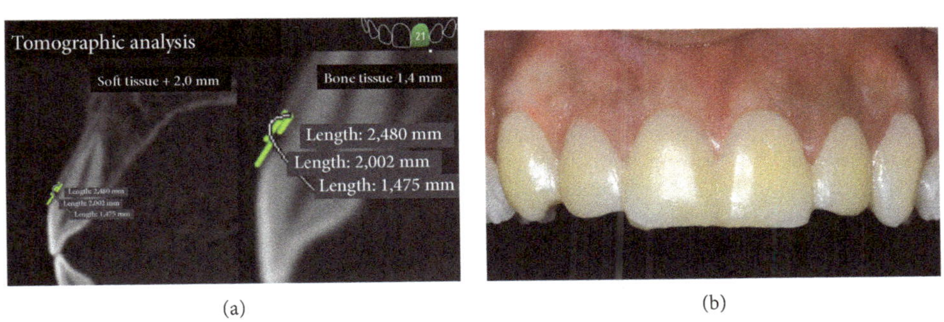

FIGURE 2: Planning the osteotomy and mockup. (a) Tomographic planning shows where the bone and gingival tissue should be removed. (b) Mockup in position that served as a guide for the removal of soft tissue from the gingival margin.

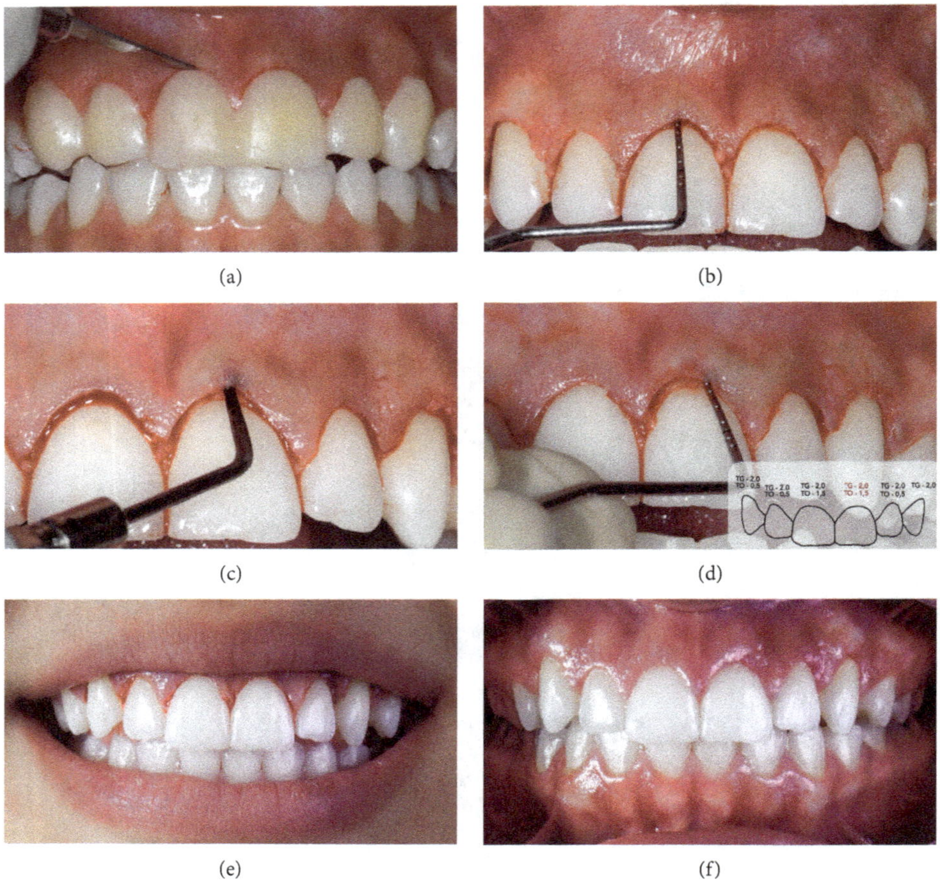

FIGURE 3: Surgical procedure. (a) Initial incision with the aid of a mockup that was used as a guide for gingival tissue removal. (b) During the probing procedure, it was verified that the distance from the gingival margin to the top of the bone crest was 1 mm, which meant that the osteotomy procedure was necessary. (c) Osteotomy was performed with piezoelectric ultrasound without flap elevation and without interference in the interdental papillae. (d) The procedure removed 1 mm of bone tissue to restore the biological space, taking into account the thin gingival phenotype presented in the patient. (e) Immediate postoperative situation where it is possible to perceive a minimally traumatic clinical condition. (f) The good postoperative condition observed 6 months after the surgical procedure: the periodontal tissue was completely healed.

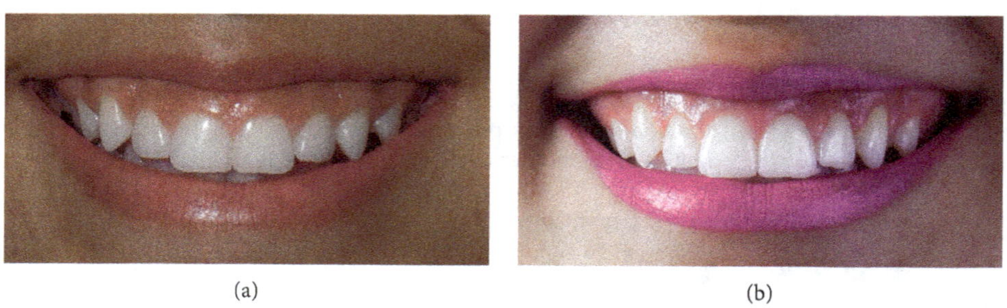

FIGURE 4: Clinical condition. (a) Before the surgical procedure. (b) Fourteen days after the surgical procedure. It is observed that the applied surgical technique promoted adequate increase in the clinical crown of the teeth and rapid recovery of periodontal tissues during the postoperative phase.

procedure, undesirable side effects, such as bleeding, inflammation, and postoperative pain, are expected [12, 13]. Thus, using a minimally invasive procedure for this type of surgical technique could have great benefits for the postoperative recovery of these patients.

The surgical technique applied in this study was based on DSD planning that allowed the production of a mockup that guided the amount of soft tissue to be removed in the primary incision [8]. For this aim, it was necessary to obtain a CT scan that allowed planning for the amount of soft tissue and bone tissue that should be removed during the surgical procedure. In addition, through the initial photographs, the original size of the teeth was predicted to assess the golden proportions [8]. The use of DSD allowed minimal removal of the soft tissue at the gingival margins without the interference of the interproximal tissue, keeping the flap closed throughout the surgical procedure.

Another important technical detail of the surgical technique was that the osteotomy procedure was performed with piezoelectric ultrasound. Hand and rotary instruments are traditionally used to perform osteotomies [10, 14, 16]; however, the flapless technique causes difficulties in the use of these traditional instruments. Rotary instruments for osteotomy procedures have been the treatment of choice in different clinical applications; however, the use of these instruments has been related to thermal damage that may alter bone tissue stability after the surgical procedure [17]. Furthermore, the use of rotatory instruments with a flapless technique may induce lesions in the soft tissues and on the root surfaces [12]. A piezoelectric ultrasound has been shown to have good efficacy in the osteotomy procedure with minimal thermal damage and reduced possibility of soft tissue and root surface injury [3, 10]. In addition, it has also been shown that sites where an osteotomy was performed with piezoelectric ultrasound have lower expressions of biological mediators of osteoclastogenesis and inflammation such as RANKL [15] and IL-1β [3], which may allow better postoperative outcomes for the patient. A limitation regarding the use of the piezoelectric ultrasound is that there is a longer clinical time required for the osteotomy procedure than the time required for osteotomies performed with rotary instruments [10, 18]; however, since the use of piezoelectric ultrasound allows for osteotomies with a flapless technique, the suture procedure is not necessary and the surgical time may be compensated for when compared to rotary instruments.

4. Conclusion

It can be concluded that using a minimally invasive clinical crown-lengthening technique was effective in repositioning the gingival margin when used with an osteotomy and presented no postoperative complications. However, randomized controlled clinical trials, with longer periods of follow-up, should be conducted to compare the effectiveness of this minimally invasive technique compared to those traditionally used for clinical crown-lengthening procedures in altered passive eruption disorders.

References

[1] P. Cortellini and M. S. Tonetti, "Improved wound stability with a modified minimally invasive surgical technique in the regenerative treatment of isolated interdental intrabony defects," *Journal of Clinical Periodontology*, vol. 36, no. 2, pp. 157–163, 2009.

[2] M. Aimetti, F. Ferrarotti, G. M. Mariani, and F. Romano, "A novel flapless approach versus minimally invasive surgery in periodontal regeneration with enamel matrix derivative proteins: a 24-month randomized controlled clinical trial," *Clinical Oral Investigations*, vol. 21, no. 1, pp. 327–337, 2017.

[3] M. Aimetti, F. Ferrarotti, L. Bergandi, L. Saksing, F. Parducci, and F. Romano, "Increase in periodontal interleukin-1β gene expression following osseous resective surgery using conventional rotary instruments compared with piezosurgery: a split-mouth randomized clinical trial," *International Journal of Periodontics and Restorative Dentistry*, vol. 36, no. 4, pp. 489–496, 2016.

[4] S. Sharma, L. F. Schneider, J. Barr et al., "Comparison of minimally invasive versus conventional open harvesting techniques for iliac bone graft in secondary alveolar cleft patients," *Plastic and Reconstructive Surgery*, vol. 128, no. 2, pp. 485–491, 2011.

[5] S. Vertuani, J. Nilsson, B. Borgman et al., "A cost-effectiveness analysis of minimally invasive versus open surgery techniques for lumbar spinal fusion in Italy and the United Kingdom," *Value in Health*, vol. 18, no. 6, pp. 810–816, 2015.

[6] S. Bittencourt, E. Del Peloso Ribeiro, E. A. Sallum, F. H. Nociti Jr., and M. Z. Casati, "Surgical microscope may enhance root coverage with subepithelial connective tissue graft: a randomized-controlled clinical trial," *Journal of Periodontology*, vol. 83, no. 6, pp. 721–730, 2012.

[7] R. A. Landázuri-Del Barrio, J. Cosyn, W. N. De Paula, H. De Bruyn, and E. Marcantonio Jr., "A prospective study on implants installed with flapless-guided surgery using the all-on-four concept in the mandible," *Clinical Oral Implants Research*, vol. 24, no. 4, pp. 428–433, 2013.

[8] C. Coachman, M. A. Calamita, and N. Sesma, "Dynamic documentation of the smile and the 2D/3D digital smile design process," *International Journal of Periodontics and Restorative Dentistry*, vol. 37, no. 2, pp. 183–193, 2017.

[9] F. V. Ribeiro, R. C. Casarin, M. A. Palma, F. H. Júnior, E. A. Sallum, and M. Z. Casati, "Clinical and patient-centered outcomes after minimally invasive non-surgical or surgical approaches for the treatment of intrabony defects: a randomized clinical trial," *Journal of Periodontology*, vol. 82, no. 9, pp. 1256–1266, 2011.

[10] T. Hanser and R. Doliveux, "MicroSaw and piezosurgery in harvesting mandibular bone blocks from the retromolar region: a randomized split-mouth prospective clinical trial," *The International Journal of Oral & Maxillofacial Implants*, vol. 33, no. 2, pp. 365–372, 2018.

[11] M. Tallarico, M. Esposito, E. Xhanari, M. Caneva, and S. M. Meloni, "Computer-guided vs freehand placement of immediately loaded dental implants: 5-year postloading results of a randomised controlled trial," *European Journal of Oral Implantology*, vol. 11, no. 2, pp. 203–213, 2018.

[12] F. V. Ribeiro, D. Y. Hirata, A. F. Reis et al., "Open-flap versus flapless esthetic crown lengthening: 12-month clinical outcomes of a randomized controlled clinical trial," *Journal of Periodontology*, vol. 85, no. 4, pp. 536–544, 2014.

[13] G. Zucchelli, P. Sharma, and I. Mounssif, "Esthetics in periodontics and implantology," *Periodontology 2000*, vol. 77, no. 1, pp. 7–18, 2018.

[14] J. C. Esteves, E. Marcantonio Jr., A. P. de Souza Faloni et al., "Dynamics of bone healing after osteotomy with piezosurgery or conventional drilling– histomorphometrical,

immunohistochemical, and molecular analysis," *Journal of Translational Medicine*, vol. 23, no. 11, article 211, 2013.

[15] G. Peker Tekdal, N. Bostanci, G. N. Belibasakis, and A. Gürkan, "The effect of piezoelectric surgery implant osteotomy on radiological and molecular parameters of peri-implant crestal bone loss: a randomized, controlled, split-mouth trial," *Clinical Oral Implants Research*, vol. 27, no. 5, pp. 535–544, 2016.

[16] K. Fugito Junior, A. R. Cortes, R. de Carvalho Destro, and M. Yoshimoto, "Comparative study on the cutting effectiveness and heat generation of rotary instruments versus piezoelectric surgery tips using scanning electron microscopy and thermal analysis," *International Journal of Oral & Maxillofacial Implants*, vol. 33, no. 2, pp. 345–350, 2018.

[17] L. Canullo, D. Peñarrocha, M. Peñarrocha, A. G. Rocio, and M. Penarrocha-Diago, "Piezoelectric vs. conventional drilling in implant site preparation: pilot controlled randomized clinical trial with crossover design," *Clinical Oral Implants Research*, vol. 25, no. 12, pp. 1336–1343, 2014.

[18] C. Stacchi, T. Vercellotti, L. Torelli, F. Furlan, and R. Di Lenarda, "Changes in implant stability using different site preparation techniques: twist drills versus piezosurgery. A single-blinded, randomized, controlled clinical trial," *Clinical Implant Dentistry and Related Research*, vol. 15, no. 2, pp. 188–197, 2013.

35

Orthognathic Surgery after Mandibular Large-Volume Osteoma Treatment

Sabit Demircan, [1] **Sabri Cemil İşler**, [2] **Aydın Gümüşdal**, [2] **and Begüm Genç** [2]

[1] *Private Practice, Beykent University Vocational School, Turkey*
[2] *Istanbul University Faculty of Dentistry Oral and Maxillofacial Surgery Department, Turkey*

Correspondence should be addressed to Sabit Demircan; sabitdemircan@hotmail.com

Academic Editor: Gianrico Spagnuolo

Osteoma is a benign asymptomatic osseous tumor. Characterization of osteoma is the proliferation of cancellous or compact bone that increases in size by continuous formation of bone. It can be seen in any craniofacial structures, usually in paranasal sinuses and jaws. In this study, we present a 17-year-old male patient with a giant osteoma in the mandibular condyle. Posttreatment post-op follow-up, post-ortho, and orthognathic surgery after dental implantation are described.

1. Introduction

Osteoma is a benign osseous tumor arising from the proliferation of cancellous or compact bone that increases in size by continuous formation of bone. It is a slow-growing, asymptomatic, and usually solitary lesion which mainly affects young adults [1, 2].

Osteomas can be central, peripheral, or extraskeletal. Central osteomas arise from the endosteum, and a peripheral osteoma from the periosteum and extraskeletal soft-tissue osteomas usually develops within the muscle [2]. The cause of slow-growing osteomas is obscure, but the tumor may arise from cartilage or osseous periosteum; whether osteomas are benign neoplasm or hamartomas is not known [3]. Osteoma occurring in either the condyle or the condylar process may result in morphologic and functional disturbances, including facial asymmetry and temporomandibular joint dysfunction [4].

There are several treatment methods for osteomas. Usually, osteomas are asymptomatic, and leaving them alone is an option. Routine radiographic controls would be enough in these cases and osteomas might fade away. In some other cases, patients might have some symptoms or asymmetry, then nonsteroidal anti-inflammatory drugs (NSAIDs) support, curettage, radiofrequency ablation, or surgical treatment can be applied [5].

In this study, we present a 17-year-old male patient with a giant osteoma in the mandibular condyle. Posttreatment post-op follow-up, post-ortho, and orthognathic surgery after dental implantation are described.

2. Case Report

A systemically healthy male patient, 17 years old, with a prominent large swelling at the left mandibular ramus area leading to facial asymmetry which had developed over the previous 4 years, had referred to the Istanbul University, Faculty of Dentistry, Department of Oral and Maxillofacial Surgery. The swelling was not painful and no orofacial infection signs were reported. The patient had a history of head trauma due to falling off from a tree at the age of 6.

On extraoral examination, a hard, subcutaneous, multinodular, and painless mass of the complete left mandibular ramus was present. Deviation of the mandible to the right during mouth-opening and the protrusion are detected. During intraoral examination, there were no signs of pathology at the left mandible or the mandibular ramus area. With the radiological examination, the panoramic radiograph showed a large lobulated radiodense mass in the left mandibular ramus area and it also appeared to have a retromandibular partition (Figure 1). These findings were suggestive of a calcified odontogenic tumor affecting the

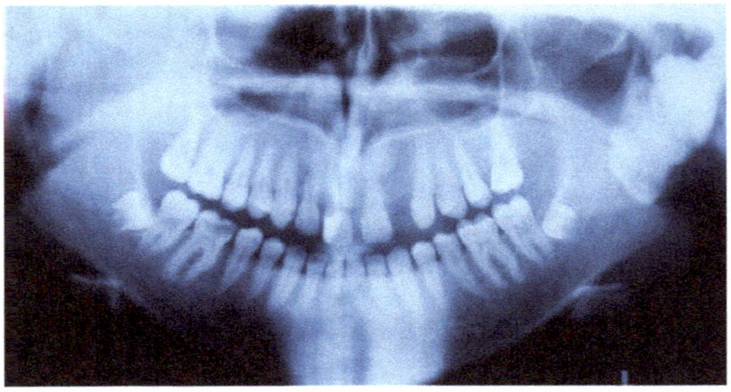

FIGURE 1: The initial panoramic radiograph of the patient.

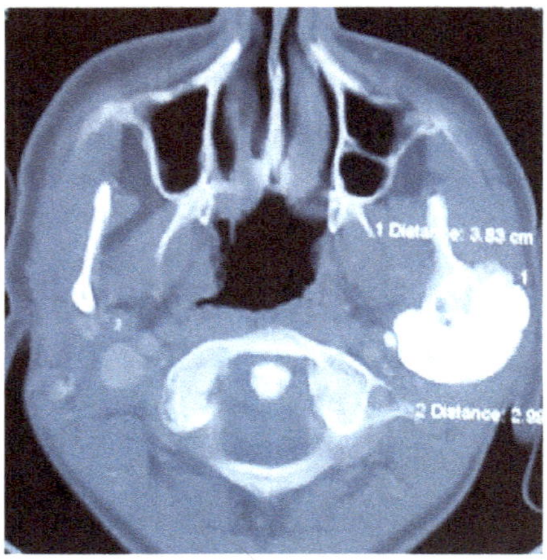

FIGURE 2: The initial CBCT of the patient.

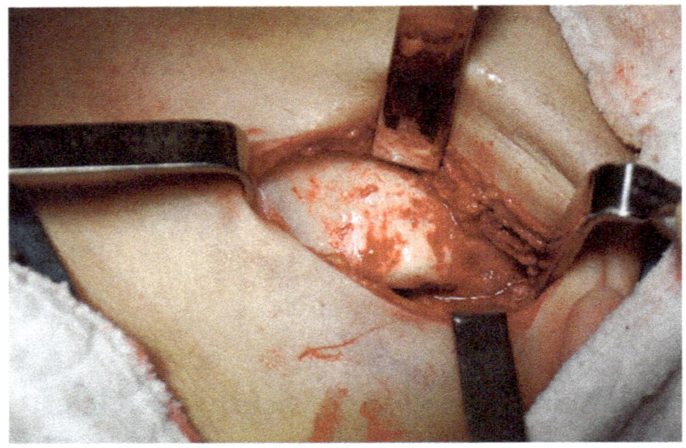

FIGURE 3: Extraoral approach to the lesion.

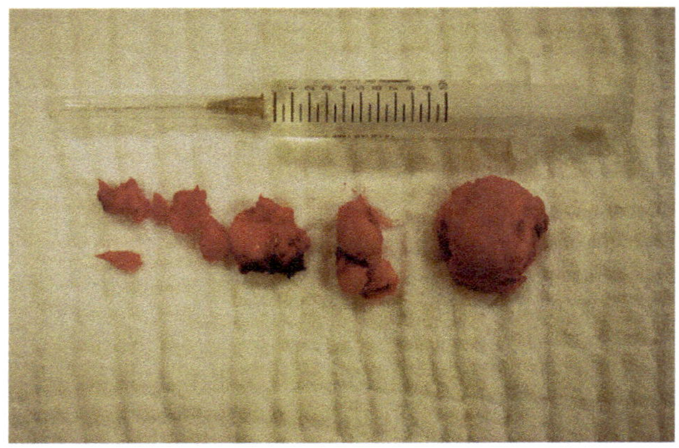

FIGURE 4: The removed lesions.

jaw bone requiring a segmental or block resection. For further evaluation of the character and extent of the mass, Cone Beam Computed Tomography (CBCT) was performed. The CBCT scan showed a diffuse enlargement measuring 4.5 × 3.5 × 3 cm in the entire left mandibular ramus extending anteriorly to the mastoid process of the parietal bone (Figure 2). Because of the actual dysphagia, the facial asymmetry, and the progression of the lesion, it was decided to perform an operative correction to the left mandible. Under general anesthesia with nasoendotracheal intubation, the mandible was approached extraorally. 6 ml of 1/100000 adrenaline containing articaine HCl was injected to control the local hemorrhage. Using a fissure bur and a chisel, the lobular part of the lateral and medial side of the ascending ramus were resected and the mandible was reshaped (Figures 3 and 4). Besides this, healing was uneventful. Postoperative follow-up in the 6th month with dental volumetric tomography scans showed no evidence of pathology with an acceptable mandibular contour. In the next 5 years follow-up, there was no recurrence.

The patient also had class III skeletal malocclusion. After cephalometric analysis and malocclusion of the skeletal class III of the patient were detected, orthodontic treatment started. Following the initial treatment, the patient's wisdom teeth were extracted. The patient was made ready for orthognathic surgery.

7 years after the osteoma surgery, orthognathic surgery was performed. The bone at the left mandibular ramus area was fully regenerated and healthy. By performing two separate surgical operations instead of one operation, a possible bad split was avoided. Patient's age became proper for the surgery and the patient went through orthodontic treatment before the surgery. Two separate surgeries were comfortable for the patient. The only disadvantage of the separate surgeries was expensiveness of the treatment process.

Maxilla Le Fort I osteotomy was performed with 3 mm anterior and 4 mm right, and mandibular bilateral sagittal split osteotomy was performed and 1 mm back and 2 mm left was taken (Figures 5–7). At the end of the first year following the operation, the patient's existing tooth deficiencies were rehabilitated by applying a dental implant (Figure 8).

3. Discussion

There is a very little understanding about the nature of osteomas, and three theories have been proposed: developmental, neoplastic, and reactive. It is unlikely that osteomas are a developmental anomaly, as most cases occur in adults and not during childhood or adolescence [3, 6]. It is also unlikely that osteomas are of a neoplastic nature, because of their very slow growth rate. The possibility of osteomas being a reactive lesion possibly resulting from local trauma is based on the

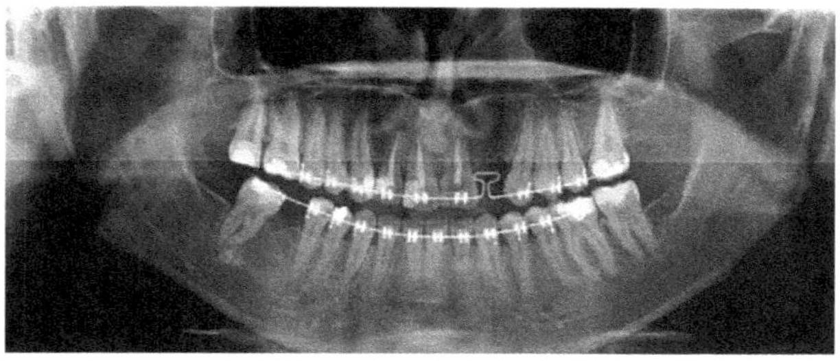

FIGURE 5: Panoramic radiograph of the patient before the orthognathic surgery.

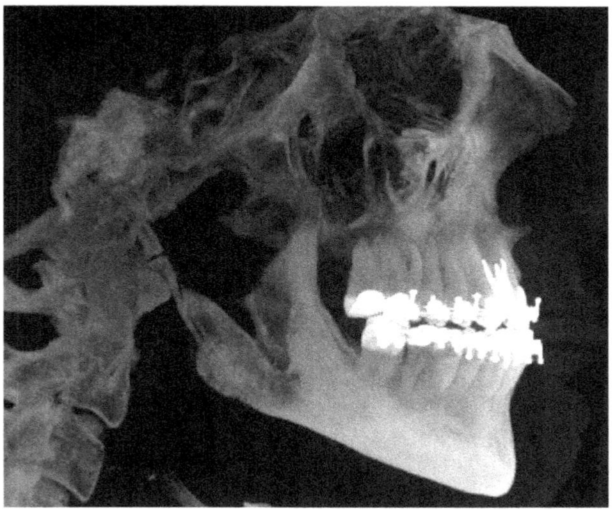

FIGURE 6: 3D view of the patient before the orthognathic surgery.

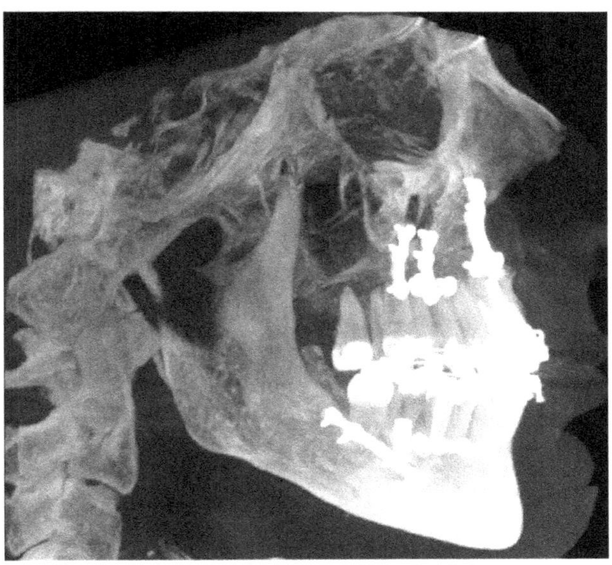

FIGURE 7: 3D view of the patient after the orthognathic surgery.

history of trauma prior for the development of the lesion in some cases. However, this can be considered only in sites that are more susceptible to trauma, such as the angle or lower border of the mandible, but not in most of the cases. As many

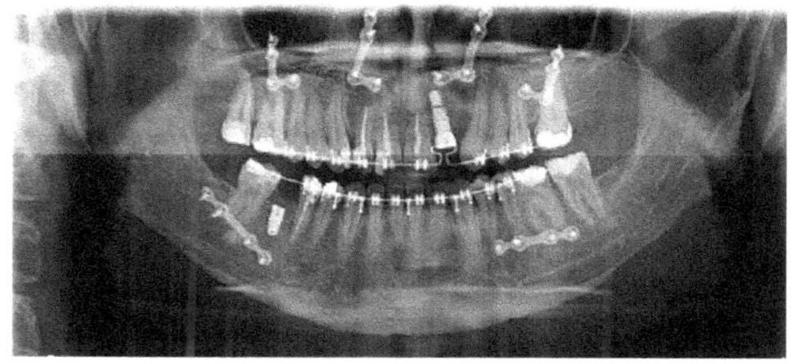

FIGURE 8: The panoramic radiograph of the patient after the implant surgery.

of the PO lesions are located in close proximity to muscle attachment (i.e., masseter, medial pterygoid, and temporalis), it is possible that muscle traction may play a role in the development of the PO [7]. The combination of trauma and muscle traction was also considered as a possible mechanism of the pathogenesis of osteomas [8, 9]. An accidental fall off a tree in the patient's history should have been considered as an etiology for this case.

Peripheral osteomas are uncommon. Clinically, the peripheral osteomas are usually asymptomatic slow-growing lesions which can produce swelling and asymmetry. The pathogenesis of peripheral osteomas is unclear [8, 10]. In the present case, the lesion was diagnosed at the age of 13. It has taken 4 years for the lesion to grow to this volume in accordance with the slow-growing characteristic.

Osteomas of the condyle may cause a slow progressive shift in occlusion with deviation of the midline of the chin towards the unaffected side and also lead to acute pain, limited mouth-opening, and malocclusion such as cross-bite [11]. Difficulties in swallowing and facial asymmetry were major complaints of the patient at the time of referral to our clinic, slow shifting of mandible to the right side was a symptom leading us to diagnose.

On radiological imaging, osteomas are well-defined radiopaque masses with distinct borders [12]. Osteomas composed solely of compact bone are uniformly opaque, while those containing cancellous bone show evidence of an internal trabecular structure [13]. They are smooth surfaced with a thin sclerotic rim. Imaging of osteomas can be achieved by traditional radiography (i.e., panoramic radiograph and Water's view) or by CT scan. The use of CT scanning with 3-D reconstruction makes it possible to achieve a better resolution and more precise localization [14, 15].

Removal of osteomas is not generally necessary. Surgery is indicated only when the lesion is symptomatic or actively growing [16, 17]. In our opinion, the surgical approach should be specific for cases. For the mandible, there are intraoral or extraoral approaches. The intraoral approach is preferable when possible, mainly for esthetic reasons [9].

During the initial few hours after general anesthesia, a temporary facial paralysis was observed due to the applied local anesthesia during the operation. This should not be misdiagnosed as a permanent facial paralysis [18].

In this case, in addition to a giant osteoma, there was also class III skeletal malocclusion. The osteoma should be removed because it caused asymmetry, and the malocculusion should be fixed by orthognathic surgery. The osteoma was very massive, and bone of the left mandibular ramus region was weak after osteoma removal. After waiting 7 years, the orthognathic surgery was performed. The separate surgeries were necessary to minimise risk of complications. With a separate surgery, bad split was avoided. The orthognathic surgery was comfortable for the patient and the surgeons. Expectedly, difficulty of elevation of the soft tissues was diagnosed. The bone of the left mandibular ramus region was totally regenerated and healthy. Performing a second surgery did not affect the degree of difficulty of the bilateral sagittal split osteotomy.

4. Conclusion

Osteomas are slowly growing pathological osseous structures; possible localizations are central, peripheral parts of bones or extraskeletaly, mostly in muscles. Osteomas in the mandibular region can cause problems such as deviation of mandible and limitation of masticator function. Treatment options vary depending on the degree of the asymmetry and functional disorders and the location and size of the lesion. Surgical approaches like blocking or total resection and corrective surgery of the lesions' contour should be considered when the "wait and see" option is inefficacious. Surgical approaches also have to be supported with histological findings. Recurrence or progress of the lesion should be examined with intermittent controls. If it is confirmed, the continuation of the dental treatment is recommended.

References

[1] J. C. M. A. Mancini, M. Woltmann, V. B. Felix, and R. R. Freitas, "Peripheral osteoma of the mandibular condyle," *International Journal of Oral and Maxillofacial Surgery*, vol. 34, no. 1, pp. 92-93, 2005.

[2] S. Tochihara, T. Sato, H. Yamamoto, K. Asada, and K. Ishibashi, "Osteoid osteoma in mandibular condyle," *International Journal of Oral and Maxillofacial Surgery*, vol. 30, no. 5, pp. 455–457, 2001.

[3] I. Kaplan, Z. Nicolaou, D. Hatuel, and S. Calderon, "Solitary central osteoma of the jaws: a diagnostic dilemma," *Oral Surgery, Oral Medicine, Oral Pathology, Oral Radiology, and Endodontics*, vol. 106, no. 3, pp. e22–e29, 2008.

[4] C. H. Siar, A. A. Jalil, S. Ram, and K. H. Ng, "Osteoma of the condyle as the cause of limited-mouth opening: a case report," *Journal of Oral Science*, vol. 46, no. 1, pp. 51–53, 2004.

[5] C. P. Cantwell, J. Obyrne, and S. Eustace, "Current trends in treatment of osteoid osteoma with an emphasis on radiofrequency ablation," *European Radiology*, vol. 14, no. 4, pp. 607–617, 2004.

[6] D. Schulze, "Radiographic diagnostics: osteoma of the left mandibular notch," *Quintessence International*, vol. 39, no. 8, pp. 702-703, 2008.

[7] A. Kerckhaert, E. Wolvius, K. V. D. Wal, and J. W. Oosterhuis, "A giant osteoma of the mandible: case report," *Journal of Cranio-Maxillo-Facial Surgery*, vol. 33, no. 4, pp. 282–285, 2005.

[8] S. K. Shetty and L. Biddappa, "Recurrence of a giant peripheral osteoma of mandible," *Journal of Maxillofacial and Oral Surgery*, vol. 14, no. S1, pp. 452–456, 2015.

[9] P. Gawande, V. Deshmukh, and J. B. Garde, "A giant osteoma of the mandible," *Journal of Maxillofacial and Oral Surgery*, vol. 14, no. 2, pp. 460–465, 2015.

[10] R. Agrawal, S. Agrawal, S. Bhargava, M. Motlani, and R. Agrawal, "An uncommon case of solitary peripheral osteoma in the mandible," *Case Reports in Dentistry*, vol. 2015, Article ID 319738, 4 pages, 2015.

[11] G. Bhatt, S. Gupta, S. Ghosh, S. Mohanty, and P. Kumar, "Central osteoma of maxilla associated with an impacted tooth: report of a rare case with literature review," *Head and Neck Pathology*, vol. 13, no. 4, pp. 554–561, 2018.

[12] W. R. Proffit, T. A. Turvey, and C. Phillips, "The hierarchy of stability and predictability in orthognathic surgery with rigid fixation: an update and extension," *Head & Face Medicine*, vol. 3, no. 1, p. 21, 2007.

[13] D. Blinder, M. Peleg, and S. Taicher, "Surgical considerations in cases of large mandibular odontomas located in the mandibular angle," *Intenational Journal of Oral & Maxillofacial Surgery*, vol. 22, no. 3, pp. 163–165, 1993.

[14] P. J. Christopher, S. Periasamy, P. Devadoss, and S. P. Kumar, "Surgical access to a complex composite odontoma via sagittal split osteotomy of the mandible," *Cureus*, vol. 9, no. 12, article 1915, 2017.

[15] G. Mensink, J. P. Verweij, P. J. J. Gooris, and M. JPRV, "Bilateral sagittal split osteotomy in a mandible previously reconstructed with a non-vascularized bone graft," *Intenational Journal of Oral & Maxitlofacial Surgery*, vol. 42, no. 7, pp. 830–834, 2013.

[16] G. B. Wong, "Surgical management of a large, complex mandibular odontoma by unilateral sagittal split osteotomy," *Journal of Oral and Maxillofacial Surgery*, vol. 47, no. 2, pp. 179–182, 1989.

[17] W. Zhang, B. Li, H. Gui, L. Zhang, X. Wang, and G. Shen, "Reconstruction of complex mandibular defect with computer-aided navigation and orthognathic surgery," *Journal of Craniofacial Surgery*, vol. 24, no. 3, pp. e229–e233, 2013.

[18] S. Rao, S. Rao, and D. S. R. Pramod, "Transoral removal of peripheral osteoma at sigmoid notch of the mandible," *Journal of Maxillofacial and Oral Surgery*, vol. 14, no. S1, pp. 255–257, 2015.

Permissions

All chapters in this book were first published by Hindawi Publishing Corporation; hereby published with permission under the Creative Commons Attribution License or equivalent. Every chapter published in this book has been scrutinized by our experts. Their significance has been extensively debated. The topics covered herein carry significant findings which will fuel the growth of the discipline. They may even be implemented as practical applications or may be referred to as a beginning point for another development.

The contributors of this book come from diverse backgrounds, making this book a truly international effort. This book will bring forth new frontiers with its revolutionizing research information and detailed analysis of the nascent developments around the world.

We would like to thank all the contributing authors for lending their expertise to make the book truly unique. They have played a crucial role in the development of this book. Without their invaluable contributions this book wouldn't have been possible. They have made vital efforts to compile up to date information on the varied aspects of this subject to make this book a valuable addition to the collection of many professionals and students.

This book was conceptualized with the vision of imparting up-to-date information and advanced data in this field. To ensure the same, a matchless editorial board was set up. Every individual on the board went through rigorous rounds of assessment to prove their worth. After which they invested a large part of their time researching and compiling the most relevant data for our readers.

The editorial board has been involved in producing this book since its inception. They have spent rigorous hours researching and exploring the diverse topics which have resulted in the successful publishing of this book. They have passed on their knowledge of decades through this book. To expedite this challenging task, the publisher supported the team at every step. A small team of assistant editors was also appointed to further simplify the editing procedure and attain best results for the readers.

Apart from the editorial board, the designing team has also invested a significant amount of their time in understanding the subject and creating the most relevant covers. They scrutinized every image to scout for the most suitable representation of the subject and create an appropriate cover for the book.

The publishing team has been an ardent support to the editorial, designing and production team. Their endless efforts to recruit the best for this project, has resulted in the accomplishment of this book. They are a veteran in the field of academics and their pool of knowledge is as vast as their experience in printing. Their expertise and guidance has proved useful at every step. Their uncompromising quality standards have made this book an exceptional effort. Their encouragement from time to time has been an inspiration for everyone.

The publisher and the editorial board hope that this book will prove to be a valuable piece of knowledge for researchers, students, practitioners and scholars across the globe.

List of Contributors

Nisha Manila
Oral and Maxillofacial Radiology, Department of Diagnostic Sciences, Louisiana State University School of Dentistry, New Orleans, Louisiana, USA

Madhu Nair
Oral and Maxillofacial Radiology, Director of Imaging Center, Texas A&M College of Dentistry, Dallas, Texas, USA

Hui Liang
Director of Oral and Maxillofacial Radiology Resident Program, Department of Diagnostic Sciences, Texas A&M College of Dentistry, Dallas Texas, USA

Abdullah Alfadda
Endodontic Division, Dental Services, Central Region, King Abdulaziz Medical City, Ministry of National Guard Health Affairs, Riyadh, Saudi Arabia

Abdulmohsen Alfadley and Ahmed Jamleh
Department of Restorative and Prosthetic Dental Sciences, College of Dentistry, King Saud Bin Abdulaziz University for Health Sciences, King Abdullah International Medical Research Center, Ministry of National Guard Health Affairs, Riyadh, Saudi Arabia

Jiao Wang, Errui Wang, Xin Yang and Lu Yuan
School of Stomatology, Lanzhou University, Lanzhou 730000, China

Zhige Li, Jie Zhang and Baoping Zhang
School of Stomatology, Lanzhou University, Lanzhou 730000, China
Department of Oral and Maxillofacial Surgery, Lanzhou University, Lanzhou 730000, China

Gerardo La Monaca
Department of Sense Organs, Sapienza University of Rome, Rome, Italy

Nicola Pranno, Giorgio Pompa and Iole Vozza
Department of Oral and Maxillo-Facial Sciences, Sapienza University of Rome, Rome, Italy

Cira Rosaria Tiziana di Gioia
Department of Radiological, Oncological and Pathological Sciences, Sapienza University of Rome, Rome, Italy

Maria Paola Cristalli
Department of Biotechnologies and Medical Surgical Sciences, Sapienza University of Rome, Rome, Italy

Gabriele Villa
Unit of Periodontology, Fondazione IRCCS Ca' Granda Ospedale Maggiore Policlinico, University of Milan, Milan, Italy
Private Practice, Biella, Italy

Gionata Bellucci and Simone Magnolo
Unit of Periodontology, Fondazione IRCCS Ca' Granda Ospedale Maggiore Policlinico, University of Milan, Milan, Italy

Farah Asa'ad
Department of Biomaterials, Institute of Clinical Sciences, The Sahlgrenska Academy, University of Gothenburg, Göteborg, Sweden

Marina Consuelo Vitale, Roberto Alcozer, Martina Minardi, Maria Francesca Sfondrini, Karin Bertino and Andrea Scribante
Unit of Orthodontics and Pediatric Dentistry, Section of Dentistry, Department of Clinical, Surgical, Diagnostic and Pediatric Sciences, University of Pavia, Pavia 27100, Italy

Maria Gloria Nardi and Matteo Pellegrini
Section of Dentistry, Department of Clinical, Surgical, Diagnostic and Pediatric Sciences, University of Pavia, Pavia 27100, Italy

Francesco Spadari and Federica Pulicari
Maxillo-Facial and Odontostomatology Unit, Fondazione IRCCS Cà Granda Ospedale Maggiore Policlinico, Milan 20122, Italy
Department of Biomedical, Surgical and Dental Sciences, University of Milan, Via Della Commenda 10, Milan 20122, Italy

Mohammad Al-Obaida
Department of Restorative Dental Sciences, King Saud University, Riyadh, Saudi Arabia

Ubiracy Gaião, Leonardo Fernandes da Cunha, Cibele de Almeida Kintopp, André Vivan Garcia, Carla Castiglia Gonzaga, Alexandre Moro and Gisele Maria Correr
School of Health Sciences, Graduate Program in Dentistry, Universidade Positivo, Curitiba, PR, Brazil

Mehrnaz Moradinejad
Department of Orthodontics, Dental School, Ahvaz Jundishapur University of Medical Sciences, Ahvaz, Iran

Alireza Hashemi Ashtiani
Department of Prosthodontics, Dental School, Ahvaz Jundishapur University of Medical Sciences, Ahvaz, Iran

Vahid Rakhshan
Department of Anatomy, Dental School, Azad University of Medical Sciences, Tehran, Iran

Hrudi Sundar Sahoo, R. Kurinji Amalavathy and D. Pavani
Department of Conservative Dentistry and Endodontics, Sathyabama Dental College, Chennai, Tamil Nadu, India

Neda Kardouni Khoozestani
Departments of Oral and Maxillofacial Pathology, Cancer Institute, Tehran University of Medical Sciences, Tehran, Iran

Farzaneh Mosavat and Ramtin Azar
Oral and Maxillofacial Radiology, School of Dentistry, Tehran University of Medical Sciences, Tehran, Iran

Mohammad Shirkhoda
Department of Onco-Surgery, Cancer Institute, Tehran University of Medical Sciences, Tehran, Iran

Sven Rinke
Dental Clinic Prof. Dr. S. Rinke, Dr. M. Jablonski & Dr. H. Ziebolz, Hanau, Germany
University Medical Center Göttingen, Department of Prosthodontics, Göttingen, Germany

Anna Metzger and Holger Ziebolz
Dental Clinic Prof. Dr. S. Rinke, Dr. M. Jablonski & Dr. H. Ziebolz, Hanau, Germany

Raffaello Viganò
DDS, Freelancer in Varese, Italy
University of Milano, Milano, Italy

Mirko Disconzi and Edoardo Bertini
University of Milano, Milano, Italy

Luca Viganò
Department of Oral Radiology, San Paolo Dental Building, University of Milano, Milano, Italy

Cinzia Casu
Private Dental Practice, Cagliari, Italy

Rim Kallala
University of Monastir, Faculty of dental Medicine, Department of dental anatomy, Monastir, Tunisia
University of Monastir, Research Laboratory of Occlusodontics and Ceramic Prostheses LR16ES15, 5000 Monastir, Tunisia
Department of Fixed Prosthodontics of the Dental Clinic of Monastir, Monastir, Tunisia

Yosra Gassara, Amani Adli, Dalenda Hadyaoui, Zohra Nouira, Belhassen Harzallah and Mounir Cherif
University of Monastir, Research Laboratory of Occlusodontics and Ceramic Prostheses LR16ES15, 5000 Monastir, Tunisia
Department of Fixed Prosthodontics of the Dental Clinic of Monastir, Monastir, Tunisia

Ines Azouzi
University of Monastir, Research Laboratory of Occlusodontics and Ceramic Prostheses LR16ES15, 5000 Monastir, Tunisia
Department of Fixed Prosthodontics of the Military Hospital of Instruction of Tunis, Tunis, Tunisia

Chiraz Baccouche
University of Monastir, Faculty of dental Medicine, Department of dental anatomy, Monastir, Tunisia

Soumaya Touzi
University of Monastir, Faculty of dental Medicine, Department of dental anatomy, Monastir, Tunisia
University of Monastir, Research Laboratory of Occlusodontics and Ceramic Prostheses LR16ES15, 5000 Monastir, Tunisia

Giorgio Serafini, Marco Lollobrigida, Lorenzo Fortunato, Giulia Mazzucchi, Luca Lamazza, Dario Di Nardo, Iole Vozza and Alberto De Biase
Department of Oral and Maxillo Facial Sciences, "Sapienza" University of Rome, Italy

Mara Riminucci
Department of Molecular Medicine, "Sapienza" University of Rome, Italy

Gabriel Magnucki
Zahnzentrum Schomaker & Magnucki, Bahnhofstrasse 16-18, 27211 Bassum, Germany

Shinsuke Yamamoto, Naoki Taniike and Toshihiko Takenobu
Department of Oral and Maxillofacial Surgery, Kobe City Medical Center General Hospital, Kobe, Hyogo 650-0047, Japan

Daisuke Yamashita
Department of Pathology, Kobe City Medical Center General Hospital, Kobe, Hyogo 650-0047, Japan

Zahra Vasegh and Mitra Ghazizadeh Ahsaie
Department of Oral and Maxillofacial Radiology, School of Dentistry, Shahid Beheshti University of Medical Sciences, Tehran, Iran

Miyako Hoshino, Michiko Nishimura, Kaoru Kusama and Kentaro Kikuchi
Division of Pathology, Department of Diagnostic and Therapeutic Sciences, Meikai University School of Dentistry, 1-1 Keyakidai, Sakado, Saitama 350-0283, Japan

Katsuyuki Inoue, Tomohisa Kaneda and Hideaki Sakashita
Second Division of Oral and Maxillofacial Surgery, Department of Diagnostic and Therapeutic Sciences, Meikai University School of Dentistry, 1-1 Keyakidai, Sakado, Saitama 350-0283, Japan

Yukiko Sato
Division of Pathology, Cancer Institute, Japanese Foundation for Cancer Research, 3-8-31 Ariake, Koto-ku, Tokyo 135-8550, Japan
Department of Pathology, Cancer Institute Hospital, Japanese Foundation for Cancer Research, 3-8-31 Ariake, Koto-ku, Tokyo 135-8550, Japan

Kengo Takeuchi
Division of Pathology, Cancer Institute, Japanese Foundation for Cancer Research, 3-8-31 Ariake, Koto-ku, Tokyo 135-8550, Japan
Department of Pathology, Cancer Institute Hospital, Japanese Foundation for Cancer Research, 3-8-31 Ariake, Koto-ku, Tokyo 135-8550, Japan
Pathology Project for Molecular Targets, Cancer Institute, Japanese Foundation for Cancer Research, 3-8-31 Ariake, Koto-ku, Tokyo 135-8550, Japan

Toshitaka Nagao
Department of Anatomic Pathology, Tokyo Medical University, 7-3-1 Hongo, Bunkyo-ku, Tokyo 113-0033, Japan

Adepitan A. Owosho
Missouri School of Dentistry and Oral Health, A.T. Still University, Kirksville, Missouri, USA

Chukwubuzor Okwuosa and Donald I. Obi
University of Nigeria Teaching Hospital, Nsukka, Enugu, Nigeria

Robinson O. Okiti
University College Hospital, Ibadan, Oyo, Nigeria

Kurt F. Summersgill
Department of Diagnostic Sciences, School of Dental Medicine, University of Pittsburgh, Pittsburgh, Pennsylvania, USA

Rim Kallala
Dental Faculty of Monastir, Tunisia
University of Monastir, Research Laboratory of Occlusodontics and Ceramic Prostheses LR16ES15, 5000 Monastir, Tunisia
Department of Dental Faculty at the Dental Faculty of Monastir, Tunisia

Mohamed Habib Chaouch
Dental Faculty of Monastir, Tunisia

Karim Nasr and Teva Courset
Faculty of Dental Surgery and University Hospital, Toulouse, France

Mokhtar Mamdouh Abdel-Latif
Maxillofacial Surgery and Diagnostic Sciences, Division of Oral Surgery, College of Dentistry, Jazan University, Jazan, Saudi Arabia

Shankargouda Patil
Maxillofacial Surgery and Diagnostic Sciences, Division of Oral Pathology, College of Dentistry, Jazan University, Jazan, Saudi Arabia

Anas Alyahya, Humam Karkoutly and Hussam Milly
Department of Conservative Dentistry and Endodontics, Dental Institute, Damascus University, Damascus, Syria

Qamar Hashem
Clinical Dental Sciences Department/Endodontic Division College of Dentistry, Princes Noura Bint Abdulrahman University, Riyadh, Saudi Arabia

Milla Huuhka
Department of Oral and Maxillofacial Diseases, Turku University Hospital, Turku, Finland

Aaro Turunen
Department of Oral and Maxillofacial Surgery, Institute of Dentistry, University of Turku, Turku, Finland

Yosuke Iijima, Nami Nakayama, Leona Kashimata, Miki Yamada, Shunsuke Hino, Takahiro Kaneko and Norio Horie
Department of Oral and Maxillofacial Surgery, Saitama Medical Center, Saitama Medical University, Saitama, Japan

Ryutaro Kawano
Department of Pathology, Saitama Medical Center, Saitama Medical University, Saitama, Japan

Albandari Bin-Rubayan
Ministry of Health (SCFHS), Prosthodontics Program (Training Center: Department of Restorative and Prosthetic Dental Sciences, College of Dentistry, Dar Al Uloom University), Riyadh, Saudi Arabia

Abdulaziz Samran
Department of Restorative and Prosthetic Dental Sciences, School of Dentistry, Dar Al-Uloom University, Riyadh, Saudi Arabia
Department of Prosthodontics, School of Dentistry, Ibb University, Yemen

Ali Alqerban
Department of Preventive Dental Sciences, College of Dentistry, Prince Sattam Bin Abdulaziz University, Alkharj, Saudi Arabia
Department of Preventive Dental Science, Dar Al Uloom University, Riyadh, Saudi Arabia

Sahani Anupama and Pilana Vithanage Kalani Shihanika Hettiarachchi
Department of Oral Medicine and Periodontology, Faculty of Dental Sciences, University of Peradeniya, Sri Lanka

Anna Lysenko
Department of Maxillofacial Surgery, Research Institute of Dentistry and Maxillofacial Surgery, Russia

Alexandra Razumova and Andrey Yaremenko
Department of Dental Surgery and Maxillofacial Surgery, First Pavlov State Medical University, Russia

Rustam Mirzakhmedov
Create Unique 3D Filters, Russia

Anna Zubareva
Department First Pavlov State Medical University, Russia

Marina Chibisova
Department of Radiology in Dentistry, Private Educational Institution SPb INSTOM, Private Educational Institution St. Petersburg Institute of Post-Graduate Dentistry, Russia

Mirlany Mendes Maciel Oliveira
Bucomaxilofacial Surgery and Traumatology Clinical Hospital of the Federal University of Uberlândia (HC-UFU), Uberlândia, Minas Gerais, Brazil

Rodrigo da Franca Acioly, Dennis Dinelly de Souza, Bruno Araújo da Silva and Daniel Do Carmo Carvalho
Buccomaxillofacial Surgery, Department of Buccomaxillofacial Surgery and Traumatology, Hospital Geral de Roraima, Boa Vista, RR, Brazil

M. Singh, I. K. Limbu, P. K. Parajuli and R. K. Singh
Department of Prosthodontics and Crown-Bridge, B P Koirala Institute of Health Sciences, Dharan, Nepal

Ahmad Y. Imam
Oral and Maxillofacial Prosthodontics Department, Faculty of Dentistry, King Abdulaziz University, Jeddah, Saudi Arabia

Raghad A. Al-Dabbagh
Oral and Maxillofacial Rehabilitation Department, Faculty of Dentistry, King Abdulaziz University, Jeddah, Saudi Arabia

Massoumeh Zargaran
Department of Oral and Maxillofacial Pathology, Faculty of Dentistry, Kurdistan University of Medical Sciences, Sanandaj, Iran

Setareh Shojaei
Department of Oral & Maxillofacial Pathology, School of Dentistry, Hamadan University of Medical Sciences, Hamadan, Iran

Ana Carolina Monachini Marcantonio, Cássio Rocha Scardueli, Camila Chiérici Marcantonio, Rosemary Adriana Chiérici Marcantonio and Elcio Marcantonio Jr.
Department of Diagnosis and Surgery, Univ. Est. Paul. - UNESP, Araraquara 14801-903, Brazil

Guilherme José Pimentel Lopes de Oliveira
Department of Periodontology/Implantology, Dental School, Federal University of Uberlândia-UFU, Uberlândia 38405-266, Brazil

Sabit Demircan
Private Practice, Beykent University Vocational School, Turkey

Sabri Cemil İşler, Aydın Gümüşdal and Begüm Genç
Istanbul University Faculty of Dentistry Oral and Maxillofacial Surgery Department, Turkey

Index

www.ingramcontent.com/pod-product-compliance
Lightning Source LLC
LaVergne TN
LVHW082230200926
848484LV00008B/2327
9798887406336